The Promise of Assistive Technology to Enhance Activity and Work Participation

Committee on the Use of Selected Assistive Products and Technologies in Eliminating or Reducing the Effects of Impairments

Alan M. Jette, Carol Mason Spicer, Jennifer Lalitha Flaubert, *Editors*

Board on Health Care Services

Health and Medicine Division

A Consensus Study Report of
The National Academies of
SCIENCES · ENGINEERING · MEDICINE

THE NATIONAL ACADEMIES PRESS
Washington, DC
www.nap.edu

THE NATIONAL ACADEMIES PRESS 500 Fifth Street, NW Washington, DC 20001

This activity was supported by Contract/Task Order No. SS00-13-60048/0007 with the U.S. Social Security Administration. Any opinions, findings, conclusions, or recommendations expressed in this publication do not necessarily reflect the views of any organization or agency that provided support for the project.

International Standard Book Number-13: 978-0-309-45784-2
International Standard Book Number-10: 0-309-45784-X
Digital Object Identifier: https://doi.org/10.17226/24740
Library of Congress Control Number: 2017944212

Additional copies of this publication are available for sale from the National Academies Press, 500 Fifth Street, NW, Keck 360, Washington, DC 20001; (800) 624-6242 or (202) 334-3313; http://www.nap.edu.

Printed in the United States of America

Suggested citation: National Academies of Sciences, Engineering, and Medicine. 2017. *The Promise of Assistive Technology to Enhance Activity and Work Participation.* Washington, DC: The National Academies Press. doi: https://doi.org/10.17226/24740.

The National Academies of

SCIENCES · ENGINEERING · MEDICINE

The **National Academy of Sciences** was established in 1863 by an Act of Congress, signed by President Lincoln, as a private, nongovernmental institution to advise the nation on issues related to science and technology. Members are elected by their peers for outstanding contributions to research. Dr. Marcia McNutt is president.

The **National Academy of Engineering** was established in 1964 under the charter of the National Academy of Sciences to bring the practices of engineering to advising the nation. Members are elected by their peers for extraordinary contributions to engineering. Dr. C. D. Mote, Jr., is president.

The **National Academy of Medicine** (formerly the Institute of Medicine) was established in 1970 under the charter of the National Academy of Sciences to advise the nation on medical and health issues. Members are elected by their peers for distinguished contributions to medicine and health. Dr. Victor J. Dzau is president.

The three Academies work together as the **National Academies of Sciences, Engineering, and Medicine** to provide independent, objective analysis and advice to the nation and conduct other activities to solve complex problems and inform public policy decisions. The National Academies also encourage education and research, recognize outstanding contributions to knowledge, and increase public understanding in matters of science, engineering, and medicine.

Learn more about the National Academies of Sciences, Engineering, and Medicine at **www.nationalacademies.org**.

COMMITTEE ON THE USE OF SELECTED ASSISTIVE PRODUCTS AND TECHNOLOGIES IN ELIMINATING OR REDUCING THE EFFECTS OF IMPAIRMENTS

ALAN M. JETTE (*Chair*), Professor, Health Law, Policy and Management, Boston University School of Public Health

FABRICIO E. BALCAZAR, Professor, Disability and Human Development, University of Illinois at Chicago

LAURA J. BALL, Speech-Language Pathologist and Director, Hearing and Speech Research, Center for Translational Research, Children's National Health System, and Professor, Pediatrics, School of Medicine and Health Sciences, The George Washington University

RORY A. COOPER, Distinguished Professor and FISA Foundation and Paralyzed Veterans of America Chair, School of Health and Rehabilitation Sciences, University of Pittsburgh, and Senior Career Scientist, VA Pittsburgh Healthcare System

JANNA L. FRIEDLY, Associate Professor, Physical Medicine and Rehabilitation, University of Washington, and Medical Director, Limb Preservation and Amputation Services, Harborview Medical Center

WALTER R. FRONTERA, Professor, Physical Medicine, Rehabilitation, and Sports Medicine and Physiology, University of Puerto Rico School of Medicine

KATYA HILL, Associate Professor, Communication Science and Disorders, University of Pittsburgh

BARBARA L. KORNBLAU, Executive Director, Coalition for Disability Health Equity, and Adjunct Professor, Florida A&M University

FRANK R. LIN, Associate Professor, Otolaryngology-Head and Neck Surgery and Geriatric Medicine, Johns Hopkins University School of Medicine

LAURA A. MILLER, Research Scientist/Prosthetist, Center for Bionic Medicine, Shirley Ryan AbilityLab, and Clinical Associate Professor, Physical Medicine and Rehabilitation, Northwestern University

KENNETH J. OTTENBACHER, Russell Shearn Moody Distinguished Chair in Neurological Rehabilitation and Director, Division of Rehabilitation Sciences, University of Texas Medical Branch at Galveston

LINDA J. RESNIK, Research Career Scientist, Providence VA Medical Center, and Professor, Health Services, Policy and Practice, Brown University

JON A. SANFORD, Director, Center for Assistive Technology and Environmental Access, and Professor of Industrial Design, Georgia Institute of Technology

STEPHANIE J. SJOBLAD, Clinical Coordinator and Professor, Hearing and Communication Center, Division of Speech and Hearing Sciences, University of North Carolina at Chapel Hill

LAWRENCE C. VOGEL, Chief of Pediatrics, Assistant Chief of Staff, Medical Director, Spinal Cord Injury Program, Chicago Shriners Hospitals for Children, and Professor of Pediatrics, Rush Medical College

Consultants

PATRICIA M. OWENS, Consultant, Health and Disability Policy and Programs

AMOL KARMARKAR, Assistant Professor, Division of Rehabilitation Sciences, University of Texas Medical Branch

MAUREEN O'CONNELL, Attorney at Law, Southern Disability Law Center

JAMES R. SHELDON, JR., Supervising Attorney, National Assistive Technology Advocacy Project, Neighborhood Legal Services, Inc.

Study Staff

CAROL MASON SPICER, Study Director

JENNIFER LALITHA FLAUBERT, Associate Program Officer

FRANK R. VALLIERE, Associate Program Officer (*until July 2016*)

LAURA VERCAMMEN, Research Associate (*October 2016-December 2016*)

NICOLE GORMLEY, Senior Program Assistant

PAMELA RAMEY-McCRAY, Administrative Assistant

DAVID A. BUTLER, Acting Director, Board on the Health of Select Populations (*July 2016-December 2016*)

FREDRICK ERDTMANN, Director, Board on the Health of Select Populations (*until July 2016*)

SHARYL J. NASS, Director, Board on Health Care Services

Reviewers

This Consensus Study Report was reviewed in draft form by individuals chosen for their diverse perspectives and technical expertise. The purpose of this independent review is to provide candid and critical comments that will assist the National Academies of Sciences, Engineering, and Medicine in making each published report as sound as possible and to ensure that it meets the institutional standards for quality, objectivity, evidence, and responsiveness to the study charge. The review comments and draft manuscript remain confidential to protect the integrity of the deliberative process.

We thank the following individuals for their review of this report:

Kendra Betz, VA National Center for Patient Safety
William R. Botten, U.S. Access Board
George Demiris, University of Washington
William A. Erickson, Cornell University
Alberto Esquenazi, MossRehab
Howard H. Goldman, University of Maryland at Baltimore
Helen Marie Hoenig, Durham VA Medical Center
Lisa I. Iezzoni, Harvard Medical School and Massachusetts General Hospital
Andrew J. Imparato, Association of University Centers on Disabilities
Susan Kapp, University of Washington
Todd Kuiken, Rehabilitation Institute of Chicago
Cathy L. Lazarus, Mount Sinai Beth Israel
Rachel McArdle, U.S. Department of Veterans Affairs

Ryan McCreery, Boys Town National Research Hospital
David McNaughton, Pennsylvania State University
Joseph J. Montano, Weil Cornell Medicine
Edward L. Myers III, Attorney at Law (Retired)
Frank A. Sloan, Duke University
Kathryn M. Yorkston, University of Washington

Although the reviewers listed above provided many constructive comments and suggestions, they were not asked to endorse the conclusions or recommendations of this report nor did they see the final draft before its release. The review of this report was overseen by **Robert S. Lawrence,** Johns Hopkins University, and **Bradford H. Gray,** Urban Institute. They were responsible for making certain that an independent examination of this report was carried out in accordance with the standards of the National Academies and that all review comments were carefully considered. Responsibility for the final content rests entirely with the authoring committee and the National Academies.

Acknowledgments

The study committee and the National Academies of Sciences, Engineering, and Medicine's Health and Medicine Division project staff take this opportunity to recognize and thank the many individuals who shared their time and expertise to support the committee's work and inform its deliberations.

This study was sponsored by the U.S. Social Security Administration (SSA). We thank McArthur Allen, Gina Clemons, Joanna Firmin, Scott Marko, Nancy Miller, and Mary Beth Rochowiak for their guidance and support, as well as Megan Butson and Thomas Mulherin for their assistance. The committee also acknowledges SSA for verifying relevant technical content for accuracy. The committee benefited greatly from discussions with the individuals who presented at and attended the committee's open sessions: Laura J. Ball, Susanne M. Bruyère, Megan Conway, Justin Creamer, Melissa Day, William A. Erickson, Bradley Flohr, Amy S. Goldman, Michelle C. Jackson, Michael Kidd, John Kramschuster, Daniel E. Kubrin, Jo Anne Materkowski, Ryan McCreery, Susan M. Miller, Penny L. Nechanicky, Patricia M. Owens, Mark Schmeler, Gerald Stark, Colleen Thoma, and Kristin Tugman. The committee is grateful to these presenters for volunteering to share their expertise, knowledge, data, and opinions not only with the committee but also with the members of the public who participated in the committee's open sessions. The committee also appreciates the efforts of numerous individuals who assisted project staff in identifying the presenters. Particular thanks go to Winthrop Cashdollar for his introductions to representatives from the private disability insurance industry.

The committee acknowledges the many staff within the Health and Medicine Division who provided support in various ways to this project, including Carol Mason Spicer (study director), Jennifer Flaubert (associate program officer), Nicole Gormley (senior program assistant), Karen Helsing (senior program officer), Frank Valliere (program officer), Laura Vercammen (research associate), and Julie Wiltshire (financial associate). The committee extends great thanks and appreciation to the Health and Medicine Division board directors who oversaw the project: Rick Erdtmann, David Butler, and Sharyl Nass. Research assistance was provided by Rebecca Morgan (senior research librarian, National Academies). Finally, Rona Brière and Alisa Decatur are to be credited for the superb editorial assistance they provided in preparing the final report.

Contents

Boxes, Figures, and Tables

BOXES

FIGURES

TABLES

Acronyms and Abbreviations

AAC	augmentative and alternative communication
ABC	American Board for Certification in Orthotics, Prosthetics and Pedorthics
ABLE	Achieving a Better Life Experience
ABN	advanced beneficiary notice
ACA	Patient Protection and Affordable Care Act
ACTA	Air Carrier Transportation Act
ADA	Americans with Disabilities Act
ADL	activity of daily living
ADMC	Advance Determination of Medical Coverage
AFP	Alternative Financing Program
AL/EL	artificial/electrolarynx
ALS	amyotrophic lateral sclerosis
APRN	advanced practice registered nurse
ASHA	American Speech-Language-Hearing Association
ASoC	Amputation System of Care
AT	assistive technology
ATP	assistive technology professional
C&P	compensation and pension
CAP	Computer/Electronic Accommodations Program
CARF	Commission on Accreditation of Rehabilitation Facilities
CDC	U.S. Centers for Disease Control and Prevention
CHIP	Children's Health Insurance Program
CMS	Centers for Medicare & Medicaid Services

CPP	Canada Pension Plan
CPT	Current Procedural Terminology
CR	cost reimbursement
DASH	Disabilities of the Arm, Shoulder, and Hand (questionnaire)
dB	decibels
DBS	disability benefits specialist
DDS	Disability Determination Services
DE	disability examiner
DM	digital modulation
DME	durable medical equipment
DME-MAC	Durable Medical Equipment-Medicare Administrative Contractor
EHLR	Education for the Handicapped Law Report
EMG	electromyographic
EN	employment network
ENT	ear, nose, and throat
EPSDT	Early and Periodic Screening, Diagnostic, and Treatment
ESS	esophageal speech
FBR	federal benefit rate
FDA	U.S. Food and Drug Administration
FFP	federal financial participation
FM	frequency modulated
FODAC	Friends of Disabled Adults and Children
FY	fiscal year
GAO	U.S. Government Accountability Office
HCBS	home- and community-based services
HCPCS	Healthcare Common Procedure Coding System
HMO	health maintenance organization
IADL	instrumental activity of daily living
ICD-9	*International Classification of Diseases*, Ninth Revision
ICF	*International Classification of Functioning, Disability and Health*
ICIDH	*International Classification of Impairments, Disabilities, and Handicaps*
IDEA	Individuals with Disabilities Education Act

IDELR	Individuals with Disabilities Education Law Report
IEP	individualized education plan
IMU	inertial measurement unit
IRS	Internal Revenue Service
ISO	International Organization for Standardization
JAN	Job Accommodation Network
LCD	Local Coverage Determination
MAE	mobility assistive equipment
MRADL	mobility-related activity of daily living
MSP	Medicare Savings Program
NAAL	National Assessment of Adult Literacy
NCART	National Coalition for Assistive and Rehab Technology
NCD	National Coverage Determination
NHANES	National Health and Nutrition Examination Survey
NHIS	National Health Interview Survey
NHIS-D	National Health Interview Survey-Disability
NIDILRR	National Institute on Disability, Independent Living, and Rehabilitation Research
OSEP	Office for Special Education Programs
P&A	protection and advocacy
PA	physician assistant
PAAT	Protection and Advocacy for Assistive Technology
PANS	Polytrauma/Amputation Network Sites
PASS	Plan to Achieve Self-Support
PC	psychological consultant
PDA	personal digital assistant
PIDA	Power Mobility Indoor Driving Assessment
PM&R	physical medicine and rehabilitation
POMS	Program Operations Manual System
POV	power operated vehicle
PRAT	Polytrauma Rehabilitation Assistive Technology Lab
PSAP	personal sound amplification product
PTSD	posttraumatic stress disorder
QDE	qualified disability expense
RAC	Regional Amputation Care Center

RERC	Rehabilitation Engineering Research Center
RESNA	Rehabilitation Engineering and Assistive Technology Society of North America
RFC	residual functional capacity
RSA	Rehabilitation Services Administration
RVSR	rating veterans service representative
SGA	substantial gainful activity
SGD	speech-generating device
SHAP	Southampton Hand Assessment Procedure
SIPP	Survey of Income and Program Participation
SLP	speech-language pathologist
SMS	seating and mobility specialist
SSA	U.S. Social Security Administration
SSDI	Social Security Disability Insurance
SSI	Supplemental Security Income
TAI	Transfer Assessment Instrument
TEP	tracheoesophageal voice prosthesis
TRS	telecommunications relay service
TSV	tracheostomy speaking valve
UCP	United Cerebral Palsy
UEP	upper-extremity prosthesis
VA	U.S. Department of Veterans Affairs
VASRD	VA Schedule for Rating Disabilities
VBA	Veterans Benefits Administration
VC	voluntary closing
VHA	Veterans Health Administration
VO	voluntary opening
VR	vocational rehabilitation
VR&E	Vocational Rehabilitation and Employment
VSC	Veterans Service Center
WHO	World Health Organization
WIOA	Workforce Innovation and Opportunity Act
wpm	words per minute
WSMD	wheeled and seated mobility device

Summary[1]

The U.S. Census Bureau has reported that 56.7 million Americans had some type of disability in 2010, which represents 18.7 percent of the civilian noninstitutionalized population included in the 2010 Survey of Income and Program Participation (SIPP). Only 41.1 percent of working-age individuals (ages 18 to 64) with a disability reported employment in the SIPP, a percentage that may be lower for individuals with impairments who could benefit from the use of products and technologies in the categories discussed in this report. By contrast, the employment rate for persons of working age without a disability was 79.1 percent. Similarly, the 2014 American Community Survey found that more than half of the U.S. population with disabilities (51.6 percent) were people aged 18 to 64, while 40.7 percent were aged 65 and older. Of those aged 18 to 64 living in the community, 34.4 percent were employed, compared with 75.4 percent of this age group without disabilities.

The U.S. Social Security Administration (SSA) provides disability benefits through the Social Security Disability Insurance (SSDI) program and the Supplemental Security Income (SSI) program. The SSDI program, established in 1956, provides benefits to adults with disabilities who have paid into the Disability Insurance Trust Fund and to their spouses and adult children who are unable to work because of severe long-term disability. Enacted in 1972, SSI is a means-tested program based on income and financial assets that provides income assistance from U.S. Treasury general funds

[1]This summary does not include references. Citations to support the text and conclusions herein are provided in the body of the report.

to adults aged 65 and older, individuals who are blind, and disabled adults and children. As of December 2015, approximately 11 million individuals were SSDI beneficiaries, and about 8 million were SSI beneficiaries.

SSA currently considers assistive devices in the nonmedical and medical areas of its program guidelines. During determinations of substantial gainful activity and income eligibility for SSI benefits, the reasonable cost of items, devices, or services that applicants need to enable them to work with their impairment is subtracted from eligible earnings, even if those items or services are used for activities of daily living in addition to work. In addition, SSA considers assistive devices in its medical disability determination process and assessment of work capacity.

In a 2012 report, the U.S. Government Accountability Office (GAO) recommended that SSA "conduct limited and focused studies on the availability and effects of considering more fully assistive devices and workplace accommodations in its disability determinations." GAO concluded that "without such efforts to study how certain assistive devices and accommodations are playing a role in helping individuals with impairments stay at work or return to work, and their costs in comparison to potentially providing years of disability benefit payments, SSA may be missing an opportunity to assist individuals with disabilities to reengage in the workforce."

Accordingly, SSA asked the Health and Medicine Division of the National Academies of Sciences, Engineering, and Medicine to convene a committee of relevant experts to provide an analysis of selected assistive products and technologies, including wheeled and seated mobility devices (WSMDs), upper-extremity prostheses (UEPs), and products and technologies selected by the committee that pertain to hearing and to communication and speech in adults. The committee's statement of task is presented in Box S-1.

STUDY APPROACH AND SCOPE

In addition to conducting an extensive review of the literature pertaining to assistive products and technologies, the committee held three public meetings and one public teleconference to hear from invited experts in areas pertinent to this study. The committee also commissioned two papers: (1) a paper on selected sources of funding or coverage for relevant assistive technologies, which forms much of the basis for Chapter 7; and (2) a summary of data pertaining to the use of relevant assistive technologies among Medicare recipients of working age with various impairments (aged 20 to 67) (see Appendix C). Collectively, these sources inform the committee's findings and conclusions presented throughout the report.

The content of this report reflects four overlapping spheres of information the committee investigated to approach its statement of task:

BOX S-1
Statement of Task

An ad hoc committee will provide an analysis of the use in adults of selected assistive products and technologies, including wheeled/seated mobility devices, upper-extremity prostheses, and committee-selected products and technologies that pertain to hearing and to communication and speech. The committee will provide definitions and explanations of relevant terms, including *assistive technology* and *workplace reasonable accommodations*.

Drawing upon existing data to the extent they are available, the committee will address the following questions:

- For the selected products and technologies
  - To what extent are they being used, and by whom?
  - What is the observed range of impairment mitigating effects?
  - How does use vary depending upon the individual, including those with other impairments or comorbidities and how does this vary for different occupations?
  - To what extent have they altered the outlook for occupational success?
  - What are typical training and adaptation times?
- To the degree possible, the committee will address
  - What information exists on access to and availability of the selected assistive products and technologies in the current health care and rehabilitation environment, including access to appropriate evaluation and training by qualified personnel?
  - Under what circumstances, if any, do employers provide access to these products and technologies as workplace reasonable accommodations?
  - What costs are associated with the product and technology acquisition, product maintenance, repair, and replacement and how do disabled individuals gain financial access to the products and technologies?
  - For young adults, what challenges exist in transitioning from a school environment to the workplace?
- To the extent information is available, the committee will describe the decision-making processes of other government or private monetary disability benefit programs regarding the use of the selected assistive products and technologies.

The report will include conclusions but not recommendations.

- The committee developed a framework based on the *International Classification of Functioning, Disability and Health* to explain how the relevant terms identified by SSA and the committee, including "assistive technology" and "workplace reasonable accommodations," relate to one another and how the products and technologies they denote can act as facilitators in mitigating the impact of various impairments and enhancing work performance and participation. This framework can serve as a guide for organizations that evaluate the effects of impairments and the impact of assistive products and technologies and other environmental interventions on reducing those effects.

- Four chapters of this report provide for the four categories of assistive products and technologies the committee was asked to address descriptions of the range of products and technologies in those categories; clinical considerations, including the range of effects on mitigating the impacts of impairments; and the prevalence of use.
- Questions of access to the selected assistive products and technologies and to appropriate evaluation and training by qualified personnel also are addressed, particularly with respect to coverage and funding for products and services. Challenges for young adults transitioning from a school environment to pathways to employment are discussed as well.
- The report includes a review of the assessment, acquisition, and use of relevant products and technologies in selected public and private disability programs that provide monetary benefits.

OVERALL CONCLUSIONS

In addition to chapter-specific findings and conclusions, the committee formulated nine overall conclusions.

The Promise of Assistive Products and Technologies

The committee's review of the literature and the expert opinions of its members and others who provided input for this study made clear that appropriate-quality assistive products and technologies in all four categories examined may mitigate the impact of impairments sufficiently to allow people with disabilities to work. In some cases, however, environmental and personal factors create barriers to employment despite the impairment-mitigating effects of these products and technologies. In addition, maximal user performance requires that individuals receive the appropriate devices for their needs, proper fitting of and training in the use of the devices, and appropriate follow-up care. Even if these conditions are met, moreover, and even given relevant technological advances, assistive products and technologies may not fully mitigate the effects of impairments or associated activity limitations. The committee emphasizes that environmental, societal, and personal factors are as important in determining individuals' overall functioning with respect to employment. For these reasons, the committee drew the following conclusions:

1. **Assistive products and technologies hold promise for partially or completely mitigating the impacts of impairments and enhancing work participation when appropriate products and technologies are available, when they are properly prescribed and fitted, when the user receives proper training in their use and appropriate follow-up, and when societal and environmental barriers are limited.**
2. **When matching individuals with appropriate assistive products and technologies, it is important to understand the complexity of factors that must be optimized to enhance function. Selecting, designing, or modifying the correct device for an individual and providing training in its use, as well as appropriate follow-up, are complex but necessary elements for maximizing function among users of assistive products and technologies.**

Access to and Coverage of Assistive Products and Technologies

Financial access to appropriate assistive products and technologies as well as qualified providers varies significantly across reimbursement and funding sources in the United States. Numerous pathways exist for accessing these products and technologies and related services, but different coverage sources vary in their missions, their eligibility requirements, and the types of assistive products and technologies and related services they cover. In some cases, a mismatch exists between the products and technologies covered and those that would best meet the needs of users to enhance their participation in work and other life roles. In some cases, there also exists a shortage or geographic imbalance of qualified providers and clinics with the knowledge, skill, and expertise to properly evaluate, fit, and train people in the use of assistive products and technologies.

In addition, socioeconomic status and education levels may affect access to coverage for assistive products and technologies and related services. Health literacy is associated with a variety of factors, including educational level. Acquisition of assistive devices may be promoted by people's knowledge of their needs, device and coverage options, and means to pursue the device(s) they need. Moreover, loss of access and coverage among youth of transition age[2] is a significant impediment to their independent living,

[2]Transition age typically encompasses the period from high school (ages 15 to 16) through young adulthood (ages 24 to 26).

transition to work, vocational readiness, or further education. The committee drew the following conclusions with respect to access and coverage:

3. **Access to appropriate assistive products and technologies and to qualified providers and teams with the knowledge, skill, and expertise necessary to properly evaluate, fit, train, and monitor people in the use of those products and technologies is frequently limited and varies considerably from case to case, state to state, district to district, urban to rural and frontier areas, and funding source to funding source.**
4. **The variability of coverage for assistive products, technologies, and related services is an important impediment to optimizing function and maintaining gainful employment among transitioning youth and adults with impairments.**

Information and Policy Concerning Assistive Products and Technologies

Individuals' knowledge about assistive product and technology options, their needs, their coverage options, and the means available to them to pursue the products and technologies they need will either promote or hinder their acquisition of the devices. However, the distribution of this knowledge varies greatly. Socioeconomic status, education level, and a variety of personal factors—including ethnic, cultural, and language barriers—may affect access to assistive products and technologies and related services even when they are covered. The committee therefore drew the following conclusion:

5. **Education regarding the availability of assistive products and technologies and knowledge and training that empower users to self-advocate or have a significant other (e.g., family member, friend, or professional) advocate for them are important elements in achieving successful access to appropriate assistive products and technologies and related services.**

The provision of assistive products and technologies, such as WSMDs, UEPs, and augmentative and alternative communication devices, is contingent largely on reimbursement policy rather than patient need. In some cases, the products and technologies that are covered by Medicare and other insurers as medically necessary are not those that would best meet the needs of users to enhance their participation in life roles. Medicare and other insurers may reject payment for devices and components that are new technologies or that they do not consider medically necessary even if prescribed by a trained professional. In addition, the relatively small numbers and/or variable distribution of providers and clinics qualified to provide relevant assistive technology services limit access to those services independently of funding or reimbursement considerations. Accordingly, the committee drew the following conclusion:

6. **Assistive products and technologies are advancing at a much faster rate relative to clinician education, regulations, and reimbursement systems, which may limit access to these devices and/or access to training in their use.**

The mission of funding sources and benefit programs affects the extent to which they provide, or help beneficiaries to obtain, appropriate assistive products and technologies and related services designed to facilitate their ability to work. Some private disability insurers provide certain assistive products and technologies in support of occupational functioning and return to work. State vocational rehabilitation agencies may provide or facilitate the acquisition of assistive products and technologies and related services to enable eligible individuals to prepare for, retain, or regain work based on their personal vocational goals. The Veterans Health Administration is an integrated health care system that provides high-quality, comprehensive, interdisciplinary care and assistive products and technologies to veterans. In addition, a few private health insurers provide integrated health care plans through which covered individuals receive clinical care, prescription drugs, and assistive products and technologies. Based on its review of selected monetary disability benefit programs and funding sources for assistive products and technologies, the committee drew the following conclusion:

7. **Some coverage and disability benefit models, such as those of the Veterans Health Administration, state vocational rehabilitation agencies, some private disability insurance carriers, and a few private health insurers, are more holistic than others, providing access to a greater range of assistive products and technologies and related services that can be appropriate to meeting individuals' needs and facilitating their ability to work.**

Evaluation of Ability to Work

The concept of disability has evolved to reflect a biopsychosocial model in which disability is perceived as the interaction between an individual's functional capacity and relevant social and physical environmental and personal factors. Although assistive products and technologies may mitigate the impacts of impairment sufficiently to allow a person to work, personal factors such as gender, race/ethnicity, age, socioeconomic status, insurance coverage, education, and previous work experience can influence how an individual experiences disability. In addition, the individual experience of disability is influenced by such environmental factors as the job market, workplace attitudes, geographic location, and the built environment. Although the committee found that a complete evaluation of a person's functioning would include the assistive products and technologies he or she normally uses, that finding needs to be tempered by the following conclusion:

8. **Professionals involved in disability determinations cannot assume that because an individual uses a particular assistive product or technology, this device is always effective for that person, that it mitigates the impact of the person's impairment, or that it enables the person to work. Environmental, societal, and personal factors also must be taken into account.**

Data on the Use and Effectiveness of Assistive Products and Technologies

The committee found that data on the prevalence of use of the assistive products and technologies discussed in this report and the extent to which they mitigate the impacts of impairments are fragmented and limited. At this time, it is difficult to quantify the impact of assistive products and technologies and related services on impairment mitigation and employability because of contextual/environmental, societal, and personal factors that affect device use and job function; the lack of data on occupational success; and unequal access to relevant products and technologies and training. The committee recognizes that limited or lack of evidence about the impact of assistive products and technologies and related rehabilitative services on activity and participation may affect decisions by funding sources about which devices and services to cover. Information from outcomes research could contribute to studies on the effectiveness or cost-effectiveness of various assistive products and technologies and thereby help to inform the development of rational resource utilization, including coverage decisions by insurers and other funding sources. Accordingly, the committee drew the following conclusion:

9. **Additional research is needed to understand how the specifications for and use of assistive technologies and products and related services impact inclusion in society and work participation for individuals with disabilities. Such research may not only enhance knowledge in these areas but also inform the development of rational resource utilization, including informing cost-benefit analyses and coverage for devices and related services.**

1

Introduction

The U.S. Census Bureau has reported that 56.7 million Americans had a disability in 2010, a figure that represents 18.7 percent of the civilian noninstitutionalized population included in the 2010 Survey of Income and Program Participation (SIPP) (Brault, 2012). Compared with 79.1 percent of working-age individuals (ages 18 to 64) without a disability that reported employment in the SIPP, only 41.1 percent of working-age individuals with a disability reported employment, a percentage that may be lower for individuals with impairments who could benefit from the use of products and technologies in the categories discussed in this report (Brault, 2012; Johnson et al., 2007; Kaye et al., 2000). Similarly, the 2014 American Community Survey found that more than half of the U.S. population with disabilities (51.6 percent) were people aged 18 to 64, while 40.7 percent were aged 65 and older. Of those aged 18 to 64 living in the community, 34.4 percent were employed, compared with 75.4 percent of this age group without disabilities (Kraus, 2015).

CONTEXT FOR THIS STUDY

Social Security Administration

The U.S. Social Security Administration (SSA) provides monetary benefits to eligible individuals with disabilities through two programs: Social Security Disability Insurance (SSDI) and Supplemental Security Income (SSI). The SSDI program, established in 1956, provides benefits to eligible adults with disabilities who have paid into the Disability Insurance Trust

Fund and to their spouses and adult children who are unable to work because of severe long-term disability. Enacted in 1972, SSI is a means-tested program based on income and financial assets that provides income assistance from U.S. Treasury general funds to eligible adults aged 65 and older, individuals who are blind, and disabled adults and children. As of December 2015, approximately 11 million individuals were SSDI beneficiaries, and about 8 million were SSI beneficiaries (SSA, 2016b).

To receive SSDI or SSI benefits, an individual must meet the definition of disability: "if he or she has a medically determinable physical or mental impairment (or combination of impairments) that prevents him or her from doing any substantial gainful activity (SGA), and has lasted or is expected to last for a continuous period of at least 12 months, or is expected to result in death" (SSA, 2012a). In determining whether the definition of disability is met, SSA uses a five-step sequential process for adults.

- In the first step, SSA field offices perform financial screens to deny claims for applicants who work and earn income above the SGA limit (Wixon and Strand, 2013). SGA is defined as "work that involves doing significant and productive physical or mental duties and is done (or intended) for pay or profit."[1] The monthly SGA amount for nonblind individuals in 2017 is $1,170 after deducting impairment-related work expenses (SSA, 2017). Impairment-related work expenses, such as certain attendant care services, medical devices, equipment, and prostheses, may be deducted from any SGA (SSA, 2015). For SSDI applicants, insured status is verified, while countable income and resources are verified to be below thresholds for SSI applicants.
- In step 2, applicants receive medical screens to determine whether they have a medically determinable severe impairment. According to SSA's Program Operations Manual System, "when medical evidence establishes only a slight abnormality or a combination of slight abnormalities which would have no more than a minimum effect on an individual's ability to work, such impairment(s) will be found 'not severe,' and a determination of 'not disabled' will be made" (SSA, 2012b). Applicants will also be denied in step 2 if their impairment is "not expected to result in death, and has neither lasted 12 months nor is expected to last for a continuous period of 12 months" (SSA, 2012a).
- In step 3, an applicant's impairment is assessed using the *Listing of Impairments*, which is a regulatory list of medical conditions and criteria created by SSA to assist in disability determination. If an

[1]20 CFR § 404.1510.

applicant's impairment "meets" or "equals" a listing and meets the duration requirement, the applicant is allowed benefits. To "meet" a listing, a claimant must have a medically determinable impairment that satisfies all of the criteria in that listing. An impairment "equals" a listing if it is "at least equal in severity and duration to the criteria of any listed impairment" (SSA, 2016c). SSA assesses an applicant's residual functional capacity (RFC) when his or her impairment is severe but does not meet or equal the medical criteria within the *Listings*. SSA defines RFC as "an individual's maximum capacity for performance taking into account the limitations resulting from his or her impairment" (SSA, 2016a).

- In step 4, SSA assesses whether an applicant's RFC allows him or her to perform past work. An applicant who is able to perform past work will be denied benefits, but applicants who are unable to do so proceed to step 5.
- At step 5, an applicant's RFC and vocational factors such as age, education, and work experience and transferrable skills are considered in determining whether he or she can perform other work in the national economy. Applicants who are determined to be unable to perform work in the national economy are allowed benefits, while those who are determined to be able to perform work are denied.

Americans with Disabilities Act

The Americans with Disabilities Act (ADA) helps individuals with disabilities in ways that differ from those of SSA. The ADA seeks to eliminate discrimination against any individual who is considered a "qualified individual with a disability." The act defines disabilities through a three-pronged approach, in which each prong is its own definition. The first prong, often referred to as the "actual disability" prong, requires having a physical or mental impairment that substantially limits one or more major life activities to be considered a person with a disability[2]:

- *Physical impairment* is defined as "any physiological disorder or condition, cosmetic disfigurement, or anatomical loss affecting one or more body systems, such as neurological, musculoskeletal, special sense organs, respiratory (including speech organs), cardiovascular, reproductive, digestive, genitourinary, immune, circulatory, hemic, lymphatic, skin, and endocrine."[3]

[2] 29 CFR § 1630.2(g).

[3] 29 CFR § 1630.2(h)(1).

- *Mental impairment* is defined as "any mental or psychological disorder, such as an intellectual disability, organic brain syndrome, emotional or mental illness, and specific learning disabilities."[4]
- *Major life activities* is broadly defined to include, but is not limited to, the following list: "caring for oneself, performing manual tasks, seeing, hearing, eating, sleeping, walking, standing, sitting, reaching, lifting, bending, speaking, breathing, learning, reading, concentrating, thinking, communicating, interacting with others, and working."[5] The following are also included in the regulations as major life activities: "the operation of a major bodily function, including functions of the immune system, special sense organs and skin; normal cell growth; and digestive, genitourinary, bowel, bladder, neurological, brain, respiratory, circulatory, cardiovascular, endocrine, hemic, lymphatic, musculoskeletal, and reproductive functions. The operation of a major bodily function includes the operation of an individual organ within a body system."[6] A person need only be substantially limited in one major life activity to have a substantially limiting impairment.[7]

The second prong, often referred to as the "record of" prong, requires that an individual have "a record of a physical or mental impairment that substantially limited a major life activity."[8] This applies to an individual who *had* a substantially limiting impairment in the past or *was misclassified as having one* in the past, but does not currently have a substantially limiting impairment.

The third prong, often referred to as the "regarded as" prong, applies to individuals whom others regard as having a substantially limiting impairment.[9] People often treat others differently if they regard them as having a substantial impairment.

The ADA mandates that "absent undue hardship," employers must make reasonable accommodations for employees who meet the "actual disability" or "record of" prong definition of disability if the employees request them.[10] Failure to do so is considered discrimination. The ADA protects individuals from discrimination in employment only if they are "qualified individuals with a disability." This means they have met "the requisite skill, experience, education and other job-related requirements of

[4]29 CFR § 1630.2(h)(2).
[5]29 CFR § 1630.2(i)(1)(i).
[6]29 CFR § 1630.2(i)(1)(ii)
[7]29 CFR § 1630.2(j)(1)(viii).
[8]29 CFR § 1630.2(g)(1)(ii).
[9]29 CFR § 1630.2(g)(1)(iii).
[10]29 CFR § 1630.9(e).

the employment position" *and*, "with or without reasonable accommodation, can perform the essential functions of such position."[11]

The ADA and SSA standards for determining disability in terms of work are different. SSA does not consider an individual's ability to work *with the assistance of reasonable accommodations* in its determination of whether that individual is disabled and unable to engage in SGA or work. Under the ADA, by contrast, a person qualifies as an individual with a disability for work purposes if he or she has a substantially limiting impairment (actual disability definition) or a record of a substantially limiting impairment (record of definition) and can perform the essential functions of a job *with or without reasonable accommodations*. Thus, under the ADA, if a person can perform his or her job with reasonable accommodations, that individual is considered disabled but able to work. However, should the person's employer fail to provide the needed reasonable accommodations or take them away, the person is still considered a qualified individual with a disability but is unable to perform the job without the reasonable accommodations. The different SSA and ADA definitions of disability create a conundrum, as evidenced by *Cleveland v. Policy Management Systems Corporation.*

Cleveland v. Policy Management Systems Corporation

In *Cleveland v. Policy Management Systems Corporation* (1999), the Supreme Court recognized that ADA determinations and disability determinations under the Social Security Act "both help individuals with disabilities, but in different ways."[12] The petitioner, Cleveland, had a stroke during employment at Policy Management Systems Corporation. "The stroke left her impaired in her concentration, memory, and language skills."[13] Cleveland applied for SSDI benefits, stating that she was "disabled" and "unable to work." After 3 months, Cleveland's condition improved, and she returned to work, reporting her return to work to SSA. SSA denied her application for SSDI, noting that she had returned to work. However, 3 months after she returned to work and 4 days after SSA denied her SSDI benefits, Policy Management Systems terminated her. Cleveland then asked SSA to reconsider its denial. She offered the following reason for requesting the reconsideration: "I was terminated [by Policy Management Systems] due to my condition and I have not been able to work since. I continue to be disabled."[14] According to the Court, "she later added that she had

---

[11] 29 CFR § 1630.2(m).
[12] 526 U.S. at 799.
[13] 526 U.S. at 796.
[14] 526 U.S. at 797.

'attempted to return to work in mid-April,' that she had 'worked for three months,' and that Policy Management Systems terminated her because she 'could no longer do the job' in light of her 'condition.'"[15]

SSA denied Cleveland's request for reconsideration. She requested an SSA hearing, "reiterating that 'I am unable to work due to my disability,' and presenting new evidence about the extent of her injuries."[16] Approximately 10 months later, SSA awarded Cleveland SSDI benefits retroactive to the date of her stroke.[17] However, the week before SSA awarded Cleveland her SSDI benefits, she filed a suit under the ADA against her former employer, Policy Management Systems Corporation, contending that it terminated her "without reasonably 'accommodat[ing] her disability.'"[18] Cleveland alleged in her ADA suit "that she requested, but was denied, accommodations such as training and additional time to complete her work," and she submitted an affidavit to support the need for the reasonable accommodations from her treating physician.[19] Rather than evaluate Cleveland's request for reasonable accommodations on the merits, the District Court granted summary judgment, noting that by applying for and receiving SSDI benefits, Cleveland "had conceded that she was totally disabled."[20] The summary judgment prevented Cleveland from presenting any testimony on the merits regarding whether she was a "qualified individual with a disability" able to perform the essential functions of the job, with or without reasonable accommodations, the key inquiry under the ADA.[21]

The Fifth Circuit Court affirmed the District Court's grant of summary judgment, stating, "The application for or the receipt of social security disability benefits creates a *rebuttable* presumption that the claimant or recipient of such benefits is judicially estopped from asserting that he is a 'qualified individual with a disability [emphasis added].'"[22] The Fifth Circuit Court further noted that it was "at least theoretically conceivable that under some limited and highly unusual set of circumstances the two claims would not necessarily be mutually exclusive."[23] However, it concluded this was not the case with Cleveland. It explained, "Cleveland consistently represented to the SSA that she was totally disabled, she has failed to raise a genuine issue of material fact rebutting the presumption that she is judicially estopped from now asserting that for the time in question she

[15] 526 U.S. at 797.
[16] 526 U.S. at 796.
[17] 526 U.S. at 796.
[18] 526 U.S. at 797.
[19] 526 U.S. at 797.
[20] 526 U.S. at 797.
[21] 526 U.S. at 805.
[22] 526 U.S. at 798.
[23] 526 U.S. at 798.

was nevertheless a 'qualified individual with a disability' for purposes of her ADA claim."[24]

The Supreme Court vacated the Fifth Circuit Court's decision and remanded the case for further proceedings in the trial court.[25] According to the Supreme Court, courts cannot apply a special negative presumption because ADA suits and disability benefit claims do not inherently conflict, explaining that "there are too many situations in which an SSDI claim and an ADA claim can comfortably exist side by side."[26] The Supreme Court noted the differences between SSA determinations and the ADA's requirements. According to the Court, "By way of contrast, when the SSA determines whether an individual is disabled for SSDI purposes, it does *not* take the possibility of 'reasonable accommodation' into account, nor need an applicant refer to the possibility of reasonable accommodation when she applies for SSDI [emphasis added]."[27] The Court compared the SSDI standards with the requirements of ADA claims, noting, "The result is that an ADA suit claiming that the plaintiff can perform her job *with* reasonable accommodation may well prove consistent with an SSDI claim that the plaintiff could not perform her own job (or other jobs) *without* it [emphasis added]."[28] The Court was persuaded by Cleveland's statement in her brief describing the discrepancy between "her SSDI statements that she was 'totally disabled' and her ADA claim, that she could 'perform the essential functions' of her job. . . . The first statements, she says, 'were made in a forum which does not consider the effect that reasonable workplace accommodations would have on the ability to work.'"[29] Thus, since SSA does not consider reasonable accommodations in determining SSDI, an ADA plaintiff's claim that she can perform the essential functions of a job with reasonable accommodations is consistent with an SSDI claim that she is unable to work *without* accommodations.

As part of its congressional oversight, the U.S. Government Accountability Office (GAO) conducted studies examining SSA's disability programs (Bertoni, 2012; GAO, 2012, 2015; Robertson, 2002). The GAO designated federal disability programs managed by SSA and the U.S. Department of Veterans Affairs as high-risk for relying on outdated criteria in determining whether individuals qualify for benefits (GAO, 2015). SSA was designated as high-risk "in part, because their programs emphasize medical conditions in assessing work capacity without adequate consideration of work opportunities afforded by advances in medicine, technology, and job demands"

[24] 526 U.S. at 798.
[25] 526 U.S. at 807.
[26] 526 U.S. at 802.
[27] 526 U.S. at 802.
[28] 526 U.S. at 802-803.
[29] 526 U.S. at 806.

(GAO, 2012). According to a 2002 report, scientific advances as well as social changes have enhanced the potential for individuals with disabilities to work (Robertson, 2002). The report asserts that the assistive products and technologies resulting from scientific advances, which include advanced wheelchair designs, a new generation of prosthetic devices, and voice recognition systems, provide more capabilities and allow for more independence for individuals with disabilities relative to the products and technologies available in the past (Robertson, 2002). The report also notes that social change has promoted the inclusion and participation of individuals with disabilities in society, which includes the work environment (Robertson, 2002). In 2012, the GAO recommended that SSA "conduct limited and focused studies on the availability and effects of considering more fully assistive devices and workplace accommodations in its disability determinations" (GAO, 2012). The GAO concluded that "without such efforts to study how certain assistive devices and accommodations are playing a role in helping individuals with impairments stay at work or return to work, and their costs in comparison to potentially providing years of disability benefit payments, SSA may be missing an opportunity to assist individuals with disabilities to reengage in the workforce" (Bertoni, 2012).

STUDY CHARGE AND SCOPE

In 2015, SSA asked the Health and Medicine Division of the National Academies of Sciences, Engineering, and Medicine to convene a committee of relevant experts to provide a comprehensive analysis of the use of assistive products and technologies, including wheeled and seated mobility devices (WSMDs), upper-extremity prostheses (UEPs), and committee-selected products and technologies that pertain to hearing and to communication and speech in adults[30] (see Box 1-1 for the committee's statement of task). The 15-member committee included experts in the areas of physical medicine and rehabilitation; speech-language pathology; augmentative and alternative communication; rehabilitation science/engineering; physical therapy; occupational therapy; workplace accommodations; disability law and policy; environmental modifications; assistive devices, including WSMDs and upper-limb prostheses; and assistive devices related to hearing and communication (see Appendix D for biographical sketches of the committee members).

In carrying out its task, the Committee on the Use of Selected Assistive Products and Technologies in Eliminating or Reducing the Effects of Impairments was asked by the sponsor to address several specific topics,

[30]These four categories of assistive products and technologies give SSA the greatest challenge (Firmin, 2016).

BOX 1-1
Statement of Task

An ad hoc committee will provide an analysis of the use in adults of selected assistive products and technologies, including wheeled/seated mobility devices, upper-extremity prostheses, and committee-selected products and technologies that pertain to hearing and to communication and speech. The committee will provide definitions and explanations of relevant terms, including *assistive technology* and *workplace reasonable accommodations.*

Drawing upon existing data to the extent they are available, the committee will address the following questions:

- For the selected products and technologies
  - To what extent are they being used, and by whom?
  - What is the observed range of impairment mitigating effects?
  - How does use vary depending upon the individual, including those with other impairments or comorbidities and how does this vary for different occupations?
  - To what extent have they altered the outlook for occupational success?
  - What are typical training and adaptation times?
- To the degree possible, the committee will address
  - What information exists on access to and availability of the selected assistive products and technologies in the current health care and rehabilitation environment, including access to appropriate evaluation and training by qualified personnel?
  - Under what circumstances, if any, do employers provide access to these products and technologies as workplace reasonable accommodations?
  - What costs are associated with the product and technology acquisition, product maintenance, repair, and replacement and how do disabled individuals gain financial access to the products and technologies?
  - For young adults, what challenges exist in transitioning from a school environment to the workplace?
- To the extent information is available, the committee will describe the decision-making processes of other government or private monetary disability benefit programs regarding the use of the selected assistive products and technologies.

The report will include conclusions but not recommendations.

including defining and explaining terms relevant to the assistive devices environment, providing an analysis of the impairment-mitigating effects of the selected assistive devices, describing the training regimen and adaptation time for the selected devices, identifying the prevalence of use of the selected devices by specific physical and mental disorders and by age, providing an analysis of access to and availability of the selected devices, providing information on consideration of the selected devices in other programs that provide monetary benefits based on disability, and describing special considerations related to use of assistive devices by young adults as they transition from high school to the workplace. The committee's task did not encompass reviewing the potential effects of regulatory and commercial policies on assistive technology outcomes research.

SSA'S CONSIDERATION OF SELECTED ASSISTIVE PRODUCTS AND TECHNOLOGIES

The following is a description of how SSA considers certain assistive products and technologies during its sequential evaluation process, which, as detailed above, includes assessment of whether an adult's impairment meets or medically equals a listing (step 3), evaluation of RFC to do past work (step 4), and consideration of RFC and vocational factors to determine the ability to do other work (step 5).

Wheeled and Seated Mobility Devices

During step 3 of SSA's sequential evaluation process, most adults who use WSMDs for ambulation have an impairment that meets or medically equals a listing because of their "inability to ambulate effectively" (SSA, 2016a). An inability to ambulate effectively is defined as "having insufficient lower extremity functioning to permit independent ambulation without the use of a hand-held assistive device(s) that limits the functioning of both upper extremities" (SSA, 2016a). Examples include the inability to walk without the use of a walker, the inability to walk a block at a reasonable pace on rough surfaces, and the inability to use standard public transportation (SSA, 2016a). Since most adults using WSMDs have an impairment that meets or medically equals a listing, SSA does not evaluate their functioning beyond step 3. Instead, policy specifies that when evaluating RFC for an individual who cannot stand or walk for the majority of a workday, SSA will focus on the individual's manipulative and visual abilities to engage in SGA (SSA, 2016a).

Upper-Extremity Prostheses

During step 3 of the sequential evaluation process, most adults who use bilateral UEPs have an impairment that meets or medically equals a listing because of their "inability to perform fine and gross movements effectively" (SSA, 2016a). Examples include the inability to prepare a simple meal and feed oneself, the inability to take care of personal hygiene, and the inability to sort and handle papers or files. In steps 4 and 5, when an individual is missing an upper extremity, RFC has been evaluated by assessing reduced strength and nonexertional capacities. An allowance is often given when standing and walking limitations are present as well. These practices were enacted when many individuals who were missing an upper limb did not use prostheses (SSA, 2016a).

Lower-Extremity Amputations

SSA policy requires that individuals with lower-limb amputations wear their prostheses when ambulation is being assessed. Medical documentation is required when an individual cannot use a prosthesis. If an individual is medically capable of wearing a prosthesis and does not have an appropriate reason for failing to do so, SSA will determine that the individual is not disabled (SSA, 2016a).

Hearing Aids

During step 3, SSA does not consider an individual's ability to hear with a hearing aid when evaluating hearing impairment (not treated by cochlear implantation). Although previous rules did require the use of a hearing aid during evaluation, many individuals did not bring one to the exam because they lacked access to such a device, had lost it, had forgotten to bring it, or had brought one that did not work. In addition, research performed in 2010 indicated that generic hearing aids were not widely available because of technological advances that allow for more highly customized hearing aids, and hearing testing in clinical practice generally was unaided (SSA, 2016a). In addition, SSA believes that evaluation with a hearing aid does not provide information on whether an individual with a hearing impairment can effectively use the device on a sustained basis or in other environments (SSA, 2016a). Therefore, SSA changed its policy to evaluate a hearing impairment at step 3 only without the use of a hearing aid to reflect the current state of practice.

When assessing RFC and ability to perform work in steps 4 and 5, SSA evaluates an individual's ability to hear with a hearing aid if the severity of his or her hearing loss does not meet or medically equal a listing. As mentioned earlier, RFC is an individual's maximum ability to perform sustained work activities; therefore, SSA assesses the maximum ability of the claimant when he or she is wearing a hearing aid. SSA policy specifies that "basic communication is all that is needed to do unskilled work" (SSA, 2016a). If an individual maintains basic communication skills, he or she can perform unskilled occupations "within the exertional RFC for which he or she has the capacity" (SSA, 2016a).

Speech Impairments

In step 3, SSA evaluates loss of speech for adults as the inability "to produce speech by any means [including] the use of mechanical or electronic devices that improve voice or articulation" (SSA, 2016a). Speech proficiency is evaluated on the basis of audibility, intelligibility, and functional efficiency. When an individual's speech impairment does not meet or medically equal a listing and assessment proceeds to steps 4 and 5, his or her RFC with respect to speech and communication limitations is assessed with consideration of the individual's vocational factors, age, education, and work experience.

STUDY APPROACH

The committee conducted an extensive review of the literature pertaining to assistive products and technologies. This review began with a search from years 2000 to 2016 of online databases including Medline, Embase, Cochrane Database of Systematic Reviews, and Lexis Nexis. Committee members and project staff identified additional literature and databases using traditional academic research methods and online searches throughout the course of the study. This literature review revealed a paucity of national data on the prevalence of use or the incidence of prescription of assistive products and technologies relevant to this study within the United States, largely because no single nationally representative source of data contains this information. In addition, there is little published research on the functional outcomes associated with the use of assistive products and technologies and associated services by individuals with disabilities, particularly with respect to work participation.

The committee used a variety of resources to supplement its literature review. Meeting in person five times, the committee held three public workshops and one public teleconference to hear from invited experts in areas pertinent to the study. Speakers at the workshops included experts in assistive devices pertaining to hearing and communication and speech recognition, WSMDs, UEPs, workplace accommodations, disability statistics, and the transition from high school to the workplace. The committee also heard from representatives of Kaiser Permanente, the Veterans Health Administration, Medicare, and state vocational rehabilitation services agencies, who addressed the coverage of relevant assistive products and technologies. Representatives from the Veterans Benefits Administration, Unum, Prudential Financial, and the Canada Pension Plan addressed disability insurance and benefit programs.

In addition, the committee commissioned two papers to provide additional critical analysis in areas relevant to its task. The first provides an analysis of financial access to (funding sources for) relevant assistive products and technologies, focusing on the following public funding sources: Medicaid, Medicare, vocational rehabilitation services, and special education programs under the Individuals with Disabilities Education Act. The other provides analysis of Centers for Medicare & Medicaid Services beneficiaries receiving support for relevant assistive devices (see Appendix C). In addition, the paper includes data on the prevalence of use of assistive devices from such sources as the National Health Interview Survey Functioning and Disability Module and the SIPP. The paper provides data and information on working-age adults aged 20-67.

The committee's work was further informed by previous National Academies reports, including *Enabling America: Assessing the Role of Rehabilitation Science and Engineering* (IOM, 1997), *The Dynamics of Disability: Workshop on Disability in America* (IOM and NRC, 2002), *Improving the Social Security Disability Decision Process* (IOM, 2007a), *The Future of Disability in America* (IOM, 2007b), and *Hearing Health Care for Adults: Priorities for Improving Access and Affordability* (NASEM, 2016).

REPORT ORGANIZATION

Chapter 2 situates terms relevant to the assistive product and technology environment within a framework developed by the committee. Chapters 3 through 6, respectively, provide for the four selected categories of assistive products and technologies—wheeled and seated mobility devices, upper-extremity prostheses, hearing devices, and augmentative and alternative communication devices—descriptions of the various products and technologies[31]; clinical considerations, including effects on mitigating the impacts of impairments; and the prevalence of use. Chapter 7 provides an overview of financial access to the relevant assistive products and technologies. Chapter 8 reviews the assessment, acquisition, and use of these products and technologies in selected disability programs that provide monetary benefits. Finally, Chapter 9 presents overarching conclusions derived from the findings and conclusions provided throughout the report.

---

[31]Chapters 3, 4, and 6 include images of a variety of assistive products and technologies. The images serve as examples of device categories only and should not be considered an endorsement of specific products or manufacturers.

REFERENCES

Bertoni, D. 2012. *SSA disability programs: Progress and challenges related to modernizing: Testimony before the Subcommittee on Social Security, Committee on Ways and Means, House of Representatives.* http://www.gao.gov/assets/650/648321.pdf (accessed January 18, 2017).

Brault, M. W. 2012. Americans with disabilities: 2010. *Current Population Reports* 7(2012): 1-131.

Firmin, J. 2016. *Social Security Administration presentations relevant to the committee's task.* Presentation to the Committee on the Use of Selected Assistive Products and Technologies in Eliminating or Reducing the Effects of Impairments, Washington, DC, March 31.

GAO (U.S. Government Accountability Office). 2012. *Modernizing SSA disability programs: Progress made, but key efforts warrant more management focus.* Report to the chairman, Subcommittee on Social Security, Committee on Ways and Means, House of Representatives. http://www.gao.gov/assets/600/591701.pdf (accessed January 18, 2017).

GAO. 2015. *High-risk series: An update.* http://www.gao.gov/assets/670/668415.pdf (accessed September 16, 2016).

IOM (Institute of Medicine). 1997. *Enabling America: Assessing the role of rehabilitation science and engineering.* Washington, DC: National Academy Press.

IOM. 2007a. *Improving the social security disability decision process.* Washington, DC: The National Academies Press.

IOM. 2007b. *The future of disability in America.* Washington, DC: The National Academies Press.

IOM and NRC (National Research Council). 2002. *The dynamics of disability: Measuring and monitoring disability for social security programs.* Washington, DC: National Academy Press.

Johnson, K. L., B. Dudgeon, C. Kuehn, and W. Walker. 2007. Assistive technology use among adolescents and young adults with spina bifida. *American Journal of Public Health* 97(2):330-336.

Kaye, H. S., T. Kang, and M. P. LaPlante. 2000. *Mobility device use in the United States.* Washington, DC: National Institute on Disability and Rehabilitation Research, U.S. Department of Education.

Kraus, L. 2015. *Disability statistics annual report.* http://www.disabilitycompendium.org/docs/default-source/2015-compendium/annualreport_2015_final.pdf (accessed October 17, 2016).

NASEM (National Academies of Sciences, Engineering, and Medicine). 2016. *Hearing health care for adults: Priorities for improving access and affordability.* Washington, DC: The National Academies Press.

Robertson, R. E. 2002. *SSA disability programs: Fully updating disability criteria has implications for program design.* http://www.gao.gov/new.items/d02919t.pdf (accessed January 18, 2017).

SSA (U.S. Social Security Administration). 2012a. *POMS DI 00115.015 Definitions of disability.* https://secure.ssa.gov/poms.nsf/lnx/0400115015 (accessed July 16, 2017).

SSA. 2012b. *POMS DI 24505.001 Individual must have a medically determinable severe impairment.* https://secure.ssa.gov/poms.nsf/lnx/0424505001 (accessed September 16, 2016).

SSA. 2015. *POMS DI 10520.001 Impairment-related work expenses (IRWE).* https://secure.ssa.gov/poms.nsf/lnx/0410520001 (accessed December 12, 2016).

SSA. 2016a (unpublished). *Background for IOM on SSA policy and processes related to assistive devices and workplace reasonable accommodations.* Baltimore, MD: SSA.

SSA. 2016b. *Fast facts and figures about Social Security, 2016*. https://www.ssa.gov/policy/docs/chartbooks/fast_facts/2016/fast_facts16.pdf (accessed September 15, 2016).

SSA. 2016c. *POMS DI 24505.015 Finding disability based on the listing of impairments*. https://secure.ssa.gov/poms.nsf/lnx/0424505015 (accessed September 15, 2016).

SSA. 2017. *Substantial gainful activity*. https://www.ssa.gov/oact/cola/sga.html (accessed January 23, 2017).

Wixon, B., and A. Strand. 2013. *Identifying SSA's sequential disability determination steps using administrative data*. https://www.ssa.gov/policy/docs/rsnotes/rsn2013-01.html (accessed January 19, 2017).

2

Environmental Facilitators Framework

As part of the statement of task for this study outlined by the U.S. Social Security Administration (SSA) (see Box 1-1 in Chapter 1), the committee was asked to "provide definitions and explanations of relevant terms, including *assistive technology* and *workplace reasonable accommodations*." To meet this objective, the committee, in addition to providing definitions of the terms identified by SSA in a glossary (see Appendix B), developed an environmental facilitators framework based on the model of disability in the *International Classification of Functioning, Disability and Health* (ICF). This chapter begins with an overview of the ICF and related models. It then provides a detailed description of the committee's environmental facilitators framework. The chapter ends with findings and conclusions.

Before proceeding, it is important to understand as context for the ICF and the committee's framework the evolution of the concept of disability over the past quarter century from a medical to a biopsychosocial model. The medical model identifies disability as a "feature of the person" caused by disease, injury, or some other health condition (WHO, 2001, 2002, p. 8; see also IOM, 1991; Kaplan, 2000). According to that model, disability is managed through medical care in the form of individual treatment or through adjustments or changes to behavior (Kaplan, 2000; WHO, 2001). Conversely, the biopsychosocial model identifies disability as a problem at the societal level, with the goal of integrating all individuals into society (Kaplan, 2000; Whiteneck, 2006; WHO, 2001). Therefore, managing disability is the collective responsibility of society to allow for the full participation of individuals with disabilities in all aspects of life (Kaplan, 2000; WHO, 2001). This evolution of the concept of disability is reflected in the

ICF, related disability models, and the committee's environmental facilitators framework.

THE *INTERNATIONAL CLASSIFICATION OF FUNCTIONING, DISABILITY AND HEALTH* AND RELATED MODELS

In 1980, the World Health Organization (WHO) issued the *International Classification of Impairments, Disabilities, and Handicaps* (ICIDH) as a tool for organizing the consequences of disease into three distinct classifications: impairment at the organ level, disability at the person level, and handicap at the societal level (WHO, 1980). However, the labeling of "handicap" at the societal level and the failure to include environmental factors created some problems in the use of the ICIDH (IOM, 2006; WHO, 1980). The latter factors are explicitly incorporated in both earlier and later models of disability. A model developed by Nagi (1965) initiated research into the environmental factors at the family, community, and society levels that affect disability as an outcome. And Fougeyrollas (1995) clarified the usefulness of a holistic model that stresses the role of environmental factors in social participation for individuals with disabilities.

In 2001, the WHO published the ICF as a revision to the ICIDH. The ICF is a classification scheme that identifies and describes the relationships among the various factors that interact to effect health and function. Its revised classifications of disability are body structure and function at the organ level, activity at the person level, and participation at the societal level. Environmental factors are incorporated into the conceptualization of disability, and the term "handicap" is eliminated to expand the scope of the model and allow for the description of positive experiences (WHO, 2001). Specifically, the ICF conceptualizes an individual's functioning as the interaction among his/her health condition, environmental factors, and personal factors.

The information in the ICF is organized into two parts: *functioning and disability* and *contextual factors*. As shown in Figure 2-1, functioning and disability (the middle tier of the figure) consist of body functions and structures and activities and participation, while contextual factors (the bottom tier) consist of both environmental and personal factors. Body functions are defined as the "physiological functions of body systems (including psychological functions)" and body structures as the "anatomical parts of the body such as organs, limbs and their components" (WHO, 2001, p. 10).

Environmental factors "refer to all aspects of the external or extrinsic world that form the context of an individual's life and, as such, have an impact on that person's functioning" (WHO, 2001, p. 213). These factors can be classified into two levels—individual and societal. The individual level encompasses the immediate environment of the individual, while the

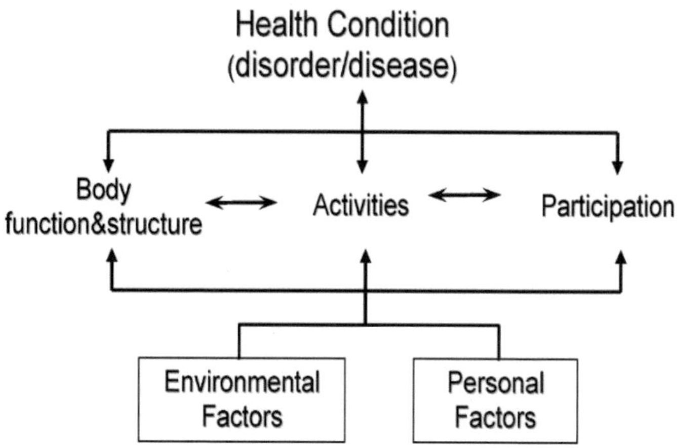

FIGURE 2-1 Organization of the *International Classification of Functioning, Disability and Health.*
SOURCE: WHO, 2001.

societal level refers to "formal and informal social structures, services, and overarching approaches or systems in the community or society that impact the individual" (WHO, 2001, p. 17). Examples of environmental factors include job market, geographic location, noise level, built environment, and transportation. Built environment encompasses all of the tools individuals need to perform work activities. Transportation is another environmental factor that is necessary for an individual to participate fully in employment.

Personal factors represent influences on functioning particular to the individual (WHO, 2013). Given the large variation in society and culture and even a lack of clarity with respect to these factors, they are not classified within the ICF (WHO, 2013). Yet, while developing a classification for personal factors can be challenging, it also represents an opportunity. Including this type of information in data collection could assist investigators in providing "empirical background for the future development of personal factors in the ICF" (WHO, 2013, p. 26), and codifying personal factors in the ICF could help in conveying "information important for a complete description of the functioning profile" (WHO, 2013, p. 40). Personal factors that may affect functioning include gender, race, ethnicity, age, social and educational background, past and current experiences and life events, behavior patterns, and psychological assets (WHO, 2013).

Both environmental and personal factors act as facilitators or barriers along the disablement pathway. As a facilitator, assistive technology is an environmental factor that can help reduce the effects of an impairment. Conversely, certain features in the built environment may act as barriers that prevent an individual with a disability from completing a task.

The biopsycho-ecological model expands on the biomedical and biopsychosocial models to encourage a more comprehensive understanding of illness, injury, activity limitation, and restriction of participation at the interface between the person and the environment (Stineman and Streim, 2010). This model operates through health environmental integration, which recognizes complex interactions beginning at the cellular level and ending at the individual's experience of the environment (Stineman and Streim, 2010).

One effort that begins to identify the role and pathways of contextual (i.e., environmental and personal) interventions in the disablement/enablement process within an ICF framework is the modification of the ICF developed by the National Health and Aging Trends Study (Freedman, 2009). This modification entails the inclusion of a new domain—"accommodations" (see Figure 2-2)—defined as behavioral responses to changes in capacity. Accommodations include the receipt of help, assistive technology, environmental modifications, and other compensatory strategies (Freedman, 2009) that act on the interactions among the ICF domains to enhance activity and participation.

ENVIRONMENTAL FACILITATORS FRAMEWORK

In the context of the evolution of the understanding of disability described above, it is evident that SSA's approach to disability is based on a medical model rather than a biopsychosocial model that stresses the importance of environmental factors. Particularly, the agency's current focus is on impairment mitigation and functional capacity as mandated by legislation. More all-encompassing definitions based on the biopsychosocial model, including those adopted by the U.S. Congress in the Americans with Disabilities Act (ADA), the WHO in the ICF, and the U.S. Centers for Disease Control and Prevention (CDC), identify disability as a problem that results from the interaction of a person's impairments and functional capacity with external factors, recognizing the significant role of the environment in contributing to disability. Specifically, the ADA recognizes that full participation of individuals with disabilities in society is dependent on the use of accessible designs to remove physical environmental barriers in public and private facilities, while reasonable accommodations are crucial for achieving full participation in the workplace (IOM, 2006). In addition, the CDC identifies the difficulty of a person with a disability to perform certain activities and interact with the surrounding world (CDC, 2016). For SSA, the importance of the biopsychosocial model is not solely in understanding disability but, more importantly, in clearly identifying environmental

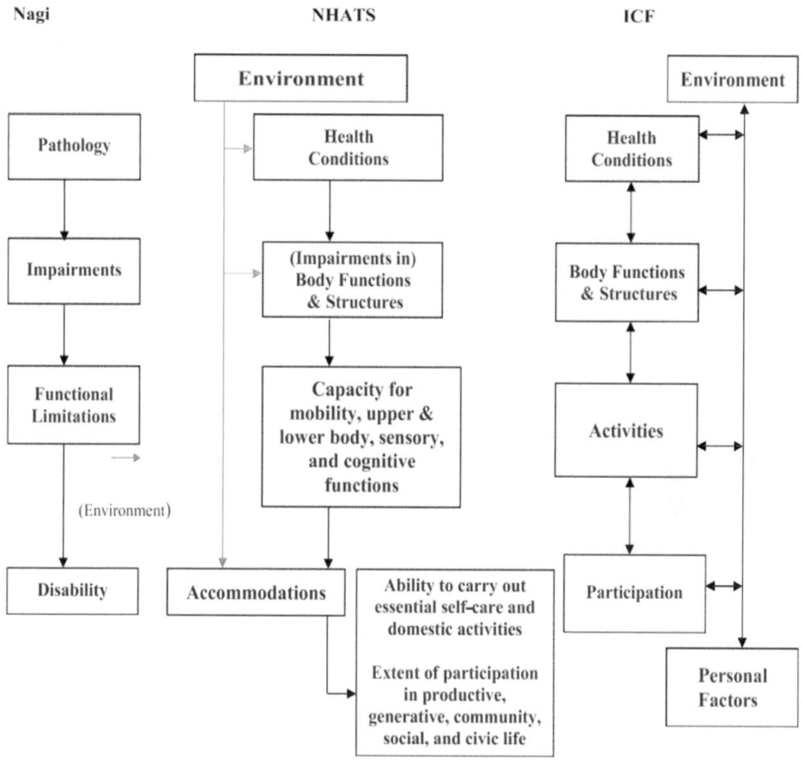

FIGURE 2-2 Comparison of the Nagi (1965), National Health and Aging Trends Study (NHATS) (Freedman, 2009), and *International Classification of Functioning, Disability and Health* (ICF) (WHO, 2001) frameworks.
SOURCE: Freedman, V. A. 2009. Adopting the ICF language for studying late-life disability: A field of dreams? *The Journals of Gerontology, Series A: Biological Sciences and Medical Sciences* 64(11):1172-1174, Published by Oxford University Press on behalf of the Gerontological Society of America.

factors as potential focal points for interventions. Accordingly, the committee developed the environmental facilitators framework depicted in Figure 2-3, based on the ICF.

Framework Description

The environmental facilitators framework illustrated in Figure 2-3 is a conceptual model showing potential relationships. It builds on the ICF to identify specific environmental interventions and the pathways along which

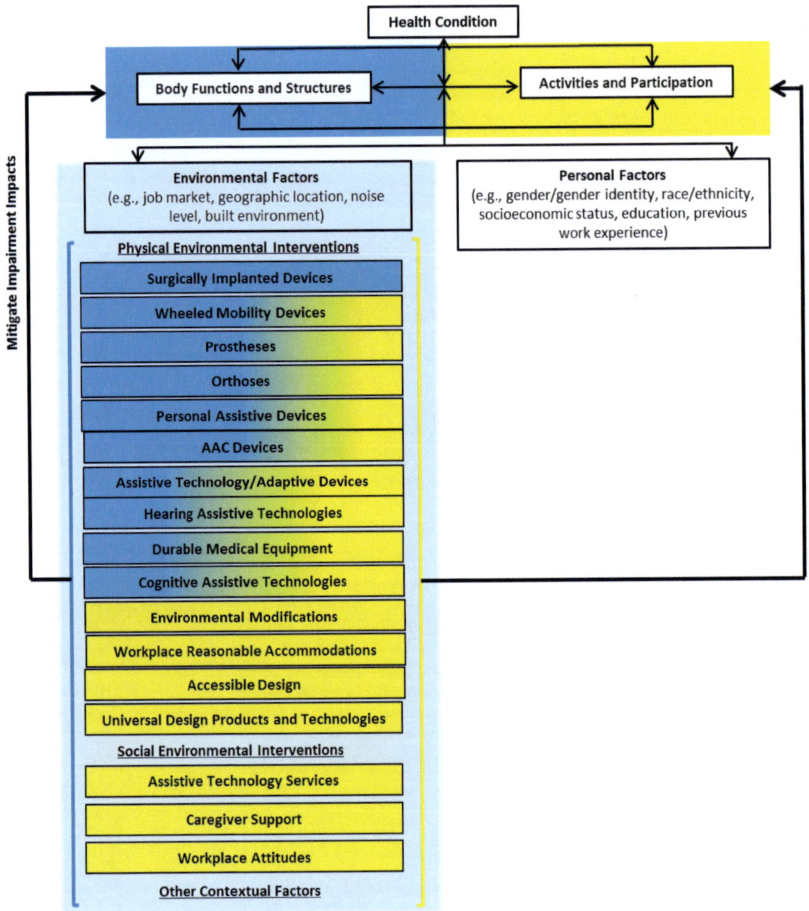

FIGURE 2-3 Environmental facilitators framework.
NOTES: The extent to which environmental interventions mitigate the impact of impairments (blue) and performance barriers (yellow) is based on the committee's expert opinion. AAC = augmentative and alternative communication.

those interventions can act either to mitigate the impact of impairment by restoring or replacing relevant body structure and/or function or to enhance activities and participation by mitigating performance barriers. The former interventions target organ system impairment(s), while the latter target contextual factors.

As shown in Figure 2-3, environmental factors include physical environmental interventions, social environmental interventions, and other contextual factors (light blue box). Assistive products and technologies are physical environmental interventions that can either mitigate the impact of impairments by restoring or replacing relevant function (shown in blue), enhance performance and activity by mitigating performance barriers (shown in yellow), or do both in varying degrees (shown in blue and yellow).

As illustrated in Figure 2-3, for example, surgically implanted devices (e.g., artificial joint, cochlear implant) solely mitigate the impact of impairment because they directly affect the individual's body functions and structures (and therefore are shown in blue). In contrast, wheeled mobility devices, prostheses, orthoses, personal assistive devices, and augmentative and alternative communication devices primarily mitigate the impact of impairment but, depending on the type of device, may also act to reduce performance barriers to participation and activity (and therefore are shown mainly in blue but also in yellow). For instance, the use of a power wheelchair may mitigate the impact of impairment by allowing individuals to have independent mobility. Whereas independent mobility may improve an individual's capacity to work, it is not directly linked to enhanced performance and participation within a workplace. On the other hand, a standing wheelchair that enables an individual to reach a counter that is required for the performance of a specific work activity is clearly aimed at mitigating a performance barrier.

The greater proportion of yellow for assistive technology/adaptive devices, hearing assistive technologies, durable medical equipment, and cognitive assistive technologies in Figure 2-3 reflects the fact that these interventions equally mitigate the impact of impairment and reduce performance barriers. For example, a hearing assistive technology such as a hearing aid or personal listening device may mitigate impairment by providing an individual with hearing loss with improved audibility of sounds, such as speech or music, regardless of the context. Alternatively, the use of an assistive listening system in the workplace is aimed at enhancing work performance by allowing an individual with hearing loss to participate in a work activity that involves listening to others.

Finally, some interventions (indicated in all yellow) serve solely to mitigate performance barriers to participation in the workplace. They include both physical environmental interventions—such as environmental modifications, workplace reasonable accommodations, accessible design, and universal design products and technologies—and social environmental interventions, including assistive technology services, caregiver support, and workplace attitudes. As mentioned earlier, personal factors also may have an impact on the outcome of interventions. These factors may include gender/gender identity, race/ethnicity, socioeconomic status, education, and previous work experience.

Implications for SSA

The environmental facilitators framework shown in Figure 2-3 can serve as a guide to assist SSA and other organizations in evaluating the effects of impairments and the impact of assistive products and technologies and other environmental interventions on mitigating those effects. It is important for such organizations to assess individuals' functional capacity when using the products and technologies they normally use to mitigate their impairments. However, capacity and performance do not necessarily imply participation, nor are they necessarily sufficient for predicting work performance. Work participation and performance are directly related to environmental factors beyond the personal assistive products and technologies individuals may use when their ability to execute a particular task or function is being assessed during a disability determination. For instance, environmental modifications and workplace reasonable accommodations are work-specific and vary from place to place, making it difficult to determine an individual's ability to participate in work activities based on the use of assistive devices alone. Even if an individual with a severe impairment could perform (with or without such devices) the tasks necessary for a particular job with appropriate environmental modifications or accommodations, there is no guarantee that those modifications or accommodations will in fact be available. In short, it is essential to consider a multitude of complex contextual (environmental and personal) factors when assessing an individual's ability to work. Moreover, environmental modifications and social acceptance are necessary to allow for the full participation of individuals with disabilities in all aspects of life. However, SSA's medical model approach positions the agency on the side of simply mitigating the impact of impairment. Accordingly, it is unreasonable to expect the agency to factor environmental interventions designed solely to enhance participation, such as environmental modifications, workplace reasonable accommodations, and accessible and universal design, or social environmental interventions, such as workplace attitudes, into its disability determinations. If SSA's mission were to evolve to encompass facilitating employment among people with disabilities, it would be necessary for the agency to take a more holistic approach that would include an assessment not only of a person's functional capacity but also the personal and environmental factors shown in Figure 2-3.

FINDINGS AND CONCLUSIONS

Findings

2-1. Some assistive products and technologies can enhance work performance or mitigate impairment, while others may do both.

2-2. The concept of disability has evolved to reflect a biopsychosocial model in which disability is perceived as the interaction between an individual's functional capacity and relevant environmental and personal factors.
2-3. Likewise, based on the *International Classification of Functioning, Disability and Health* model, understanding a person's ability to participate in work includes not only the person's functional capacity but also relevant environmental and personal factors.
2-4. Environmental factors such as job market, geographic location, and built environment can influence how an individual experiences disability.
2-5. Personal factors such as gender/gender identity, race/ethnicity, age, socioeconomic status, insurance coverage, education, and previous work experience can influence how an individual experiences disability.
2-6. A complete evaluation of a person's functioning would include assistive products and technologies that mitigate the person's impairments.
2-7. The Social Security Administration's (SSA's) current focus is on impairment mitigation and functional capacity as mandated by legislation. Accordingly, the agency's emphasis is on understanding the role of interventions that mitigate the impact of impairments by restoring or replacing body structure and/or function.

Conclusions

2-1. Assistive products and technologies may mitigate the impact of an impairment sufficiently to allow a person to work. In some cases, however, environmental and personal factors create barriers to employment despite those impairment-mitigating effects. [Finding 2-1]
2-2. Assessment of work participation requires consideration of an individual's functional capacity plus a multitude of complex environmental and personal factors. [Findings 2-2, 2-3, 2-4, 2-5]
2-3. If SSA's mission were to evolve to encompass facilitating employment among people with disabilities, a holistic approach that would include an assessment not only of a person's functional capacity but also of personal and environmental factors would be necessary. [Findings 2-2, 2-3]
2-4. To assess the effects of impairments on a person's ability to work, it is important to evaluate the person's functional capacity while using the assistive products and technologies he or she normally uses. [Finding 2-6]

2-5. Given SSA's current mission, it is unreasonable to expect the agency to factor into its disability determinations environmental interventions designed solely to mitigate performance barriers. [Finding 2-7]

REFERENCES

CDC (U.S. Centers for Disease Control and Prevention). 2016. *Disability overview*. https://www.cdc.gov/ncbddd/disabilityandhealth/disability.html (accessed March 21, 2017).

Fougeyrollas, P. 1995. Documenting environmental factors for preventing the handicap creation process: Quebec contributions relating to ICIDH and social participation of people with functional differences. *Disability and Rehabilitation* 17(3-4):145-153.

Freedman, V. A. 2009. Adopting the ICF language for studying late-life disability: A field of dreams? *The Journals of Gerontology, Series A: Biological Sciences and Medical Sciences* 64(11):1172-1174.

IOM (Institute of Medicine). 1991. *Disability in America: Toward a national agenda for prevention*. Washington, DC: National Academy Press.

IOM. 2006. *Workshop on disability in America: A new look*. Washington, DC: The National Academies Press.

Kaplan, D. 2000. The definition of disability: Perspective of the disability community. *Journal of Health Care Law and Policy* 3(2):352-364.

Nagi, S. 1965. Some conceptual issues in disability and rehabilitation. In *Sociology and Rehabilitation*, edited by M. B. Sussman. Washington, DC: American Sociological Association.

Stineman, M. G., and J. E. Streim. 2010. The biopsycho-ecological paradigm: A foundational theory for medicine. *Physical Medicine and Rehabilitation* 2(11):1035-1045.

Whiteneck, G. 2006. Conceptual models of disability: Past, present, and future. In *Workshop on disability in America: A new look*, edited by M. J. Field, A. M. Jette, and L. Martin. Washington, DC: The National Academies Press. Pp. 50-66.

WHO (World Health Organization). 1980. *International Classification of Impairments, Disabilities, and Handicaps: A manual of classification relating to the consequences of disease*. Geneva, Switzerland, and Albany, NY: WHO.

WHO. 2001. *International Classification of Functioning, Disability and Health*. Geneva, Switzerland: WHO.

WHO. 2002. *Towards a common language for functioning, disability and health: ICF*. Geneva, Switzerland: WHO.

WHO. 2013. *How to use the ICF: A practical manual for using the International Classification of Functioning, Disability and Health*. Geneva, Switzerland: WHO.

3

Wheeled and Seated Mobility Devices

Wheeled and seated mobility devices (WSMDs) are medical devices that are intended to provide mobility and function for persons with restricted or no ability to ambulate without assistance from technology. This chapter begins with an overview of the use of WSMDs and a detailed taxonomy of the various types of these devices. The chapter next reviews the use of WSMDs and clinical considerations in the choice of a WSMD for a particular individual. Evaluation and monitoring, training and adaptation, and access and availability are then addressed in turn. The chapter ends with findings and conclusions.

OVERVIEW OF THE USE OF WHEELED AND SEATED MOBILITY DEVICES

The Survey of Income and Program Participation (SIPP), conducted by the U.S. Census Bureau, is a population-based source of information for overall use of WSMDs in the United States (U.S. Census Bureau, 2016). In 2010, the SIPP found that 1.5 percent of the population aged 15 and older (3.6 million people) used a WSMD (wheelchair or scooter) (U.S. Census Bureau, 2016). A study using the Canadian Survey on Disability, conducted in 2012, found the prevalence of wheelchair and scooter use among community-living Canadians aged 15 and older to be approximately 1.0 percent of the total population (Smith et al., 2016). The difference between these prevalence rates for the U.S. and Canadian populations is not discussed by the authors.

Figure 3-1 projects the number of wheelchair users over a 25-year

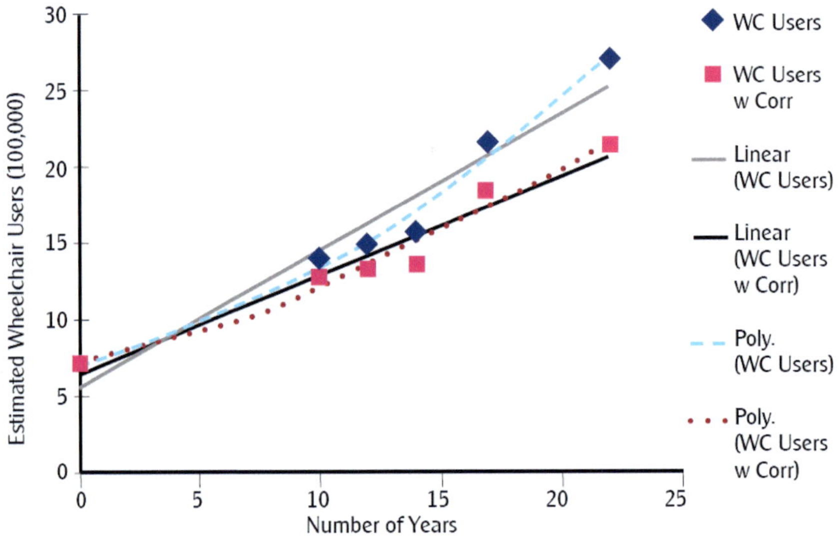

FIGURE 3-1 Projected number of wheelchair users (linear and polynomial model). SOURCE: Flagg, J. 2009. Wheeled mobility demographics. In *The industry profile on wheeled mobility*, edited by S. M. Bauer and M. E. Bunning. Buffalo, NY: Rehabilitation Engineering Research Center on Technology Transfer. Pp. 7-29.

period beginning in 2005 based on data from both the National Health Interview Survey-Disability (NHIS-D) and the SIPP (CDC, 2016; Flagg, 2009; U.S. Census Bureau, 2016). These estimates include both correction for population growth ("WC Users w Corr") and no correction for population growth ("WC Users") (Flagg, 2009). The figure suggests a quadrupling of the estimated number of wheelchair users into the next decade.

Obtaining population-based prevalence information related to access, user characteristics, cost, and evaluation of outcomes for working-age users of WSMDs is challenging. The challenge is related to the fact that in the United States, multiple agencies and service providers are responsible for determining the need for assistive devices, providing the devices, delivering the training in their use, monitoring their use, and assessing outcomes (Crane and Minkel, 2009). This fragmented approach to the delivery of assistive device–related health care services is discussed in detail elsewhere in this report. As a result of this fragmentation, no single public-use data source includes prevalence information related to use of WSMDs specifically among individuals of working age (20-67).

TAXONOMY[1]

WSMDs can improve function, independence, home and community integration, activity, participation, comfort, and quality of life (Chaves et al., 2004; Davies et al., 2003; Edwards and McCluskey, 2010; Laferrier et al., 2010; Salminen et al., 2009; Scherer, 2002; Trefler et al., 2004). Many different types of such devices exist. In 2005, through the National Coverage Determination (NCD) process, the Centers for Medicare & Medicaid Services (CMS) issued function-based criteria for mobility assistive equipment (MAE), which entail an algorithmic process called the "Clinical Criteria for MAE Coverage."

Because, as reviewed in subsequent sections of this chapter, so many such devices exist and individual needs are complex, the process for choosing and customizing the appropriate devices for a person encompasses many steps (Arledge et al., 2011). Several types of devices may serve various needs for an individual throughout the day in different contexts, especially in and around work (Iezzoni et al., 2009). A common example is the scooters used by grocery store customers. Likewise, standing wheelchairs or scooters are commonly used as workplace accommodations. Moreover, given the need for regular maintenance and repair, it is important to have a back-up WSMD to reduce or avoid maintenance- or repair-related "sick days."

The most appropriate primary manual wheelchairs for individuals with such conditions as paraplegia due to spinal cord injury are customizable and of the lightest weight possible. The most appropriate primary powered wheelchairs are customizable and have programmable controls (Paralyzed Veterans of America Constorium for Spinal Cord Medicine, 2005). Customizable manual wheelchairs have been shown to be more durable, cost-effective, and comfortable than noncustomizable manual wheelchairs (Cooper et al., 1999; DiGiovine et al., 2000; Fitzgerald et al., 2001). Likewise, customizable powered wheelchairs have been shown to improve function, to prevent wheelchair-associated injuries, and to have significantly better durability compared with standard powered wheelchairs (Cooper, 2001; Fass et al., 2004; Worobey et al., 2012). In general, less customizable wheelchairs are more likely to fail on standardized fatigability and durability testing (DiGiovine et al., 2000).

Employment is most likely among people with good upper-body strength, coordination, and endurance who use customized or well-fitted ultra-light manual wheelchairs, sometimes with power assist devices. For individuals with impaired upper-body strength, coordination, or endurance,

[1]The images in this section serve as examples of device categories only and should not be considered an endorsement of specific products or manufacturers.

BOX 3-1
Summary of Wheeled and Seated Mobility Devices

Rollator: A wheeled mobility device used by individuals who have the ability to ambulate but require assistance with balance and may need to have a seat readily available to address fatigue.

Standard Manual Wheelchair (K0001): A wheelchair that relies on manual propulsion; a readily available wheeled mobility device intended for short-term/temporary use. The standard manual wheelchair may be used by individuals who can stand or walk to some degree. It weighs 60-80 pounds and has few adjustable features.

Standard Hemi-Wheelchair (K0002): Includes features similar to those of a standard wheelchair (K0001). It is intended primarily for individuals who are of short stature or who need to place their feet on the ground for propulsion.

High-Strength Lightweight Model Wheelchair (K0004): Has minimal adjustable features, which commonly include a small range of rear axle adjustment, arm rest positioning, and leg rest length. They are used longer term primarily by people who travel very short distances in indoor environments, and they are self-propelled.

Ultra-Lightweight Model Wheelchair (K0005): Includes all of the essential adjustments or custom fittings required to meet the needs of long-term (greater than 3 months) wheelchair use as the primary means of mobility (at least 2 hours per day). This wheelchair is durable, easy to propel, and fitted to the individual user's needs and environment.

Power Operated Vehicle (POV): Also known as a scooter. POVs are three- to four-wheeled mobility devices that are manually steered and provide control for speed/braking. They serve as a supplemental form of mobility for those who can stand and ambulate to some degree.

Group 1 Powered Wheelchair: Basic units without specialized or custom seating and with standard programmable joystick controls. This device uses differential

a powered wheelchair with powered seating functions is most helpful for supporting employability. Powered seat elevation and powered standing are among the most important features used to increase function related to employment. Unfortunately, neither is covered by CMS.

steering, which allows the wheels to turn at different speeds depending on signals from the control interface (or joystick). Designed for flat, smooth, firm, and stable indoor surfaces, as well as institutional settings.

Group 2 Powered Wheelchair: Suitable for long-term use by users who can independently weight shift or transfer. Intended primarily for indoor use within home environments and is suitable for driving short distances outside of the home within Americans with Disabilities Act (ADA)-compliant environments. Power seat functions, such as seat tilt, seat recline, and leg rest elevation, may be included. There are four basic categories: (1) power base with captain seat, (2) power base or integrated powered wheelchair with rehabilitation seating, (3) power base with single power seating option, and (4) power base with multiple power seating option.

Group 3 Powered Wheelchair: Intended for long-term use by users who cannot independently weight shift or transfer. Coverage requires meeting the following criteria: (1) the person requires alternative controls; (2) a specialized seating system is deemed necessary by a qualified clinical professional; and (3) the person requires a more durable or active user-powered wheelchair because of his or her home environment. These wheelchairs are suitable for indoor use and for outdoor use in ADA-compliant environments.

Group 4 Powered Wheelchair: Intended for long-term use by users who cannot independently weight shift or transfer. Better designed for use outside of the home relative to above devices and are ideal for active users. This mobility device includes additional capabilities that are not necessary for use within the home (e.g., speed 6 mph, curb climb 75 mm, range 16 miles/charge).

Power Assist Wheelchair: Hybrid device that has some of the attributes of manual wheelchairs and some of the benefits of powered wheelchairs. The power to propel the wheelchair comes from a combination of the user's arms and a power source (typically a battery) and motors (either integrated into the wheels or using a separate wheel or set of wheels).

Standing Wheelchair: Can be manual, powered, or some combination thereof. It either promotes passive standing in a stationary position or provides some mobility on level surfaces.

The following subsections describe the various types of WSMDs. A summary of these descriptions is provided in Box 3-1. More detailed information on the features and functionality of these devices is provided in Annex Tables 3-1 and 3-2, respectively, at the end of this chapter.

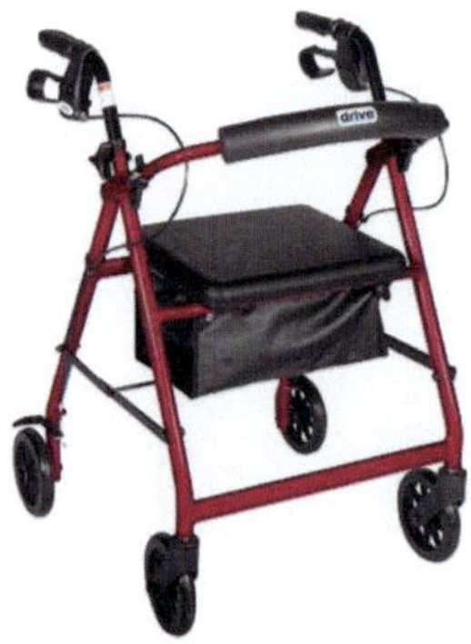

FIGURE 3-2 Rollator example.
SOURCE: Rollator Walker with Fold Up and Removable Back Support and Padded Seat. Material used with permission from Drive DeVilbiss Healthcare.

Rollators

Rollators (see Figure 3-2) are WSMDs used by individuals who have the ability to ambulate but require assistance with balance and may need to have a seat readily available to address fatigue. Rollators are most commonly used by individuals with severe cardiopulmonary limitations, those with cerebral palsy, and those who have had a cerebral vascular incident. Rollators may be covered by insurance or purchased from any number of retail outlets. They commonly cost from $100 to $150 but may cost more depending on their features. They provide very limited support for seating balance and positioning, and they require gross motor function of both the upper and lower extremities. Minimally, they extend range of reaching, lifting, and carrying. For individuals with the ability to ambulate, rollators may improve mobility, which in turn improves participation in activities of daily living (ADLs), community integration, and employment.

Manual Wheelchairs

The wide variety of manual wheelchairs can be divided into two general categories: (1) those intended to be propelled by an assistant, and (2) those intended to be propelled by the user. Within these broad categories are multiple subcategories and many options and combinations. Describing all the different varieties, styles, and options of manual wheelchairs is not feasible; therefore, only broad groupings based on Medicare coding are included here. It is worth noting that outside of the United States, most countries use a coding scheme based on International Organization for Standardization (ISO) 9999. Relative to the ultra-lightweight manual wheelchair (K0005), other manual wheelchairs tend to be larger and heavier, which makes them difficult to self-propel (especially over such surfaces as carpet or on ramps) and heavy (making them difficult to load in a vehicle), and they require large turning radii, which, for example, makes it difficult to turn from a hallway into a bathroom within the home. Clinical practice guidelines and many research studies have shown that ultra-lightweight manual wheelchairs last longer, require less maintenance, and induce fewer injuries to the upper extremities compared with other types of manual wheelchairs (Paralyzed Veterans of America Constorium for Spinal Cord Medicine, 2005).

Standard Manual Wheelchairs (K0001, K0003, K0006, K0007)

The K0001standard manual wheelchair (see Figure 3-3) has few adjustable features and is intended primarily for short-term or temporary use, commonly defined as less than 3 months. The weight of such wheelchairs is typically in the range of 60-80 pounds. These devices are not suitable for individuals whose primary means of mobility will be a wheelchair. They tend to be difficult to propel by the user and to function well only on smooth, firm, flat indoor surfaces. These wheelchairs also provide limited support for seating balance and positioning and require gross motor function of the upper extremities. Their fixed seating does not extend range of reaching, lifting, and carrying. Prices range from a low of $150 to a high of $1,000, depending on the configuration and accessories. A K0003 is nearly the same as a K0001 but lighter in weight. It is intended for individuals who cannot adequately propel a K0001. Either a K0001 or a K0003 may be equipped with a reclining backrest (E1226) if required. Wheelchairs coded K0006 are for individuals who weigh more than 250 pounds, while those coded K0007 are intended for individuals who weigh more than 300 pounds. Large individuals tend to be better served by powered wheelchairs because of the strain on their upper extremities that results from their propelling a manual wheelchair. All of these wheelchairs provide minimal

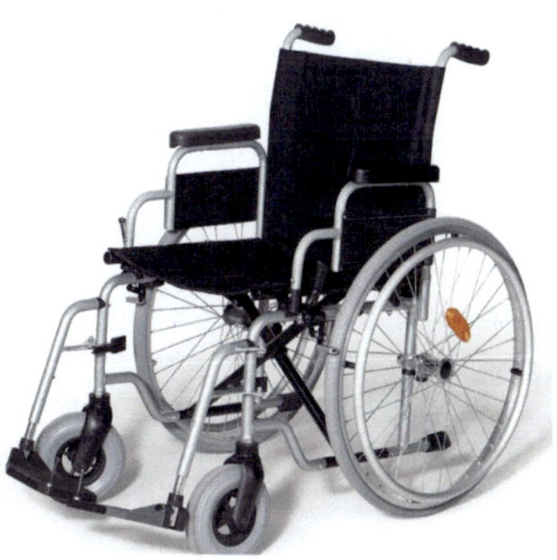

FIGURE 3-3 Example of a standard manual wheelchair.
SOURCE: iStock.com/prill.

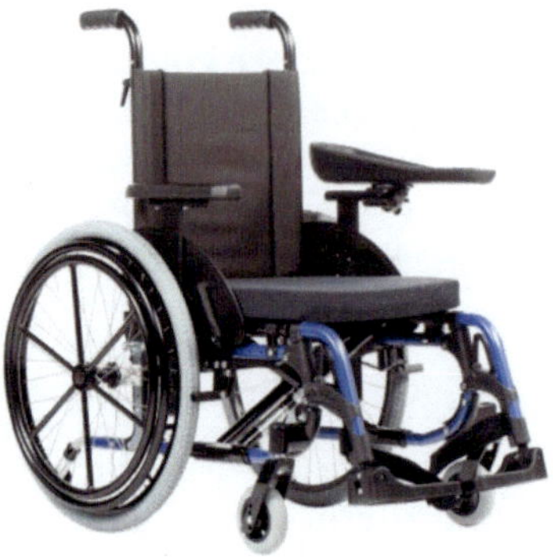

FIGURE 3-4 Example of a standard hemi-wheelchair.
SOURCE: Start M3 Hemi. Courtesy of Ottobock.

mobility, which severely limits participation in ADLs, community integration, and employment.

Standard Hemi-Wheelchair (K0002)

Like the standard manual wheelchairs described above, the standard hemi-wheelchair (K0002), depicted in Figure 3-4, typically has few adjustable features and is intended primarily for short-term or temporary use, commonly defined as less than 3 months. These wheelchairs are intended primarily for individuals who are of short stature or who need to place their feet on the ground for propulsion. Otherwise, many of their features are similar to those of a standard manual wheelchair (K0001). They provide limited support for seating balance and positioning; they require gross motor function of the upper extremities; and their fixed seating does not extend range of reaching, lifting, and carrying. These chairs also provide minimal mobility, which severely limits participation in ADLs, community integration, and employment.

High-Strength Lightweight Model Wheelchair (K0004)

The high-strength lightweight model wheelchair (K0004), depicted in Figure 3-5, has minimal adjustable features, which commonly include a small range of rear axle adjustment, arm rest positioning, and leg rest length. K0004 wheelchairs are used longer term relative to the standard manual wheelchairs and standard hemi-wheelchairs described above, primarily by people who travel very short distances in indoor environments. Individuals who use K0004 wheelchairs typically use them at least 2 hours per day; self-propel; and according to Medicare guidelines, which are followed by

A

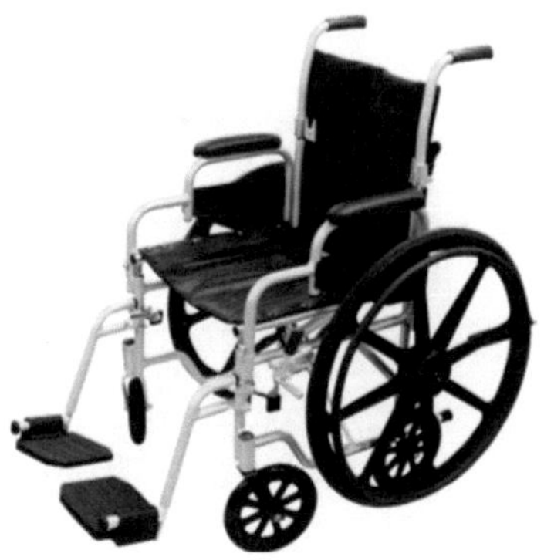

B

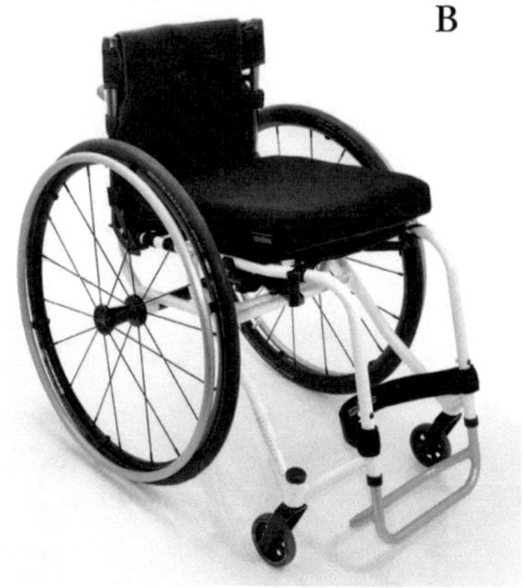

FIGURE 3-5 Examples of high-strength lightweight model wheelchairs.
SOURCES: A. Poly Fly Light Weight Transport Chair Wheelchair with Swing away Footrest. Material used with permission from Drive DeVilbiss Healthcare; B. PANTHERA X. Courtesy of Panthera.

most insurers, require such a wheelchair for at least one mobility-related ADL. K0004 wheelchairs are acceptable for short-distance mobility over flat, firm, and stable surfaces. However, they provide limited support for seating balance and positioning; they require gross motor function of the upper extremities; and their fixed seating does not extend range of reaching, lifting, and carrying. These chairs also provide minimal mobility, which severely limits participation in ADLs, community integration, and employment. Costs for K0004 wheelchairs range between $250 and $5,000. There are some challenges related to the K0004 coding, as there are large disparities in the quality of these wheelchairs and their suitability for meeting various users' needs. They range, for example, from low-cost steel wheelchairs that are similar to K0003 wheelchairs in nearly every respect to very high-performance carbon fiber wheelchairs designed with minimal adjustments for experienced and skilled users.

Ultra-Lightweight Model Wheelchair (K0005)

The ultra-lightweight model wheelchair (K0005) (see Figure 3-6) includes all of the essential adjustable features or custom fittings required to meet the needs of long-term (greater than 3 months) wheelchair use as the primary means of mobility (defined as at least 2 hours per day). Relative to the wheelchairs described above, K0005 wheelchairs have been shown to be more durable, to require less maintenance, and to be safer for

A B

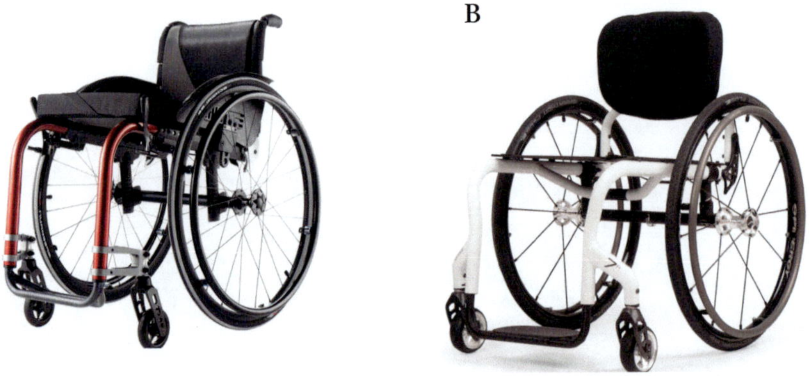

FIGURE 3-6 Examples of ultra-lightweight wheelchairs.
SOURCES: A. Küschall® Advance™. © Invacare Corporation. Used with permission; B. QUICKIE 7R. Photo courtesy of Sunrise Medical® and the QUICKIE® brand.

most long-term manual wheelchair users. Clinical practice guidelines for individuals with spinal cord injury, which are relevant to other diagnoses, recommend K0005 wheelchairs. These wheelchairs are fitted to suit individual user needs and the environment in which the user lives. They are easier to propel than the other classes of wheelchairs and are suitable for all indoor environments and for common Americans with Disabilities Act (ADA)-compliant outdoor environments. The cost for a K0005 wheelchair ranges from $1,000 to $8,000. These wheelchairs vary widely in style, form, weight, and function. They provide preferred support for seating balance and positioning; they require gross motor function of the upper extremities; and their custom or adjustable seating extends range of reaching, lifting, and carrying. These wheelchairs provide functional mobility with minimal limitations for participation in ADLs, community integration, and employment.

Powered Wheeled and Seated Mobility Devices

Although there are many different types of powered WSMDs, they fall into three broad categories: (1) those that are manually steered with speed/braking control; (2) those that are manually propelled with power assist; and (3) those that have power steering and speed/braking. According to Medicare guidelines, a person who qualifies for coverage of a powered WSMD must meet the following conditions:

> (A) the person must have a mobility limitation that significantly impairs his or her ability to participate in one or more Mobility-Related Activities of Daily Living (MRADLs) in customary locations in the home; (B) the person's mobility limitation cannot be sufficiently and safely resolved by using an appropriately fitted cane or walker; and (C) the patient does not have sufficient upper extremity function to self-propel an optimally configured manual wheelchair in the home to perform MRADLs during a typical day. (CMS, 2009)

The U.S. Department of Veterans Affairs (VA) applies broader criteria that include the veteran's participating in his or her health care and the prevention or treatment of further injury. There are numerous types of powered WSMDs, including a number of devices in use that are not regulated by the U.S. Food and Drug Administration or covered by Medicare and other insurance companies. Examples include the Segway and similar products that are used as mobility devices without modification of their original equipment manufacturer design, as well as versions that have been radically modified (see Figure 3-7) either by the person using the device or in some cases by an after-market manufacturer. There are also devices that use tracks or clusters of wheels for specialized purposes, such as outdoor mobility over unfinished terrain (see Figure 3-8) or climbing stairs. These devices have their place in the market and meet the needs of their users, in some cases including vocational needs. For someone who works on

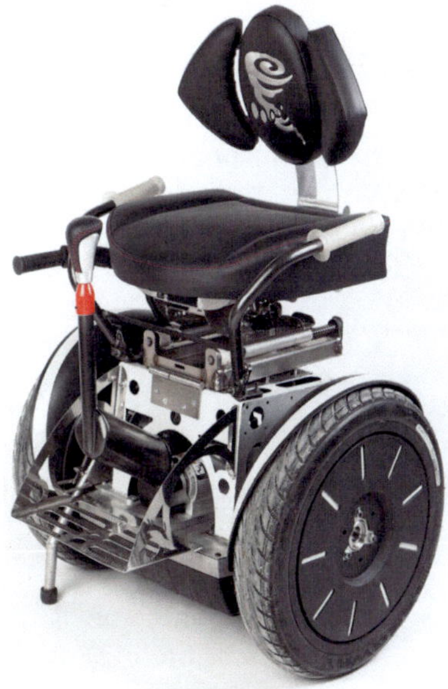

FIGURE 3-7 Segway modified to serve as a wheelchair.
NOTE: The seat is identified as the Sui Generis Seat.
SOURCE: Sui Generis Seat, 2015.

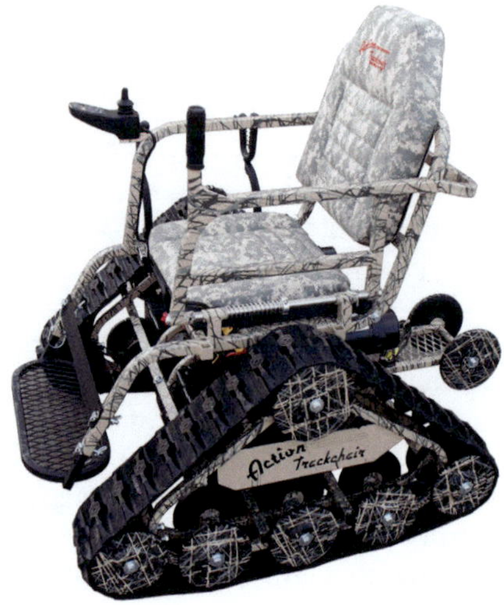

FIGURE 3-8 Action Trackchair for outdoor use.
SOURCE: Action Trackchair. Courtesy of Action Manufacturing.

construction sites or outdoors as a park employee, for example, an outdoor wheelchair may be entirely appropriate. Several classes of powered WSMDs are described below. Group 5 devices are primarily for pediatric use and are intended for individuals who weigh less than 125 pounds and are expected to grow.

Power Operated Vehicles

Power operated vehicles (POVs) (see Figure 3-9), also known as scooters, are three- or four-wheeled mobility devices that are manually steered and provide control for speed/braking. According to Medicare guidelines, to be eligible for coverage of a POV, a person must meet the general criteria described previously and also meet the following criteria:

- The person must be able to transfer safely to and from a POV.
- The person must be able to operate the manual tiller steering system.
- The person must be able to maintain postural stability and position while operating the POV in the home.
- The person's mental and physical capabilities must be sufficient for safe mobility using a POV in the home.
- The person's weight must be less than or equal to the weight capacity of the POV and greater than or equal to 95 percent of the weight capacity of the next-lower-weight class of POV.

- The person's home must provide adequate access between rooms, maneuvering space, and surfaces for the operation of the POV.
- Using a POV will significantly improve the person's ability to participate in MRADLs, and the person will use the POV in the home.
- The person has not expressed unwillingness to use a POV in the home. (CMS, 2015b)

POVs generally provide limited seating options, typically only height and minimal seat-to-backrest angle adjustment. Specialized seating and pressure-relieving cushions usually are not options. Because of their length and manual tiller steering, POVs tend to have larger turning radii relative to wheelchairs. They are intuitive to operate and frequently are used by individuals with cardiorespiratory or standing balance issues. Ranging in cost from about $500 to $5,000, these devices are intended primarily for outdoor use in ADA-compliant environments, although some small models provide indoor mobility within the home; however, caution must be exercised when using a high-seat-height and narrow-footprint POV outdoors. These wheelchairs provide limited support for seating balance and positioning; they require gross motor function of the upper extremities; and their fixed seating does not extend range of reaching, lifting, and carrying. These chairs also provide minimal mobility, which severely limits participation in ADLs, community integration, and employment.

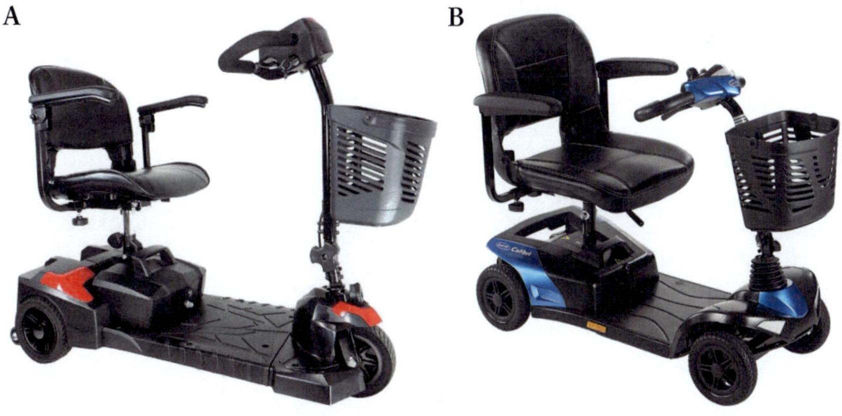

FIGURE 3-9 Examples of three- and four-wheel power operated vehicles.
SOURCES: A. Spitfire Scout 3 Wheel Travel Power Scooter. Material used with permission from Drive DeVilbiss Healthcare; B. Invacare® Colibri Scooter. © Invacare Corporation. Used with permission.

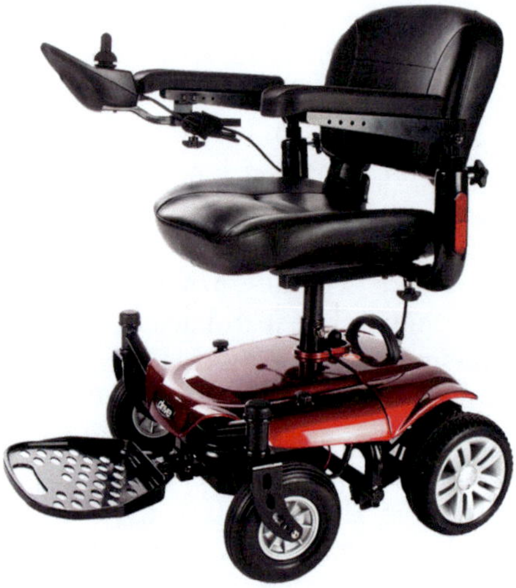

FIGURE 3-10 Example of a powered wheelchair in Medicare Group 1. SOURCE: Cobalt X16 Transportable Power Wheelchair Rear-Wheel Drive. Material used with permission from Drive DeVilbiss Healthcare.

Group 1 Powered Wheelchairs

Powered wheelchairs in Group 1 (see Figure 3-10) are basic units without specialized or custom seating and with standard programmable joystick controls. Powered wheelchairs use differential steering, which basically means that the powered wheels turn at different speeds depending on the signals from the joystick (or other user control interface) used to turn the wheelchair. Group 1 powered wheelchairs are used by individuals whose needs are not adequately met by a manual wheelchair or a POV but who do not require a powered wheelchair from Group 3 or 4. Group 1 powered wheelchairs are designed primarily for flat, smooth, firm, and stable indoor surfaces, although minimal slopes can be negotiated. The cost of Group 1 powered wheelchairs varies from about $1,200 to $5,000. These devices are used primarily in institutional settings. They provide limited support for seating balance and positioning; they require fine motor function of the upper extremities; and their fixed seating does not extend range of reaching, lifting, and carrying. These chairs provide minimal mobility, which severely limits participation in ADLs, community integration, and employment.

Group 2 Powered Wheelchairs

There are many different types of Group 2 powered wheelchairs (see Figure 3-11), which fall into four basic categories: (1) power base with captain seat, (2) power base or integrated powered wheelchair with rehabilitation seating, (3) power base with single power seating option, and

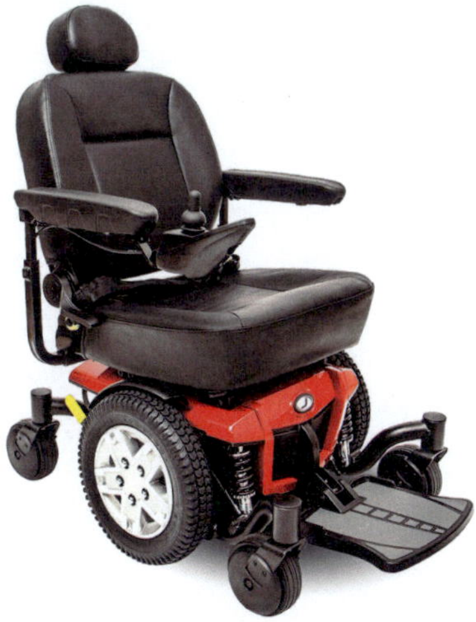

FIGURE 3-11 Example of a powered wheelchair in Medicare Group 2. SOURCE: Jazzy® 600 ES. Photo courtesy of Pride Mobility Inc.

(4) power base with multiple power seating option. Rehabilitation seating is used to help prevent pressure ulcers and/or to accommodate postural asymmetries and for individuals with impaired sensation. Group 2 powered wheelchairs are intended primarily for indoor use within home environments, but they are suitable for use over short distances outside of the home in ADA-compliant environments. Their durability is modest, as they last about 3 years before replacement or significant repair becomes necessary. Power seat functions may be included in Group 2 powered wheelchairs, including seat tilt, seat recline, and leg rest elevation. Medicare does not currently cover seat elevation; however, the VA and some other providers do. Seat elevation has been shown to improve the user's ability to transfer safely, to improve functional reach, and to increase the usable workspace (Arva et al., 2009). Group 2 powered wheelchairs range in price from about \$2,000 to \$12,000. They provide limited to moderate support for seating balance and positioning; they require fine motor function of the upper extremities; and their seating may to a limited degree extend range of reaching, lifting, and carrying. These chairs also provide minimal mobility, which limits participation in ADLs, community integration, and employment.

Group 3 Powered Wheelchairs

Powered wheelchairs in Group 3 (see Figure 3-12) are similar to those in Group 2 in many respects. They include rehabilitation seating and, in many cases, at least one powered seat function. Three primary factors differentiate a Group 3 wheelchair: (1) the person requires alternative

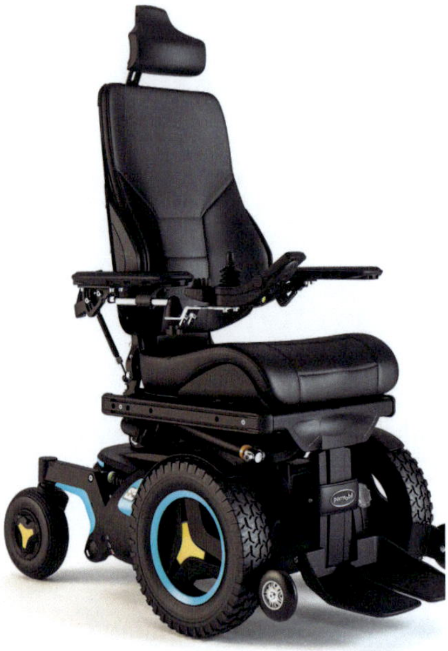

FIGURE 3-12 Example of a powered wheelchair in Medicare Group 3.
SOURCE: F3 Corpus. Copyright © 2017 Permobil.

controls, (2) a qualified clinical professional deems a specialized seating system necessary, and (3) the person requires a more durable or active user-powered wheelchair because of his or her home environment. Group 3 powered wheelchairs are suitable for indoor use and for outdoor use in ADA-compliant environments. Their durability is about 5 years with regular maintenance, with the frequency of maintenance increasing with the usage of power seat functions and alternative controls. Group 3 powered wheelchairs have a range of about 10 to 12 miles on a single charge under optimal conditions. Their cost ranges from $5,000 to $30,000, depending on the features required. These wheelchairs provide support for seating balance and positioning; alternative controls are available for individuals without fine motor function of the upper extremities; and their seating may extend range of reaching, lifting, and carrying. These chairs also provide mobility that permits participation in ADLs, community integration, and employment.

Group 4 Powered Wheelchairs

Medicare does not cover Group 4 powered wheelchairs (see Figure 3-13) because it considers them to have additional capabilities that are not necessary for use within the home (e.g., speed of 6 mph, curb climb of 75 mm, range of 16 miles/charge). The VA and other providers do cover Group 4 devices. The difference is due primarily to Medicare's focus on in-home usage, whereas the VA and state vocational rehabilitation programs have a broader mandate that includes participation in health management and return to work or school.

Some Group 4 devices would probably be better classified as Group 3 or otherwise covered because they offer the same features as Group 3 devices but have higher performance, durability, or safety; are appropriate for use in the home; and would better meet users' health and mobility needs. In other cases, the Group 4 classification provides little guidance because Medicare, as well as insurers that take their lead from Medicare coding experts, has tended to use this category to encompass "all other wheeled mobility devices." Some Group 4 devices are the most appropriate mobility device for particular users given their level of activity, their functional performance needs, and their environment. For example, college students need to be able to travel across campus to participate in their education.

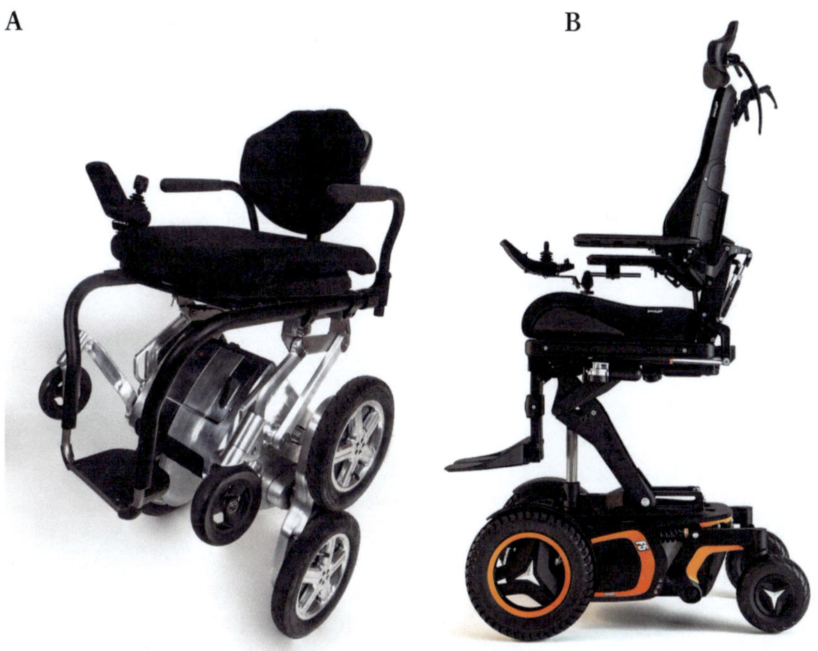

FIGURE 3-13 Examples of powered wheelchairs in Medicare Group 4.
SOURCES: A. Prototype Next Generation iBOT Base. Photo is copyright DEKA Research & Development Corp. Used with permission; B. F5 Corpus. Copyright © 2017 Permobil.

Thus, they require year-round indoor and outdoor mobility, including the ability to travel more than several miles per day. As another example, a person may wish to return to work as a construction site manager or civil engineer and be able to negotiate uneven terrain over unfinished surfaces. In some cases, a Group 4 device may simply be needed to attend appointments with health care professionals within a large medical complex that requires negotiating hills or longer distances. Given the broad range of devices encompassed by Group 4, prices range from about $6,000 to $50,000, depending on the features and capabilities. These wheelchairs provide significant support for seating balance and positioning; alternative controls are available for individuals without fine motor function of the upper extremities; and their seating may extend range of reaching, lifting, and carrying. These chairs also provide mobility that permits participation in ADLs, community integration, and employment.

Power Assist Wheelchairs

Power assist wheelchairs (see Figure 3-14) are hybrid devices that have some of the attributes of manual wheelchairs and some of the benefits of powered wheelchairs. The power to propel the wheelchair comes from a combination of the user's arms and a power source (typically a battery) and motors (either integrated into the wheels or using a separate wheel or set of wheels). Power assist wheelchairs do not have all of the features of powered wheelchairs and cannot accommodate some impairments; however, they offer an alternative to a powered wheelchair for individuals who could otherwise use a manual wheelchair but lack the ability to propel a manual wheelchair effectively because of strength or endurance limitations

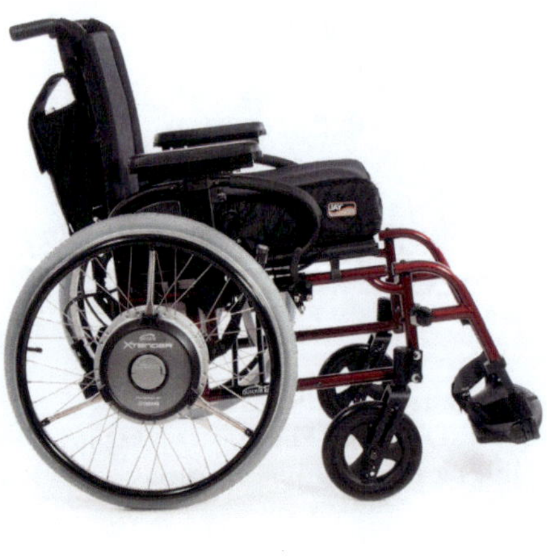

FIGURE 3-14 Example of a power assist wheelchair.
SOURCE: Quickie Xtender on a Quickie 2 wheelchair. Photo courtesy of Sunrise Medical® and the QUICKIE® brand.

or pain. Power assist wheelchairs are intended primarily for indoor use and for outdoor use in ADA-compliant environments. Their cost ranges from $4,000 to $10,000. These wheelchairs generally provide support for seating balance and positioning; they require some degree of gross motor function of the upper extremities; and their custom or adjustable seating extends range of reaching, lifting, and carrying. These chairs also provide functional mobility with minimal limitations that permits participation in ADLs, community integration, and employment.

Standing Wheelchairs

Standing wheelchairs may be manual, powered, or some combination thereof. They either promote passive standing in a stationary position (normally the case with manual devices) or provide some mobility on level surfaces. There are many physiological benefits to standing, but one of the most important is extended reach and range of motion that support employment-related activities. Standing wheelchairs may be used, for example, by health care professionals to perform medical procedures, by technicians to operate machines, and by teachers to access laboratory equipment and whiteboards. Powered wheelchairs with powered standing features are most commonly used for employment as they provide a stable and mobile platform. These wheelchairs extend range of reaching, and they may improve participation in ADLs, community integration, and employment.

THE USE OF WHEELED AND SEATED MOBILITY DEVICES

The committee used three data sources to examine WSMD use, including the association among diagnosis, impairment, and type of device used by working-age adults: (1) the SIPP (U.S. Census Bureau, 2016); (2) the National Center for Health Statistics' National Health Interview Survey (NHIS) and NHIS-D (CDC, 2016); and (3) CMS's Durable Medical Equipment (DME) files (CMS, 2013). The SIPP, NHIS, and NHIS-D include data on the civilian noninstitutionalized population and use similar methodologies for data collection and reporting. Differences include variations in years of study, sampling, scope, and level of detail gathered. The CMS DME files used in the analyses presented below are based on a random sample of the Medicare beneficiary population. Of particular interest to the committee are individuals aged 20-67 who receive Social Security Disability Insurance (SSDI). Table 3-1 highlights characteristics of the SIPP; the NHIS, including the NHIS-D; and the CMS DME.

Other sources of national-level data on WSMDs include the VA health care system, databases of state departments or offices of vocational rehabilitation, and data files of large health care systems (e.g., Kaiser Permanente).

TABLE 3-1
Characteristics of the SIPP, NHIS/NHIS-D, and CMS DME Data Sources

Characteristic	SIPP	NHIS/NHIS-D[a]	CMS-DME
Population	Noninstitutionalized U.S. population (does not include nursing homes)	Noninstitutionalized U.S. population (does not include nursing homes)	Medicare beneficiaries
Level of Device Detail	Single category for manual or electric wheelchair or electric scooter	Separate categories for manual wheelchair, electric wheelchair, and scooter	Healthcare Common Procedure Coding System for Durable Medical Equipment—wheelchairs (manual and powered) and scooters
Definition of Wheelchair Users	Participants stated that they used a wheelchair at the time of the survey	Must have been, or must be expected to be, using the device for 12 months or longer	Diagnosis and approved provider prescription for medical necessity using CMS codes
Date (years)	Panels 1984-2008	1957-2013 NHIS 1994-1997 NHIS-D[a]	2010-2014

NOTE: CMS = Centers for Medicare & Medicaid Services; DME = Durable Medical Equipment; NHIS = National Health Interview Survey; NHIS-D = National Health Interview Survey-Disability; SIPP = Survey of Income and Program Participation.

[a]Represents a separate more detailed survey with additional questions and information on persons with a disability.

SOURCES: CDC, 2016; CMS, 2013; U.S. Census Bureau, 2016.

A study by Hubbard and colleagues (2007), for example, is the first to investigate Veterans Health Administration costs for providing wheelchairs and scooters and to compare regional prescription patterns. However, the committee did not attempt to review data from these sources to determine the association between disability diagnoses and WSMD use for two reasons: first, the extent to which these data sources are representative of the working population is not known; and second, the data are restricted, proprietary, or not available as public-use files for analyses.

The analyses and figures presented below are based on information included in the CMS DME files (see Appendix C for a detailed description of the analysis methods). The DME files include a level of detail and number of variables not available in government-funded population-based surveys. For example, information on health conditions and medical diagnoses can be compared with the prescription and purchase of specific types of WSMDs. Likewise, the geographic location, distribution, and cost of WSMDs can be related to individual characteristics (age, gender, race/ethnicity), medical diagnosis (*International Classification of Diseases*, Ninth Revision [ICD-9] codes), and facility factors (urban versus rural, nonprofit versus profit).

Moreover, national surveys that collect WSMD information employ inconsistent methodologies, which makes it difficult to combine the data and identify trends and growth (Flagg, 2009). For example, the surveys use different criteria for determining a WSMD user, as well as for determining device use. As shown earlier in Table 3-1, the NHIS-D has separate categories for manual wheelchairs, electric wheelchairs, and scooters; the CMS DME files contain categories for manual wheelchairs, powered wheelchairs, and scooters. However, the SIPP contains a single category that includes manual wheelchairs, electric wheelchairs, and electric scooters. In addition, few surveys contain data on the magnitude and growth of wheelchair sales and use (Flagg, 2009). In particular, data are limited on who buys, rents, and uses powered wheelchairs (Edwards and McCluskey, 2010). There is also limited research on mobility scooters (Mortenson and Kim, 2016). According to Flagg (2009), few studies analyze the relationship between wheelchair use and gender. Furthermore, there are limited data showing the relationship between individual users' medical conditions and health (e.g., comorbidities) and/or sociodemographic characteristics and the specific types of WSMDs they use.

The DME files contain fee-for-service claims submitted by DME suppliers. DME includes a wide range of devices and services for persons with illness, injury, or chronic health conditions. Examples include crutches, hospital beds, and oxygen equipment, as well as WSMDs. The files include medical diagnoses (ICD-9 codes), comorbidities, services/devices provided as defined by the CMS Healthcare Common Procedure Coding System (HCPCS), dates of service, reimbursement amounts, and beneficiary demographic information.

It is important to identify and understand the limitations[2] of the DME files to interpret the information presented below. Since the committee's focus was on the working-age population, only persons aged 20-67 were included in the analyses. Participants under age 65 were receiving benefits from SSDI or the Medicare End-Stage Renal Disease program. Individuals who qualify for SSDI are automatically enrolled in Medicare after receiving disability benefits for 2 years. In 2015, more than 5 million Medicare beneficiaries were under age 65 and qualified for SSDI (CMS, 2015a). In 2013, more than 380,000 beneficiaries qualified for the fee-for-service Medicare

[2]Further information on data limitations is given in Appendix C.

TABLE 3-2
Demographic Characteristics of Users of Wheeled and Seated Mobility Devices by Gender

Variable	Female	Male	Total
DME Sample (5%): number (percent)	10,691 (56.3%)	8,303 (43.7%)	18,994
Age: mean (standard deviation)	57.31 (9.56)	56.20 (10.04)	56.83 (9.79)
Age: number (percent)			
20–45	1,346 (51.6%)	1,261 (48.4%)	2,607
46–55	2,246 (54%)	1,917 (46%)	4,163
56–64	3,900 (56.7%)	2,974 (43.3%)	6,874
65–67	3,199 (59.8%)	2,151 (40.2%)	5,350
Race: number (percent)			
White	7,206 (56.4%)	5,571 (43.6%)	12,777
Black	2,228 (58.7%)	1,565 (41.3%)	3,793
Hispanic	894 (52.7%)	803 (47.3%)	1,697
Other	363 (49.9%)	364 (50.1%)	727

NOTE: Information from 5 percent random sample of 2013-2014 Durable Medical Equipment (DME) Medicare beneficiaries aged 20–67.

SOURCE: DME Research Identifiable File, Centers for Medicare & Medicaid Services.

End-Stage Renal Disease program; approximately 19 percent of them were under age 65 (CMS, 2013).

Table 3-2 includes demographic information for a 5 percent random sample of beneficiaries from the Medicare DME files. This sample was used to estimate WSMD use and address issues identified for this study by the U.S. Social Security Administration (see Chapter 1), including the number of selected devices by the characteristics of users; the availability of the devices; and variation in their use across settings, age groups, and different diagnostic conditions and impairments. The data presented in all of the following tables are unadjusted for beneficiaries' sociodemographic and clinical characteristics.

Table 3-3 shows the numbers of various types of WSMDs among the DME sample displayed in Table 3-2. Medicare classifies WSMDs using the HCPCS codes.

The standard and lightweight wheelchairs accounted for about 49 percent of the WSMDs used by Medicare beneficiaries in the DME files for 2013 and 2014. (See the descriptions of these devices in the previous

TABLE 3-3
Estimated Number of Wheeled and Seated Mobility Devices by Healthcare Common Procedure Coding System (HCPCS) Codes

HCPCS Description[a]	Number	Percent	Cumulative Number	Cumulative Percent[b]
Standard wheelchair	6,579	34.6	6,579	34.6
Lightweight wheelchair	2,798	14.7	9,377	49.4
Powered wheelchair, Group 2 standard, captains chair, patient weight capacity up to and including 300 pounds	2,229	11.7	11,606	61.1
High-strength, lightweight wheelchair	1,720	9.1	13,326	70.2
Heavy-duty wheelchair	858	4.5	14,184	74.7
Extra-heavy-duty wheelchair	769	4.0	14,953	78.7
Powered wheelchair, Group 2 heavy-duty, captains chair, patient weight capacity 301 to 450 pounds	590	3.1	15,543	81.8
Powered wheelchair, Group 3 standard, multiple power option, sling/solid seat/back, patient weight capacity up to and including 300 pounds	555	2.9	16,098	84.8
Ultra-lightweight wheelchair	504	2.7	16,602	87.4
Manual adult-size wheelchair, includes tilt-in-space	428	2.3	17,030	89.7
Powered wheelchair, Group 2 standard, sling/solid seat/back, patient weight capacity up to and including 300 pounds	340	1.8	17,370	91.4
Powered wheelchair, Group 3 standard, single power option, sling/solid seat/back, patient weight capacity up to and including 300 pounds	334	1.8	17,704	93.2
Transport chair, adult size, patient weight capacity up to and including 300 pounds	323	1.7	18,027	94.9
Standard hemi (low-seat)-wheelchair	206	1.1	18,233	96.0
Power operated vehicle, Group 1 standard, patient weight capacity up to and including 300 pounds	150	0.8	18,383	96.8

continued

TABLE 3-3
Continued

HCPCS Description[a]	Number	Percent	Cumulative Number	Cumulative Percent[b]
Powered wheelchair, Group 3 standard, sling/solid seat/back, patient weight capacity up to and including 300 pounds	78	0.4	18,461	97.2
Powered wheelchair, Group 2 heavy duty, sling/solid seat/back, patient weight capacity 301 to 450 pounds	62	0.3	18,523	97.5
Powered wheelchair, Group 1 standard, captains chair, patient weight capacity up to and including 300 pounds	57	0.3	18,580	97.8
Powered wheelchair, Group 2 very heavy duty, captains chair, patient weight capacity 451 to 600 pounds	54	0.3	18,634	98.1
Powered wheelchair, Group 3 standard, captains chair, patient weight capacity up to and including 300 pounds	46	0.2	18,680	98.3
Powered wheelchair, Group 3 heavy-duty, multiple power option, sling/solid seat/back, patient weight capacity 301 to 450 pounds	41	0.2	18,721	98.6
Powered wheelchair, Group 2 standard, single power option, sling/solid seat/back, patient weight capacity up to and including 300 pounds	37	0.2	18,758	98.8
Powered wheelchair, Group 2 standard, portable, captains chair, patient weight capacity up to and including 300 pounds	35	0.2	18,793	98.9
Powered operated vehicle, Group 1 heavy-duty, patient weight capacity 301 to 450 pounds	34	0.2	18,827	99.1
Manual wheelchair accessory, push-activated power assist	24	0.1	18,851	99.2

NOTE: Information from 5 percent random sample (n = 18,994) of 2013–2014 Durable Medical Equipment (DME) Medicare beneficiaries aged 20–67.

[a]Data not shown for HCPCS wheelchairs with cell sizes <20.
[b]Percentages may not total because of rounding.

SOURCE: DME Research Identifiable File, Centers for Medicare & Medicaid Services.

TABLE 3-4
Use of Manual Versus Powered Wheelchairs by Age and Race/Ethnicity

Age Category	Wheelchair Type: Number (Percent)		
	Manual Wheelchair	Powered Wheelchair	Total[a]
20-45	1,991 10.48%	616 3.24%	2,607 13.73%
46-55	2,998 15.78%	1,165 6.13%	4,163 21.92%
56-64	4,970 26.17%	1,904 10.02%	6,874 36.19%
65-67	4,280 22.53%	1,070 5.63%	5,350 28.17%
Total	14,239 74.97%	4,755 25.03%	18,994 100.00%
Race/Ethnicity	**Wheelchair Type: Number (Percent)**		
	Manual Wheelchair	**Power Wheelchair**	**Total[a]**
White	9,456 49.78%	3,321 17.48%	12,777 67.27%
Black	2,798 14.73%	995 5.24%	3,793 19.97%
Hispanic	1,406 7.40%	291 1.53%	1,697 8.93%
Other	579 3.05%	148 0.78%	727 3.83%
Total	14,239 74.97%	4,755 25.03%	18,994 100.00%

NOTE: Information from 5 percent random sample (n = 18,994) of 2013-2014 Durable Medical Equipment (DME) Medicare beneficiaries aged 20-67.

[a]Percentages may not total because of rounding.

SOURCE: DME Research Identifiable File, Centers for Medicare & Medicaid Services.

section.) Seventy-five percent (14,239) of the wheelchairs in the DME sample were classified as manual and 25 percent (4,755) as powered.

Table 3-4 shows a breakdown of the use of manual versus powered wheelchairs among the 5 percent DME sample by age and race/ethnicity. In this sample of 18,994, approximately 36 percent of all WSMDs were used by persons aged 56-64. Powered wheelchairs were used by only 3.2 percent of the persons in the sample aged 20-45. Consistent with the demography of race and ethnicity in the United States, approximately 67 percent of WSMDs were used by non-Hispanic whites, 20 percent by blacks, and 9 percent by Hispanics. Powered wheelchairs were used substantially less across all racial and ethnic groups. Only 1.5 percent of powered wheelchairs were used by Hispanics.

The number of WSMDs was higher for females (56.3 percent, n = 10,691) than for males (43.7 percent, n = 8,303). The use of powered wheelchairs also was higher for females (13.5 percent) than for males (11.5 percent) in the sample (data not shown).

The number of WSMDs varies by primary medical diagnoses (see Table 3-5). The primary diagnoses are classified based on the system CMS uses to aggregate primary diagnoses for the Basic Stand Alone DME Public Use Files. The Data Dictionary and Codebook for this system is available from CMS (2013). The committee used the diagnostic categories available in the DME public-use files because they allow comparison with information that is publicly available without the need for a data use agreement or completion of other Medicare privacy-related requirements.

Table 3-5 indicates that approximately 33 percent of all users of WSMDs included in the Medicare DME sample were in the diagnostic categories of diseases of the nervous system and diseases of the musculoskeletal system and connective tissue. The category diseases of the nervous system (ICD-9 codes 320-359) includes the following subcategories: inflammatory diseases of the central nervous system, hereditary and degenerative diseases of the central nervous system, pain, headache syndromes, disorders of the central nervous system, and disorders of the peripheral nervous system. The category diseases of the musculoskeletal system and connective tissue (ICD-9 codes 710-739) includes the following subcategories: arthropathies and related disorders, dorsopathies, rheumatism (excluding the back), osteopathies, chondropathies, and acquired musculoskeletal deformities. The first six primary diagnostic categories in Table 3-5 account for almost 79 percent of all users of WSMDs included in the Medicare DME sample.

CLINICAL CONSIDERATIONS

Factors Affecting Wheeled and Seated Mobility Device Selection

The types of WSMDs that are most appropriate for particular individuals and the extent of their use depend on a number of factors, including body function and activity and environmental and personal factors (Cooper et al., 2015; Dicianno et al., 2011; Paralyzed Veterans of American Consortium for Spinal Cord Medicine, 2005). Body function and activity factors include physical and cognitive abilities and secondary health conditions/comorbidities, and the types of devices used by individuals need to be adjusted to changes in these factors resulting from maturation (transitioning from adolescence to adulthood, as well as aging) and disease progression, which may be accompanied by deterioration of physical and cognitive

TABLE 3-5
Estimated Number of Wheeled and Seated Mobility Devices by CMS Diagnostic Categories

Primary Diagnosis[a]	ICD-9 Codes	Number	Percent	Cumulative Number	Cumulative Percent[b]
Diseases of the nervous system	320-359	3,181	16.7	3,181	16.7
Diseases of the musculoskeletal system and connective tissue	710-739	3,054	16.1	6,235	32.8
Endocrine, nutritional and metabolic, and immunity disorders	240-279	2,471	13.0	8,706	45.8
Injury and poisoning	800-999	2,145	11.3	10,851	57.1
Diseases of the circulatory system	390-459	2,130	11.2	12,981	68.3
Diseases of the respiratory system	460-519	1,962	10.3	14,943	78.7
Symptoms, signs, and ill-defined conditions	780-799	1,453	7.6	16,396	86.3
External causes of injury and supplemental classification	E and V codes	686	3.6	17,082	89.9
Neoplasms	140-239	446	2.3	17,528	92.3
Diseases of the skin and subcutaneous tissue	680-709	384	2.0	17,912	94.3
Diseases of the genitourinary system	580-629	364	1.9	18,276	96.2
Congenital anomalies	740-759	227	1.2	18,503	97.4
Mental disorders	290-319	220	1.2	18,723	98.6
Infectious and parasitic diseases	001-139	119	0.6	18,842	99.2
Diseases of the digestive system	520-579	93	0.5	18,935	99.7
Diseases of the blood and blood-forming organs	280-289	26	0.1	18,961	99.8

NOTES: Information from 5 percent random sample (n = 18,994) of 2013-2014 Durable Medical Equipment (DME) Medicare beneficiaries aged 20-67. ICD-9 = *International Classification of Diseases*, Ninth Revision.

[a]Data not shown for primary diagnostic categories with cell sizes ≤20.
[b]Percentages may not total because of rounding.

SOURCE: DME Research Identifiable File, Centers for Medicare & Medicaid Services.

function. Other body function and activity factors include specific work or personal activities. A wide range of environmental factors also impact the types and extent of use of WSMDs, including weather, topography (terrain), geography (rural or urban), political/economic factors (funding sources, availability, and costs/accessibility), social factors (attitudinal barriers), and home/school/work environments (accessibility, maneuverability). Personal factors that impact the choice and use of WSMDs may include personal preferences, cultural and spiritual issues, and cosmetic concerns. Lastly, because of the need for physical and/or occupational therapists to evaluate the fit and seating systems of WSMDs and train individuals in their proper use, users need to have the time and money to make use of these services.

Physical Environment

The physical environment encompasses topography, geography, and weather, all of which impact the types of WSMDs that are most appropriate for individuals and the potential need for multiple types of WSMDs for a particular person. Environments that are flat, have paved surfaces, and are free from snow are suitable for all WSMDs. In contrast, if the environment is hilly and/or snow-covered, the use of a manual device may be limited, such that a powered WSMD is needed; however, those who use primarily a manual wheelchair may be able to navigate these more challenging environments using a power assist device or tire adaptions without having to have more than one WSMD.

Functional Capacity

A WSMD needs to be suited to an individual's physical and cognitive abilities (Cooper, et al., 2015; Dicianno et al., 2011; Paralyzed Veterans of American Consortium for Spinal Cord Medicine, 2000, 2005). The use of a manual wheelchair requires both adequate strength and endurance of the upper extremities and the absence of significant pain, spasticity, or contractures in the upper or lower extremities. Individuals who are at risk of pressure ulcers (such as those with spinal cord injury, spina bifida, or vascular compromise) must be capable of independently performing pressure relieves. Propelling a manual wheelchair requires at a minimum antigravity strength in the shoulders, elbow flexors, and wrist extensors. Individuals with full strength in all upper-extremity muscle groups relative to those with less upper-extremity muscle function are more likely to have relatively unlimited community mobility, including such higher-level wheelchair skills as negotiating curbs, inclines, and declines and independently performing even and uneven transfers. Individuals with full strength in all upper-extremity muscle groups relative to those with less upper-extremity muscle function also are less likely to have overuse syndrome with premature aging and upper-extremity pain. In addition, these individuals are more capable of carrying items on their lap and accessing items in backpacks or other storage devices attached to their wheelchair. Those with less than full strength in their upper extremities, especially those with weak elbow extensors, may have limited ability to transfer independently without a sliding board and/or some assistance.

For individuals who are unable to use a manual wheelchair and who have no or limited ability to ambulate, a powered wheelchair or a manual wheelchair with power assist may be appropriate. Wheelchairs with power assist, either integrated into the wheel itself or as an add-on, are appropriate for individuals with upper-extremity function that allows them to hand propel the wheelchair to some extent. For those with less upper-extremity function, a powered wheelchair may be more appropriate. The appropriate control mechanism depends on the individual's upper-extremity function and ranges from a joystick for those with adequate arm function (minimum of biceps function) to chin control, head array, or sip and puff for those with lesser arm function. For individuals with sensory loss or vascular compromise, a powered wheelchair should be equipped with power tilt-in-space and/or power recline to enable the performance of pressure relieves. Powered wheelchairs with power standing or elevating seat functions allow the user to access items, tabletops, and cabinets above the normal sitting height and to be at eye level with other individuals. A major limitation of powered wheelchairs is their size and weight, which requires the use of a van with a wheelchair lift when the user is traveling in a motor vehicle. In addition, because of the size, weight, and maneuverability of powered wheelchairs, the home and work environments must allow accessibility throughout, as well as have accessible entries/exits. When powered wheelchairs are malfunctioning, moreover, they are generally unusable, so that a back-up manual or powered wheelchair is needed.

A scooter may be appropriate for individuals who have some ambulatory ability but require a WSMD in their home, school, or work environment or in the community and are unable to use a manual wheelchair because of endurance limitations. To use a scooter, an individual must be able to sit independently and not be susceptible to pressure ulcers because of the limited seating options. Scooters may be equipped with a power elevating seat function that allows the user to access items, tabletops, and cabinets above the normal sitting height and to be at eye level with other individuals. Major limitations of scooters include their limited maneuverability and their weight, which requires that a motor vehicle used by an individual have a dedicated carrier.

There are several reasons why an individual may need more than one wheelchair and/or progress from one type of wheelchair to another. For those who use a manual or powered wheelchair, a back-up wheelchair is needed in the event that their primary wheelchair is not usable. For those who use primarily a manual wheelchair, a power assist option (integrated into the wheels or as an add-on) may be required for longer-distance mobility. For example, an adolescent with a C6 spinal cord injury who uses a manual wheelchair may require power assist when he or she attends college or becomes employed and must negotiate greater distances on campus or to and from the workplace. Because of aging and overuse of their upper extremities, individuals who utilize primarily a manual wheelchair may need to add a power assist option to that wheelchair or progress to a powered wheelchair. Individuals with disorders characterized by progressive deterioration in their motor control, muscle strength, or endurance may need to progress sequentially from manual to power assist to powered wheelchairs, and those whose course is rapidly progressive may benefit from using a power assist or powered wheelchair earlier on.

All individuals who are at risk of pressure ulcers—for example, because of spinal cord injury, spina bifida, or vascular compromise—need to have pressure-reducing seating systems guided by pressure mapping and prescribed by a knowledgeable and experienced clinician (Paralyzed Veterans of America Consortium for Spinal Cord Medicine, 2014). These seating systems need to include a pressure-reducing cushion and, as appropriate, a pressure-reducing back. For individuals who are at risk of pressure ulcers and who are not capable of independently performing pressure relieves, a powered wheelchair equipped with power tilt-in-space and/or power recline is needed to accomplish pressure relieves. For individuals with inadequate trunk and/or neck support, seating systems need to provide adequate support for sitting, which may include side bolsters, head rests, contoured seat backs, or customized seating systems. Individuals who are at risk of pressure ulcers and who transfer to a standard chair need to utilize an appropriate pressure-reducing seating device whenever they are sitting in a standard chair. Individuals with pressure ulcers that are in contact with the surface of their WSMD, such as ischial or sacral ulcers, ideally should remain off of their pressure ulcers and hence should not be sitting.

A manual or powered wheelchair needs to be appropriate for the individual's weight and body dimensions (Dicianno et al., 2011). Bariatric chairs are available for those weighing more than 300 pounds. The key dimensions of a wheelchair are the width, length, and dump of the seat and the position of the foot plate so that in the absence of significant contractures, the person is sitting with the hips, knees, and ankles in a neutral position. The dump of the seat needs to allow the individual to sit comfortably with adequate trunk support. Evaluations of the WSMD and seating system need to be conducted at least annually because of changing needs, as well as fluctuations in weight and dimensions due to pregnancy, weight gain, or weight loss as a result of illness. In the event of a decline in cognition, the type of WSMD may need to be changed or additional safeguards instituted.

For individuals who utilize augmentative communication devices, these devices need to be mounted appropriately on the WSMD and readily accessible to the individual. A removable lap tray for the WSMD may be needed by those in powered wheelchairs that cannot fit easily under standard desks and tables.

Another clinical consideration is the existence of comorbid impairments. Major comorbid impairments (secondary health conditions) that affect and impact the functioning, including sustained work activity, of many individuals who require a WSMD are musculoskeletal issues, including pain, contractures, spasticity, osteoporosis, and fractures. These musculoskeletal issues may affect an individual's ability to propel a manual or power assist wheelchair, control a powered wheelchair, and perform transfers, and they limit the amount of time that the person can remain in a seated position. In addition, spasticity may make sitting in a WSMD or standard chair unsafe if the person experiences severe muscle spasms.

Autonomic dysfunction, such as orthostatic hypotension or autonomic dysreflexia (e.g., spinal cord injury), may impact functioning, including sustained work activity. Individuals who are susceptible to orthostatic hypotension may benefit from a WSMD that reclines.

Individuals with pulmonary compromise, such as high tetraplegic spinal cord injuries, amyotrophic lateral sclerosis (ALS), or muscular dystrophy, may require ventilator support from a portable ventilator, which requires that the person's WSMD, which generally is a powered wheelchair, can accommodate the ventilator. The presence of a neurogenic bladder and bowel, such as in individuals with spinal cord injuries, spina bifida, or multiple sclerosis, may impact functioning, including sustained work activity. Wheelchair-accessible restrooms must be available and conveniently located. For those who are not independent in performing their bladder and bowel program, an assistant is required. Individuals who use a WSMD and have concomitant cognitive or visual impairments or movement/coordination disorders need to have individualized evaluation of their ability to use their WSMD with respect to their own safety and that of others. These evaluations need to be performed periodically depending on the severity and specifics of the cognitive deficits and the potential for cognitive deterioration.

Factors Associated with Use of Wheeled and Seated Mobility Devices

Even when an individual is appropriately matched to a WSMD, there are multiple factors that affect activity and participation. In the physical environment, all residential settings need to be accessible for entry and exit, including emergency contingencies. In addition, the interior rooms of residential settings—whether they are permanent or temporary, private homes/apartments or hotels/motels or nursing homes—must be accessible to WSMDs for both entry/exit and maneuverability; this requirement must be met for all sleeping, dining, and living rooms as well as for work areas, bathrooms, and kitchens. The surfaces of all pathways into and within the residential setting must be suitable for WSMDs and ideally should be flat and hard without thresholds. Interior features of the residential or work setting need to be compatible with WSMD use both for progression throughout the setting and for maneuvering. This requirement encompasses furniture as well as more permanent structures such as hallways, landings, bathrooms, and kitchens. For powered WSMDs, proper and accessible power outlets/charging stations are needed in appropriate locations.

In addition, transportation is necessary for individuals to participate fully in their community, including leisure/recreation activities, employment, social activities, health care services, and shopping. Full access to one's community may range from the neighborhood level, to an entire community, to the world beyond. Forms of transportation that facilitate participation range from personal motor vehicles (such as cars, trucks, and vans) to mass transportation (such as buses, trains, boats, and airplanes). To utilize all of these modes of community transportation, users of a WSMD require accessible ingress/egress for the WSMD; sufficient space to navigate within the vehicle; and adequate safety restraints for the individual, which may include appropriate wheelchair tie-downs (van Roosmalen et al., 2002). Transportation of wheelchairs and/or wheelchair users to workplaces may require such additional assistive equipment as ramps, lifts, adapted vehicles, and other WSMDs. For individuals who transfer from their WSMD to a seat, appropriate seating must be available to avoid skin breakdown for those who are susceptible to this condition as a consequence of sensory loss or vascular compromise. The transportation also needs to be readily accessible in a timely and reliable fashion and to provide expedient passage comparable to that provided for those who do not require a WSMD.

As described elsewhere in this report, the ADA makes it unlawful to discriminate against a qualified individual with a disability in such employment practices as recruitment, pay, hiring, firing, promotion, job assignments, training, leave, and benefits. To be protected under the ADA, an individual must have a substantial impairment—one that significantly limits or restricts a major life activity, such as hearing, seeing, speaking, breathing, performing manual tasks, walking, caring for oneself, learning, or working.[3] To be protected by the ADA, an individual with a disability also must be qualified to perform the "essential functions" of the job with

[3]42 U.S. 12102 (1990).

or without reasonable accommodation.[4] (See Chapter 7 for additional information regarding the ADA.)

Individuals using WSMDs may face additional challenges even when they are able to perform the formal essential functions associated with a position and have been provided an accommodation by the employer. For instance, they may need to be provided an appropriate and usable (e.g., snow being removed during the winter) ramp for entering the workplace building. In addition, employees must get from their home to the workplace, which may involve complex issues related to driving and/or other transportation. After arriving at the workplace parking lot or garage, employees using WSMDs must be able to use the parking garage elevator and/or navigate from the parking lot to the office building and negotiate the ramp. To do so, they may have to travel over uneven terrain, slopes, curbs, gravel, or unpaved areas. Once in the building, they may face additional barriers related to such tasks as reaching heights and managing doors and filing cabinets that require a level of coordination, balance, and dexterity that can be challenging and may not have been included among the essential functions associated with the actual job. Ensuring that these employees have easy access to the restroom facility is also a major workplace concern. These factors and job requirements must be considered both by individuals with a disability and by the members of their rehabilitation team (Boles et al., 2004; Goetzel et al., 2004).

EVALUATION AND MONITORING

Individuals who require a WSMD need to be evaluated periodically: in general, not less frequently than annually. A thorough evaluation focuses on the individual's physical condition; the functioning and fitting of the WSMD and associated seating system; the individual's current ability to utilize the WSMD (ergonomics and safety); the individual's satisfaction with the WSMD; the individual's underlying disorder and associated secondary health conditions/impairments; and assessment of past, current, and future functional needs at home, in the community, and in the workplace. With respect to the individual's work environment, it is important to take a thorough inventory of the person's functional needs; workspace layout, including accessibility of restrooms, break room, and meeting rooms; and access into and out of the workplace, including emergency exits and/or contingency plans suitable for an individual in a WSMD. Also important is assessment of the individual's current and future transportation to and from the workplace, workplace-related activities, the home, and community venues, such as the need to travel to multiple work sites.

---

[4]42 U.S. 12111 (1990).

During periodic evaluations, it may also be advisable to consider changing to a technology that might improve an individual's functioning, reduce secondary health conditions, and increase satisfaction in the workplace. Such technology changes include not only those related to the WSMD but also other technologies that would enhance the person's ability to perform his or her work duties or would reduce secondary heath conditions, such as overuse (e.g., carpal tunnel syndrome).

TRAINING AND ADAPTATION

If the user is to benefit from a WSMD, the device must be properly fitted to the body and accommodate the person's environment, and the user must be properly trained in its use and maintenance. Providing inappropriate WSMDs can have unintended consequences, such as elevated risk for trips, falls, and collisions; pain due to excessive vibration exposure; injuries due to component failures; soft-tissue injuries, including pressure ulcers; and repetitive strain injuries, such carpal tunnel syndrome, elbow tendinitis, and rotator cuff injuries. A WSMD needs to serve as an extension of the user, becoming integrated into the person's life and facilitating independence and community participation. To this end, it is essential that WSMDs be tuned for their users and that users receive training in using the features of their devices in the specific environments to be encountered. A personalized approach to this training and adaptation is important to the user's experience and can prevent dissatisfaction with and abandonment of the device. According to Galvin and Scherer (1996), failure to consider the user's opinions and preferences in device selection is the most significant factor associated with abandonment (see also the section on clinical considerations above). Poor feature matching, which can include wheelchair design, size, weight, and maneuverability, is a major factor contributing to the failure of wheelchairs to meet users' functional needs and allow them to participate in community roles (Kittel et al., 2002). Although there is a dearth of literature on the adaptation time for WSMD use, it is important to note that the process can take place over a period of years (Barker et al., 2004; Bates et al., 1993). To be able to use a WSMD safely and effectively, each person needs training in a variety of skills.

Transfer Training

The user's ability to safely enter and exit his or her WSMD is essential for health and community participation. Transfers can be independent, assisted by technology, assisted by a human, or assisted by a person using technology. The most appropriate means of transfer depends on the person being transferred, the environment (e.g., space available in which to align the WSMD with the transfer surface), the type and features of the WSMD (e.g., size, presence of a seat elevator, leg rest type), and the surface to be transferred to/from (e.g., toilet, tub, shower bench, vehicle). Studies have shown that even people who are trained and can transfer independently typically are constrained to very limited ranges of horizontal and vertical separation between the two surfaces (Crytzer et al., 2017).

Transfers, along with wheelchair propulsion, weight relief, and overhead reaching, have been identified as key activities leading to the development of shoulder pain and injury. In a survey of individuals with spinal cord injury, 65 percent reported that pain interfered with their ability to transfer (Kankipati et al., 2015). Transfer skills also are important to a wheelchair user's safety; of the falls reported to the Consumer Product Safety Commission between 1973 and 1987, 8.1 percent were related to transfers (Koontz et al., 2012). Performing sideways transfers without a sliding board is one factor associated with increased risk of accidents and falls (Toro et al., 2013).

When they first require a WSMD, many people participate in some form of rehabilitation that includes training in how to perform a safe and efficient transfer. Gaining independence with transfers often is a goal of both WSMD users and therapists because transfers are required to perform many essential functional activities. Even with the emphasis placed on transfers, however, the amount and type of training provided vary greatly, and there is no uniform way to evaluate transfer quality.

Clinicians can use the Transfer Assessment Instrument (TAI) to evaluate transfer quality and a patient's adherence to transfer training (McClure et al., 2011). The TAI assesses conservation of upper-limb function, safety, and the ability of WSMD users to direct an assistant to help them with a transfer as necessary. Items on the TAI are based on clinical practice guidelines, available transfer literature, and techniques applied in clinical training (Paralyzed Veterans of America Constorium for Spinal Cord Medicine, 2005). The TAI can be used to evaluate independent transfers, modified independent transfers (with the use of assistive devices), human-assisted transfers, and dependent transfers (using only human assistance or human assistance and technology).

Wheelchair Skills Training

To use a wheelchair safely and effectively requires mobility training. Operating a wheelchair requires the integration of multiple senses and coordinated control of multiple actions. For manual wheelchairs, strength, flexibility, and motor coordination are necessary to perform common mobility and functional ADLs. Users of powered wheelchairs must be able to operate the controls safely and judge the device's capabilities given their environment and skill set. While nearly all wheelchair users receive some training, this training usually is insufficient.

Kirby and colleagues (2004) have developed and extensively studied the Wheelchair Skills Training Program, which involves teaching a wide variety of skills in a clinical (inpatient or outpatient) or community-based setting. Demonstrated to be safe, practical, and effective, this program incorporates common motor-learning principles into a rehabilitation setting and can improve wheelchair skills in about 2 hours.

Some instruments have been developed for use in assessing wheelchair skills. The Functional Mobility Assessment is a self-report outcomes tool designed to measure the effectiveness of WSMD interventions for people with disabilities. Test-retest reliability scores for all items and participants were found to be above the acceptable value for a clinical assessment tool (Kumar et al., 2013). The Functioning Everyday with a Wheelchair questionnaire is designed to measure perceived user function related to wheelchair and scooter use (Mills et al., 2007).

A few clinical tools are available to aid clinicians in evaluating people for power mobility. However, these tools simply record whether drivers can complete certain tasks; they cannot detect the specific motor, sensory, or cognitive impairments that are related to safe and effective driving—information needed to determine not only whether individuals are capable of ultimately learning to drive but also the type and amount of training they may need. Routhier and colleagues (2003) assert the need for a controlled-environment outcome measure using a standardized obstacle course for measuring driving skills, a need not met by existing instruments for evaluating powered wheelchair driving. The Power Mobility Indoor Driving Assessment (PIDA) and the Power-Mobility Community Driving Assessment were developed not as screening tools but as a means of identifying general areas in which more training is needed (e.g., parking under a table) or in which modifications to the powered wheelchair or environment are necessary (Letts et al., 2007). Scoring is subjective such that the evaluator rates how independently a driver can perform a given task, such as approaching a closet. However, only the PIDA evaluates indoor driving. Kirby and colleagues published a Wheelchair Skills Test (MacPhee et al., 2004). And Massengale and colleagues (2005) developed the Power Mobility Road Test, which incorporates portions of the PIDA and other wheelchair driving courses used in research settings. A driver is rated on 12 structured tasks entailing basic driving and 5 unstructured tasks involving moving obstacles. These tests are useful clinically to test proficiency at performing common wheelchair skills; they do not help identify specific motor, sensory, or cognitive impairments that may be contributing to unsafe driving. The latter information is crucial in planning the type and amount of training needed for an individual to become a skilled driver. To address these gaps,

Dicianno and colleagues developed the Power Mobility Screening Tool and the Power Mobility Clinical Driving Assessment Tool, which build on the foundation of the assessment and training used for adaptive motor vehicle assessments (Kamaraj et al., 2016).

Wheelchair Maintenance Training

Wheelchair breakdowns are one cause of users being injured or stranded, and the incidence of these breakdowns is increasing. Evidence suggests that wheelchair users who routinely maintain their devices are less likely to be injured. In one study, 62 percent (n = 616) of U.S. wheelchair users with spinal cord injury reported needing ≥1 repairs within a 6-month period; 27.4 percent experienced an adverse consequence as a result of the needed repair; 7.1 percent did not complete the repair; and most repairs were completed by a vendor for powered wheelchairs and by users themselves for manual wheelchairs (Worobey, 2016). The importance of routine maintenance is increased by poor wheelchair reliability. Many wheelchairs in the United States fail to meet minimum performance and durability standards (Fitzgerald et al., 1999). While higher-cost wheelchairs tend to do better in standards testing, they still fail early. A recent meta-analysis confirms these findings and provides further evidence that manufacturers are not producing wheelchairs that comply with standards, making attention to maintenance that much more important (Wang et al., 2010).

Several resources provide information on how to maintain wheelchairs. First, as required by American National Standards Institute (ANSI)/Rehabilitation Engineering and Assistive Technology Society of North America (RESNA) Wheelchair Standards Section 15 (ANSI/RESNA, 2009), wheelchair manufacturers are required to include maintenance instructions in the user manual provided with the device. Second, maintenance checklists are available online (Cooper, 2013; Denison, 2006), including some at Spinlife,[5] a popular online wheelchair retailer (Koontz, n.d.). Rehabilitation engineering books also dedicate sections to wheelchair maintenance (Cooper, 1998; Cooper et al., 2006). In fact, the book *Wheelchair Selection and Configuration* was translated into Turkish, Romanian, and Bulgarian and used to train wheelchair users in group settings in wheelchair maintenance (Cooper, 1998; Soydan et al., 2012). The course, however, was not openly available online. Third, professional organizations' wheelchair provision and prescription guides recommend discussing maintenance as a vital component of wheelchair provision and include brief maintenance checklists for clinician (Arledge et al., 2011; Lukersmith et al., 2013).

[5]See http://www.spinlife.com/en/caringformanualwheelchairs2.cfm (accessed July 18, 2017).

In addition, the World Health Organization (WHO) has launched the Wheelchair Service Training Package, which includes a section on wheelchair maintenance training (Khasnabis and Mines, 2012). This package is designed to train wheelchair service providers, such as clinicians, in six basic wheelchair maintenance and repair skills, although it covers only manual wheelchairs. The training curriculum includes PowerPoint slides, a video of a live demonstration, and an in-person demonstration. It explains why each maintenance task should be done, how often, and how. Finally, the Wheelchair Maintenance Training Program was created as a project of the Spinal Cord Injury Model System to help address the need for wheelchair maintenance training (Worobey et al., 2016).

In addition, the WHO has released Guidelines on the Provision of Manual Wheelchairs in Less Resourced Settings, which are aimed at enhancing the quality of life of wheelchair users. The guidelines in the service delivery section focus on "good practice at all stages of the service delivery process, from referral to assessment and prescription, funding, ordering, product preparation, fitting, user training and maintenance" (WHO, 2008, p. 10). According to a study by Toro and colleagues (2016), following the WHO's guidelines has a range of positive outcomes, including increased satisfaction with the device and better quality of life.

Although these resources are available, routine wheelchair maintenance is not commonly performed by either wheelchair users or caregivers. In a study assessing wheelchair durability and its effect on user satisfaction, 26 percent of wheelchair users reported completing wheelchair repairs and 16 percent general maintenance in the past 6 months (Fitzgerald et al., 2005). And a study that assessed hospital wheelchairs showed that only 23 percent were safe and in good working condition (Young et al., 1985). Preventive maintenance services are uncommon, and users have reported seeking professional intervention only when the needed repairs have reached crisis levels (Nosek and Krouskop, 1995).

Seating and Positioning

The WSMD seating surface, including cushions and back support, is critical for comfort, safety, and prevention of such complications as pressure ulcers. Yet, while devices are available for clinical assessment of pressure distribution, as are cushions effective in distributing pressure, there remains a tremendous problem with wheelchair users incurring pressure ulcers. People who are active sitters (change their seated posture frequently) and/or perform regular pressure relief (lifting the buttocks off of the seat or dramatically changing posture by, for example, lying on the thighs) tend to be at lower risk of developing pressure ulcers. Educational tools (e.g., user guides, oral instruction, websites, apps) have proven effective in increasing knowledge of the risk of pressure ulcers among wheelchair users, but they do little to improve compliance (Schofield et al., 2013). Reminders based on timers or simple pressure or contact switches have proven only modestly effective (Griffin et al., 2007). Research has shown promise for the Virtual Seating Coach from Permobil, Inc. in increasing compliance among users of powered wheelchairs who use power seat functions (Liu et al., 2010, 2012).

Training in performing pressure relief or dynamic repositioning is usually provided in a clinic with oral instructions, perhaps with feedback from a pressure mapping system, with minimal practice because of time limitations (Griffin et al., 2007). Given the need for new users to learn how to operate and maintain their device and to propel it safely, the challenges of learning to manage seated pressure can be overwhelming, and training often requires frequent reinforcement. And, given the numerous activities and tasks in which users must engage every day, it is easy to lose track of time and forget to perform pressure reliefs even for those who are aware of the importance of preventing pressure ulcers.

ACCESS AND AVAILABILITY

Availability of Wheeled and Seated Mobility Devices

WSMDs are made available through a complex network that involves a chain of professional providers, funding sources, and manufacturers. The *Manual of Wheelchair Market Shares, Strategies, and Forecasts, Worldwide, 2012 to 2018*, published in 2012, provides a comprehensive review of the multiple factors driving the demand for and availability of WSMDs (WinterGreen Research, 2012).

Two key factors influencing the availability of these devices are the level of the person's functional limitations and his or her access to reimbursement. Discrepancies among various reimbursement and funding sources for WSMDs in the United States impact the availability of various types of these devices, as well as accessories and opportunities for training and education offered to both providers and users (Crane and Minkel, 2009). As discussed previously, for example, CMS classifies WSMDs as DME, defined under CMS rules as equipment that (1) can withstand repeated use, (2) is used to serve a medical purpose, (3) is not useful to a person in the absence of an illness or injury, and (4) is appropriate for use in the home. All of these requirements must be met to qualify for Medicare reimbursement. Thus, current Medicare policy determines the need for a manual or powered wheelchair based on the individual's need for the device inside the home. This policy is an impediment to achieving gainful employment. It also shows that a mismatch exists between the types of WSMDs covered by Medicare and those required to maximize individuals' functioning based on their diagnosis and treatment.

In addition to affecting the availability of WSMDs at the level of the individual user, current Medicare policy impacts the production and distribution of these devices by manufacturers. Medicare is the largest funding source for WSMDs in the United States. Therefore, a significant portion of sales of these devices depends on Medicare beneficiaries (Crane and Minkel, 2009), and the production of WSMDs in the United States and the types produced are directly influenced by the Medicare reimbursement system (WinterGreen Research, 2012). The net effect is to make it less likely that the devices produced will facilitate productive work outside of the home.

In contrast to the CMS DME program, the VA has a consumer-friendly program, particularly for veterans who are of working age. A veteran who meets the enrollment criteria for VA benefits is assigned to one of eight numbered, priority groups. Qualified veterans are eligible to receive WSMDs to allow them to participate in tasks of daily living in the home, community, and work environments. Qualified individuals who use a manual wheelchair for primary mobility are eligible for a custom-configured ultra-lightweight model with options and accessories when appropriately justified, and individuals who use powered wheelchairs are provided with a back-up manual device. The differences in payment policies for WSMDs between the CMS DME program and the VA program (Hubbard et al., 2007) also have a significant impact on the availability of these devices in the United States. (Models of reimbursement for assistive technology [AT], including WSMDs, are described in detail in Chapter 7.)

Issues associated with access, availability, and service delivery are important modifiers of consumer outcomes. Factors within the service delivery process, such as wait times for appointments and assessments and the range of devices and accessories available, vary across providers and programs. Groah and colleagues (2014) found that standards of care for the provision of high-quality powered wheelchairs for individuals with spinal cord injury were not being met across payer sources, except at the VA. However, no payer source, including the VA, fully met standards of care for manual wheelchairs. The VA did outperform other payers on a variety of metrics. One study of 471 veterans with traumatic amputations found that use of two or more types of WSMD together improved rehabilitation outcomes and function (Laferrier et al., 2010). Another study of 723 individuals with spinal cord injury showed that those who received their wheelchair through the VA, compared with other payers, had fewer breakdown and repair issues (Worobey et al., 2012). However, this study also showed that the incidence and adverse consequences of repairs appeared to be increasing in the United States.

Clinician Expertise in Provision of Wheeled Mobility Devices

Whether an individual receives an appropriate or effective WSMD and experiences subsequent beneficial outcomes depends on a variety of other proximal variables, including factors related to the client, provider, payer, supplier, and health care system (Eggers et al., 2009). Since the development of the assistive technology professional (ATP) certification (described below), attention has been focused on such provider factors as training and credentialing, but little research has examined the relationship between credentialing and WSMD service delivery outcomes, despite evidence suggesting that expertise and training may be important modifiers of these outcomes (Hausmann et al., 2015).

The level of clinical experience related to seating assessment, training, and follow-up evaluation depends on the severity of the user's functional limitations (physical and cognitive), the complexity of the technology, and the user's physical and social environments. When the complexity of these factors is low, rehabilitation professionals, including occupational and physical therapists, with the appropriate clinical experience are qualified to conduct assessments and provide basic WSMD training and follow-up evaluation. As the severity of the users' functional limitations becomes more profound and the complexity of the technology and the environment increases, the need for specialized training and coordinated team-based skills increases as well.

An example of the complexity associated with WSMDs is seen in standard ISO 7176-26, Wheelchairs—Part 26 (ISO, 2007). The standard classifies wheelchairs by their method of propulsion (manual or powered) and further by tilt and recline and the ability of the user (or assistant) to adjust the tilt or recline (ISO, 2007). Separate classification systems exist for seating. The Edinburgh classification of wheelchair seating equipment, for example, includes three levels of complexity (low, medium, and high) in which are nested eight levels of seating systems (Dolan and Henderson, 2013). The seating systems range in complexity from sling seat and sling back with or without a seating cushion (low), to foam carved, interlocking components or molded solid seat and/or solid back support shaped to match the user with or without additional postural support devices (high). The more complex WSMDs and seating systems require a level of specialized knowledge and skill beyond that of the typical rehabilitation professional. This level of expertise is available only in specialty rehabilitation hospitals and centers, particularly those with expertise in treating spinal cord injuries and cerebral palsy. Ensuring that complex WSMDs are properly configured and their users are adequately trained requires a coordinated interprofessional team approach to service delivery. The availability of experienced and knowledgeable clinicians is discussed below. It involves the availability of academic training programs and the collaboration of rehabilitation centers and facilities with a clinical training mission to help ensure that customized WSMDs are properly configured and users are adequately trained in their use.

Access to Trained Clinicians

Most of the credentialing bodies for the professionals referred to above include education in WSMDs in their professional requirements. While the number of hours varies, the depth of training specifically related to these devices provides only fundamental knowledge, and postprofessional continuing education combined with professional experience is required to achieve a high level of proficiency. Among health care professionals who practice primarily within the field of AT, it is generally agreed that a team approach involving a therapist, an engineer, a physician, an AT supplier, and the client is optimal. The participation of other health care professionals and family members can further enhance the team.

The U.S. Bureau of Labor Statistics reports that there are more than 200,000 physical therapists and 110,000 occupational therapists in the United States (BLS, 2016a,b), while there are fewer than 10,000 certified orthotists and/or prosthetists and approximately 8,874 physicians board-certified in physical medicine and rehabilitation (PM&R).[6] Physical therapy and physiatry require a doctoral degree before an individual qualifies for their board examination; occupational therapy currently requires a master's degree but is transitioning toward a doctoral degree; and programs in orthotics and prosthetics require a master's degree.

Degree-granting educational programs, however, represent only the beginning of the learning process necessary to maintain occupational and professional excellence in a rapidly expanding field such as rehabilitation AT. RESNA, an international, interdisciplinary organization with a commitment to technology for persons with a disability (RESNA, 2016b), provides professional development and training with approved continuing education credits, leading to certification as an ATP or seating and mobility specialist (SMS). Educational courses include Fundamentals in Assistive Technology and Advanced Seating Workshop, offered in conjunction with regular webinars related to AT. RESNA also is the home for *Assistive Technology*, the society's official journal and a major source of scientific innovation for researchers, developers, clinicians, educators, and consumers involved in advancing AT.

---

[6]As of January 4, 2017, this was the number of board-certified PM&R diplomates in the United States aged 65 or younger.

The ATP certification recognizes competence in analyzing the needs of WSMD users, helping with the selection of appropriate AT, and providing training in the use of the selected devices (RESNA, 2016c). The SMS certification is a specialty certification for professionals working in seating and mobility (RESNA, 2016c). Both certifications require an exam. The ATP exam is broad based, covering all major areas of AT while the SMS exam is focused specifically on seating, positioning, and mobility (RESNA, 2016c). To take the exam for ATP certification, candidates must meet both educational and work experience requirements (RESNA, 2016a). The education and training levels for individuals with ATP and SMS certifications differ greatly, resulting in a high degree of variability in the quality of services provided. Certified prothetists and orthotists have a scope of practice similar to that of those with ATP/SMS certification, but with formal education and training that includes obtaining a degree from an accredited program. The ATP/SMS certification could benefit from a similar model, perhaps achieving a higher standard of practice. Of course, higher standards could reduce access temporarily; in the long run, however, they could improve quality of service and access through recognition of the profession.

Another important resource for expanding professional knowledge and skill development in AT and WSMDs is the National Coalition for Assistive and Rehab Technology (NCART), a national association of suppliers and manufacturers of complex rehabilitation technology products and services that are used by individuals with significant disabilities and medical conditions (NCART, 2016). NCART's mission is to ensure that federal, state, and private coverage and reimbursement policies allow individuals with significant disabilities to have appropriate access to specialized and individually configured products and services (NCART, 2016). WSMDs account for many of the complex rehabilitation technology products and services supported by NCART advocacy.

An important professional development and educational resource directly relevant to WSMDs is the International Seating Symposium, held biannually in the United States. This symposium is one of the premier meetings in the world dedicated to clinicians, researchers, manufacturers, and others who work to improve seating and mobility among people with disabilities (ISS, 2016). The symposium includes scientific and clinical papers, in-depth workshops, special topic sessions, poster sessions, and an extensive exhibit hall. Program objectives are to identify seating and mobility interventions for people with physical disabilities, discuss service delivery practices, explore current research, and understand the features and clinical impact of seating mobility technologies (ISS, 2016). Instructional courses are provided, with associated continuing education credits.

A major source for prompting and supporting research, continuing education, professional development, and the advancement of AT science and evidence-based wheeled and mobility practice is the National Institute on Disability, Independent Living, and Rehabilitation Research (NIDILRR). NIDILRR is a federal agency in the Administration on Community Living in the U.S. Department of Health and Human Services that provides leadership and grant support for a comprehensive program of scholarly activity related to the rehabilitation of individuals with disabilities. NIDILRR's extramural research is conducted through a network of research projects and centers located throughout the country. Among its largest funding programs are Rehabilitation Engineering Research Centers (RERCs), Disability Rehabilitation Research Program grants, and the Model Systems Centers of Excellence program. The Model Systems Centers of Excellence are focused on various diagnostic groups. The Model Systems Centers of Excellence in Spinal Cord Injury are particularly important resources for advanced training in state-of-the-art technology development, clinical practice, and research related to WSMDs.

Most insurance providers, including Medicare, require a physician's prescription for a WSMD, for a therapist's assessment for the specification of a device for long-term use due to a permanent disability, and for training in its safe and effective use. Medicare and other insurers may also require that the wheelchair be provided by a supplier or a manufacturer representative who is credentialed by RESNA as an ATP. The results of a cohort study examining patterns of ownership and use of mobility aids among working-age individuals with multiple sclerosis showed variation in access to reimbursement for WSMDs as well as in training in use of the devices (Iezzoni et al., 2010). Among users of powered wheelchairs, only 37 percent were reimbursed by insurance for any part of the cost, and only 41 percent received training in the device's use (Iezzoni et al., 2010); almost 69 percent of this training was provided by the vendor and not a rehabilitation professional. Among manual wheelchair users, only 23 percent were reimbursed by insurance for any part of the cost (Iezzoni et al., 2010); 18 percent of users received training, 44 percent of them from the vendor and 44 percent from the rehabilitation provider (Iezzoni et al., 2010). Among scooter users, only 17 percent were reimbursed by insurance for any part of the cost (Iezzoni et al., 2010); only 24 percent received training in use of the device, primarily from the vendor (82 percent) and not a rehabilitation provider (Iezzoni et al., 2010). These variations have a significant impact on the types of WSMDs individuals receive, as do geographic variations in the availability of experienced and knowledgeable clinicians.

The distribution of ATP and SMS certified practitioners across the United States is depicted in Figure 3-15. As this figure illustrates, a disparity exists in the availability of practitioners holding both ATP and SMS certifications, with most being clustered around major urban areas and large medical

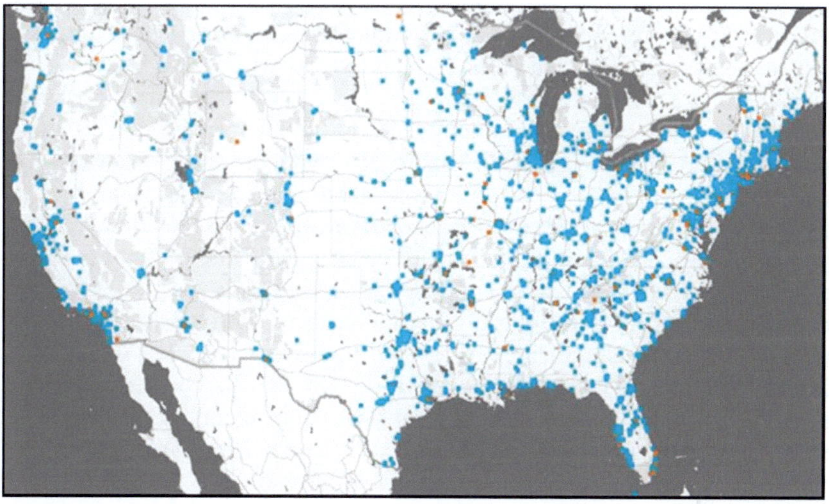

FIGURE 3-15 Distribution of ATP and SMS certified professionals.*

NOTES: ● = ATP certified ● = SMS certified.

*Data provided by the Rehabilitation Engineering and Assistive Technology Society of North America. Data mapped by the University of Pittsburgh, School of Health and Rehabilitation Sciences, Department of Rehabilitation Science and Technology. This figure was created with the assistance of Mark Schmeler and Vince Schiappa at the University of Pittsburgh. Dr. Schmeler was one of the committee's guest speakers.

centers. RESNA maintains a directory of certified practitioners (RESNA, 2016a), showing that currently 3,871 practitioners hold an ATP certification and 167 hold an SMS certification; a practitioner can hold both certifications. The majority of practitioners who are ATP certified identify seating, positioning, and mobility as a practice area. The number of ATP and SMS certified practitioners is small considering the need for their services.

Access to Clinics That Provide Wheelchairs

As noted above, the provision of a wheelchair generally involves a physician who writes a prescription, a therapist who conducts an assessment and generates a recommendation, and a supplier or a manufacturer representative. Some clinics employ a team approach to wheelchair provision and are capable of meeting the complex needs of individuals with severe disabilities. Unfortunately, there is no registry of such clinics, but there are ways to identify at least some of them. There are currently 24 VA Spinal

Cord Injuries and Disorders Centers located throughout the United States that provide comprehensive care to qualified veterans with spinal cord injuries, multiple sclerosis, and ALS. To decrease disparities and improve standards of care for WSMD service delivery, the VA established the Polytrauma Rehabilitation Assistive Technology (PRAT) Lab. The PRAT Lab currently provides consultation and resources to 27 VA facilities in 18 states.[7] This network began with the five Polytrauma Rehabilitation Centers and has expanded to Polytrauma Network Sites, Polytrauma Support Clinical Teams, and other VA Centers interested in or currently implementing AT interventions and services. The PRAT Lab standardized the WSMD service delivery process across sites by using published, evidence-based guidelines for conducting assessments, and they developed a checklist to assist therapists in implementing these guidelines (Ambrosio et al., 2007). The VA has created clinical rehabilitation engineering positions requiring a relevant degree and the ATP credential. This model helps meet the need for formalized education and credentialing of rehabilitation engineers and AT providers.

For individuals who are not veterans, access to clinics that provide WSMDs generally is very limited. The 14 NIDILRR Model Systems Centers of Excellence in Spinal Cord Injury provide comprehensive care to individuals with spinal cord injuries, including the provision of complex wheelchairs and seating systems. This program also has contributed to several survey components on wheelchair mobility, including wheelchair service delivery models, what causes disparities, and whether providers' prescriptions are appropriate. In addition, the Commission on Accreditation of Rehabilitation Facilities (CARF), an independent, nonprofit organization focused on advancing the quality of rehabilitation services, states on its website that there are 51 accredited AT clinics located throughout the United States. This list on the CARF website is not comprehensive as there are clinics that provide wheelchairs to a high standard but are not within the family of CARF-accredited facilities.

FINDINGS AND CONCLUSIONS

Findings

Access to Wheeled and Seated Mobility Devices

3-1. Persons in the neurological diagnostic group (e.g., spinal cord injury, multiple sclerosis) tend to use lightweight high-strength wheelchairs,

[7] California, Colorado, Florida, Illinois, Iowa, Massachusetts, Michigan, Minnesota, Nebraska, New Mexico, New York, North Carolina, Ohio, Pennsylvania, Texas, Utah, Virginia, and Washington.

whereas those in the obesity diagnostic group use primarily heavy- and extra-heavy-duty wheelchairs.

3-2. Well-fitted, good-quality seating helps prevent secondary health conditions such as pressure sores and overuse injuries in people using wheelchairs.

3-3. Customizable powered wheelchairs have been shown to improve functioning.

3-4. The type of wheeled and seated mobility device (WSMD) that is most appropriate for an individual depends on a number of factors, including body functions and activity, as well as environmental and personal factors.

3-5. The variable dependability and availability of WSMDs impact individuals' functioning and activity and their ability to be employed.

3-6. Access to WSMDs varies significantly across reimbursement and funding sources in the United States.

3-7. A mismatch exists between the types of WSMDs covered by Medicare and those required to maximize individuals' functioning based on their diagnosis and treatment.

Access to Highly Qualified Providers

3-8. Even though wheelchairs are ubiquitous, they do not replace all of the complex functions of the lower extremities; in addition, proper fitting and training are complex but necessary elements of maximizing users' performance, work potential, and health maintenance.

3-9. In the United States, multiple agencies and service providers are responsible for determining the need for WSMDs, providing the products and technologies, delivering the training, monitoring use of the products and technologies, and assessing outcomes.

3-10. The distribution of providers and clinics with the knowledge, skills, and expertise to properly evaluate, prescribe, and train people in the use of WSMDs varies greatly throughout the United States.

3-11. Providers of WSMDs vary in their level of knowledge, skills, and expertise.

Availability of Data

3-12. Data on the prevalence of use of WSMDs are fragmented and limited.

3-13. Factors affecting the ability to work for individuals using WSMDs include the ability to get ready for work, transportation to work, and access to the workplace.

3-14. There are limited data showing the relationship between individual users' medical conditions and health (e.g., comorbidities) and/or sociodemographic characteristics and the specific types of WSMDs they use.

3-15. The current fragmented approach to the delivery of WSMDs means that no single public-use data source includes information on the prevalence of these devices with a focus on persons of working age (ages 20-67).

Conclusions

Access to Wheeled and Seated Mobility Devices

3-1. The variation in reimbursement and funding sources and access to qualified professionals in the United States has a significant impact on the types of WSMDs individuals receive. [Findings 3-6, 3-7]

3-2. Medicare's policy limiting coverage of WSMDs to those needed for home use is an impediment to achieving gainful employment. [Findings 3-5, 3-7]

3-3. Medicare policy affects manufacturers' production and distribution of WSMDs. [Finding 3-7]

Access to Highly Qualified Providers

3-4. More qualified providers and clinics with the knowledge, skills, and expertise to properly evaluate, prescribe, and train people in the use of WSMDs are needed. [Findings 3-8, 3-10, 3-11]

3-5. A higher level of certification/training than the current assistive technology professional credential could improve the qualifications of providers in terms of the knowledge, skill, and expertise necessary to properly evaluate, prescribe, and train people in the use of WSMDs. The degree requirement from an accredited program and certification process for prosthetists and orthotists could serve as a good model for WSMD suppliers and technicians. [Finding 3-8]

Availability of Data

3-6. Information showing the relationship between individual users' medical conditions and health and/or sociodemographic characteristics and the specific types of WSMDs they use would be useful for payers, providers, and consumers to support future planning for treatment programs, the production of technologies, the training of providers, and the allocation of resources for these assistive devices. [Finding 3-14]

3-7. Although wheelchairs are ubiquitous, advances in these devices have been stifled by reimbursement policies and a lack of professional training and research investment. These barriers have limited realization of the full potential of wheelchairs, such as the introduction of new materials and the integration of robotics technology for navigation, safety, and obstacle negotiation. These types of features could further expand the population of people with independent wheeled mobility, increase safety, and prolong independent mobility as people age. [Finding 3-7]

3-8. The U.S. Census Bureau's Survey of Income and Program Participation is the best population-based source of information on the overall use of WSMDs in the United States. [Finding 3-12]

REFERENCES

Ambrosio, F., M. L. Boninger, S. G. Fitzgerald, S. L. Hubbard, S. R. Schwid, and R. A. Cooper. 2007. Comparison of mobility device delivery within Department of Veterans Affairs for individuals with multiple sclerosis versus spinal cord injury. *Journal of Rehabilitation Research & Development* 44(5):693-701.

ANSI/RESNA (American National Standards Institute/Rehabilitation Engineering and Assistive Technology Society of North America). 2009. RESNA American National Standard for Wheelchairs—Volume 1: Requirements and test methods for wheelchairs (including scooters). In *Section 15: Requirements for information disclosure, documentation and labeling*. Arlington, VA: RESNA.

Arledge, S., W. Armstrong, M. Babinec, B. E. Dicianno, C. Digiovine, T. Dyson-Hudson, J. Pederson, J. Piriano, T. Plummer, L. Rosen, M. Schmeler, M. Shea, and J. Stogner. 2011. *RESNA wheelchair service provision guide*. Arlington, VA: RESNA. http://www.resna.org/sites/default/files/legacy/resources/position-papers/RESNAWheelchairServiceProvisionGuide.pdf (accessed January 21, 2017).

Arva, J., M. R. Schmeler, M. L. Lange, D. D. Lipka, and L. E. Rosen. 2009. RESNA position on the application of seat-elevating devices for wheelchair users. *Assistive Technology* 21(2):69-72.

Barker, D. J., D. Reid, and C. Cott. 2004. Acceptance and meanings of wheelchair use in senior stroke survivors. *American Journal of Occupational Therapy* 58(2):221-230.

Bates, P. S., J. C. Spencer, M. E. Young, and D. H. Rintala. 1993. Assistive technology and the newly disabled adult: Adaptation to wheelchair use. *American Journal of Occupational Therapy* 47(11):1014-1021.

BLS (U.S. Bureau of Labor Statistics). 2016a. *Occupational outlook handbook 2016-17 edition: Occupational therapists*. https://www.bls.gov/ooh/healthcare/occupational-therapists.htm (accessed December 22, 2016).

BLS. 2016b. *Occupational outlook handbook 2016-17 edition: Physical therapists*. https://www.bls.gov/ooh/healthcare/physical-therapists.htm (accessed December 22, 2016).

Boles, M., B. Pelletier, and W. Lynch. 2004. The relationships between health risks and work productivity. *Journal of Occupational and Environmental Medicine* 46(7):737-745.

CDC (U.S. Centers for Disease Control and Prevention). 2016. *National Health Interview Survey 2015 data release*. https://www.cdc.gov/nchs/nhis/nhis_2015_data_release.htm (accessed July 30, 2016).

Chaves, E. S., M. L. Boninger, R. Cooper, S. G. Fitzgerald, D. B. Gray, and R. A. Cooper. 2004. Assessing the influence of wheelchair technology on perception of participation in spinal cord injury. *Archives of Physical Medicine and Rehabilitation* 85(11):1854-1858.

CMS (Centers for Medicare & Medicaid Services). 2009. *Medicare coverage of power mobility devices (PMDs): Power wheelchairs and power operated vehicles (POVs).* https://www.cms.gov/Outreach-and-Education/Medicare-Learning-Network-MLN/MLNProducts/downloads/PMDFactSheet07_Quark19.pdf (accessed January 25, 2017).

CMS. 2013. *Basic stand alone DME public use files.* https://www.cms.gov/Research-Statistics-Data-and-Systems/Statistics-Trends-and-Reports/BSAPUFS/BSA_DME_Line_Items_PUF.html (accessed August 1, 2016).

CMS. 2015a. *CMS research statistics data and systems/statistics trends and reports.* https://www.cms.gov/Research-Statistics-Data-and-Systems/Statistics-Trends-and-Reports/CMS-Statistics-Reference-Booklet/2015.html (accessed November 8, 2016).

CMS. 2015b. *Power mobility devices: Complying with documentation and coverage requirements.* https://www.cms.gov/Outreach-and-Education/Medicare-Learning-Network-MLN/MLNProducts/downloads/pmd_DocCvg_FactSheet_ICN905063.pdf (accessed September 7, 2016).

Cooper, R. A. 1998. *Wheelchair selection and configuration.* New York: Demos.

Cooper, R. A. 2001. Advances in wheelchair and related technologies. *Medical Engineering & Physics* 23(4):iii-iv.

Cooper, R. A. 2013. The basics of manual wheelchair maintenance. *PN Online*, September 12.

Cooper, R. A., M. L. Boninger, and A. Rentschler. 1999. Evaluation of selected ultralight manual wheelchairs using ANSI/RESNA standards. *Archives of Physical Medicine and Rehabilitation* 80(4):462-467.

Cooper, R. A., H. Ohnabe, and D. A. Hobson. 2006. *An introduction to rehabilitation engineering.* Boca Raton, FL: CRC Press.

Cooper, R., R. A. Cooper, M. L. T. Hernandez, T. M. Crytzer, T. Bobish, R. Mankowski, J. Mankowski, J. Coltellaro, B. McCormick, E. C. Ferretti, M. A. F. de Mello, and N. Upadhyay. 2015. Assistive technology: An international approach to the comprehensive management (Chapter 38). In *ISCoS textbook on comprehensive management of spinal cord injuries*, edited by H. S. Chhabra. New Delhi, India: Wolters Kluwer. Pp. 594-612.

Crane, B., and J. Minkel. 2009. Legislation and funding. In *Industry profile on wheeled mobility*, edited by S. Bauer and M. E. Buning. Buffalo, NY: University at Buffalo. Pp. 50-78.

Crytzer, T. M., R. Cooper, G. Jerome, and A. Koontz. 2017. Identifying research needs for wheelchair transfers in the built environment. *Disability and Rehabilitation: Assistive Technology* 12(2):121-127.

Davies, A., L. H. De Souza, and A. O. Frank. 2003. Changes in the quality of life in severely disabled people following provision of powered indoor/outdoor chairs. *Disability and Rehabilitation* 25(6):286-290.

Denison, I. 2006. *Wheelchair maintenance series.* http://www.assistive-technology.ca/studies/wm_full.pdf (accessed August 29, 2013).

Dicianno, B. E., M. Schmeler, and B. Y. Liu. 2011. Wheelchairs/adaptive mobility equipment and seating. In *Spinal cord medicine*, edited by S. Kirshblum and D. I. Campagnolo. Philadelphia, PA: Lippincott Williams & Wilkins. Pp. 341-358.

DiGiovine, M. M., R. A. Cooper, M. L. Boninger, B. M. Lawrence, D. P. VanSickle, and A. J. Rentschler. 2000. User assessment of manual wheelchair ride comfort and ergonomics. *Archives of Physical Medicine and Rehabilitation* 81(4):490-494.

Dolan, M. J., and G. I. Henderson. 2013. Patient and equipment profile for wheelchair seating clinic provision. *Disability and Rehabilitation: Assistive Technology* 9(2):136-143.

Edwards, K., and A. McCluskey. 2010. A survey of adult power wheelchair and scooter users. *Disability and Rehabilitation: Assistive Technology* 5(6):411-419.

Eggers, S. L., L. Myaskovsky, K. H. Burkitt, M. Tolerico, G. E. Switzer, M. J. Fine, and M. L. Boninger. 2009. A preliminary model of wheelchair service delivery. *Archives of Physical Medicine and Rehabilitation* 90(6):1030-1038.

Fass, M. V., R. A. Cooper, S. G. Fitzgerald, M. Schmeler, M. L. Boninger, S. D. Algood, W. A. Ammer, A. J. Rentschler, and J. Duncan. 2004. Durability, value, and reliability of selected electric powered wheelchairs. *Archives of Physical Medicine and Rehabilitation* 85(5):805-814.

Fitzgerald, S., R. A. Cooper, A. Rentschler, and M. Boninger. 1999. Comparison of fatigue life for three types of manual wheelchairs. *Proceedings of the First Joint BMES/EMBS Conference* 601(1):606.

Fitzgerald, S. G., R. A. Cooper, M. L. Boninger, and A. J. Rentschler. 2001. Comparison of fatigue life for 3 types of manual wheelchairs. *Archives of Physical Medicine and Rehabilitation* 82(10):1484-1488.

Fitzgerald, S., D. Collins, R. Cooper, M. Tolerico, A. Kelleher, P. Hunt, S. Martin, B. Impink, and R. Cooper. 2005. Issues in the maintenance and repairs of wheelchairs: A pilot study. *Journal of Rehabilitation Research & Development* 42(6):853-862.

Flagg, J. L. 2009. Wheeled mobility demographics. In *Industry profile on wheeled mobility*, edited by S. Bauer and M. E. Buning. Buffalo, NY: University at Buffalo. Pp. 7-29.

Galvin, J. C., and M. J. Scherer. 1996. *Evaluating, selecting, and using appropriate assistive technology*. Gaithersburg, MD: Aspen Publishers Inc.

Goetzel, R. Z., S. R. Long, R. J. Ozminkowski, K. Hawkins, S. Wang, and W. Lynch. 2004. Health, absence, disability, and presenteeism cost estimates of certain physical and mental health conditions affecting U.S. employers. *Journal of Occupational and Environmental Medicine* 46(4):398-412.

Griffin, B., H. Cooper, C. Horack, M. Klyber, and D. Schimmelpfenning. 2007. Best-practice protocols: Reducing harm from pressure ulcers. *Nursing Management* 38(9):29-32.

Groah, S. L., I. Ljungberg, A. Lichy, M. Oyster, and M. L. Boninger. 2014. Disparities in wheelchair procurement by payer among people with spinal cord injury. *PM&R* 6(5):412-417.

Hausmann, L. R., L. Myaskovsky, C. Niyonkuru, M. L. Oyster, G. E. Switzer, K. H. Burkitt, M. J. Fine, S. Gao, and M. L. Boninger. 2015. Examining implicit bias of physicians who care for individuals with spinal cord injury: A pilot study and future directions. *The Journal of Spinal Cord Medicine* 38(1):102-110.

Hubbard, S. L., S. G. Fitzgerald, B. Vogel, D. M. Reker, R. A. Cooper, and M. L. Boninger. 2007. Distribution and cost of wheelchairs and scooters provided by Veterans Health Administration. *Journal of Rehabilitation Research & Development* 44(4):581-592.

Iezzoni, L., S. R. Rao, and R. P. Kinkel. 2009. Patterns of mobility aid use among working-age persons with multiple sclerosis living in the community in the United States. *Disability and Health Journal* 2(2):67-76.

Iezzoni, L. I., S. R. Rao, and R. P. Kinkel. 2010. Experiences acquiring and using mobility aids among working-age persons with multiple sclerosis living in communities in the United States. *American Journal of Physical Medicine and Rehabilitation* 89(12):1010-1023.

ISO (International Organization for Standardization). 2007. *ISO 7176-26:2007 Wheelchairs—part 26: Vocabulary*. http://www.iso.org/iso/home/store/catalogue_tc/catalogue_detail.htm?csnumber=44224 (accessed August 31, 2016).

ISS (International Seating Symposium). 2016. *About the 2017 ISS*. http://www.iss.pitt.edu/ISS2017/ISS2017about.html (accessed July 29, 2016).

Kamaraj, D. C., B. E. Dicianno, H. P. Mahajan, A. M. Buhari, and R. A. Cooper. 2016. Interrater reliability of the power mobility road test in the virtual reality-based simulator-2. *Archives of Physical Medicine and Rehabilitation* 97(7):1078-1084.

Kankipati, P., M. L. Boninger, D. Gagnon, R. A. Cooper, and A. M. Koontz. 2015. Upper limb joint kinetics of three sitting pivot wheelchair transfer techniques in individuals with spinal cord injury. *The Journal of Spinal Cord Medicine* 38(4):485-497.

Khasnabis, C., and K. Mines. 2012. *Wheelchair service training package basic level.* Geneva, Switzerland: WHO.

Kirby, R. L., N. J. Mifflen, D. L. Thibault, C. Smith, K. L. Best, K. J. Thompson, and D. A. MacLeod. 2004. The manual wheelchair-handling skills of caregivers and the effect of training. *Archives of Physical Medicine and Rehabilitation* 85(12):2011-2019.

Kittel, A., A. D. Marco, and H. Stewart. 2002. Factors influencing the decision to abandon manual wheelchairs for three individuals with a spinal cord injury. *Disability and Rehabilitation* 24(1-3):106-114.

Koontz, A. M. n.d. *Manual wheelchair maintenance.* http://www.spinlife.com/spintips/details/k/Manual%20Wheelchair%20Maintenance/a/116/c/2 (accessed August 28, 2013).

Koontz, A. M., M. Toro, P. Kankipati, M. Naber, and R. Cooper. 2012. An expert review of the scientific literature on independent wheelchair transfers. *Disability and Rehabilitation: Assistive Technology* 7(1):20-29.

Kumar, A., M. R. Schmeler, A. M. Karmarkar, D. M. Collins, R. Cooper, R. A. Cooper, H. Shin, and M. B. Holm. 2013. Test-retest reliability of the functional mobility assessment (FMA): A pilot study. *Disability and Rehabilitation: Assistive Technology* 8(3):213-219.

Laferrier, J. Z., L. V. McFarland, M. L. Boninger, R. A. Cooper, and G. E. Reiber. 2010. Wheeled mobility: Factors influencing mobility and assistive technology in veterans and servicemembers with major traumatic limb loss from Vietnam War and OIF/OEF conflicts. *Journal of Rehabilitation Research & Development* 47(4):349-360.

Letts, L., D. Dawson, I. Bretholz, E. Kaiserman-Goldenstein, J. Gleason, E. McLellan, L. Norton, and C. Roth. 2007. Reliability and validity of the power-mobility community driving assessment. *Assistive Technology* 19(3):154-163.

Liu, H.-Y., R. Cooper, R. Cooper, A. Smailagic, D. Siewiorek, D. Ding, and F.-C. Chuang. 2010. Seating virtual coach: A smart reminder for power seat function usage. *Technology and Disability* 22(1, 2):53-60.

Liu, H.-Y., G. Grindle, A. Kelleher, R. Cooper, R. Cooper, F. C. Chuang, D. Siewiorek, and A. Smailagic. 2012. A survey of feedback modalities for wheelchair power seat functions. *IEEE Pervasive Computing* 11(3):54-62.

Lukersmith, S., L. Radbron, and K. Hopman. 2013. Development of clinical guidelines for the prescription of a seated wheelchair or mobility scooter for people with traumatic brain injury or spinal cord injury. *Australian Occupational Therapy Journal* 60(6):378-386.

MacPhee, A. H., R. L. Kirby, A. L. Coolen, C. Smith, D. A. MacLeod, and D. J. Dupuis. 2004. Wheelchair skills training program: A randomized clinical trial of wheelchair users undergoing initial rehabilitation. *Archives of Physical Medicine and Rehabilitation* 85(1):41-50.

Massengale, S., D. Folden, P. McConnell, L. Stratton, and V. Whitehead. 2005. Effect of visual perception, visual function, cognition, and personality on power wheelchair use in adults. *Assistive Technology* 17(2):108-121.

McClure, L. A., M. L. Boninger, H. Ozawa, and A. Koontz. 2011. Reliability and validity analysis of the transfer assessment instrument. *Archives of Physical Medicine and Rehabilitation* 92(3):499-508.

Mills, T. L., M. B. Holm, and M. Schmeler. 2007. Test-retest reliability and cross validation of the functioning everyday with a wheelchair instrument. *Assistive Technology* 19(2):61-77.

Mortenson, W. B., and J. Kim. 2016. Scoping review of mobility scooter-related research studies. *Journal of Rehabilitation Research & Development* 53(5):531-540.

NCART (National Coalition for Assistive and Rehabilitation Technology). 2016. *National Coalition for Assistive and Rehab Technology: Protecting and promoting access to complex rehab technology*. http://www.ncart.us (accessed July 30, 2016).

Nosek, M. A., and T. A. Krouskop. 1995. Demonstrating a model approach to independent living center-based assistive technology services. *Assistive Technology* 7(1):48-54.

Paralyzed Veterans of America Consortium for Spinal Cord Medicine. 2000. Outcomes following traumatic spinal cord injury: Clinical practice guidelines for health-care professionals. *The Journal of Spinal Cord Medicine* 23(4):289-316.

Paralyzed Veterans of America Consortium for Spinal Cord Medicine. 2005. *Preservation of upper limb function following spinal cord injury: A clinical practice guideline for health-care professionals*. Washington, DC: Consortium for Spinal Cord Medicine.

Paralyzed Veterans of America Consortium for Spinal Cord Medicine. 2014. *Pressure ulcer prevention and treatment following spinal cord injury: A clinical practice guideline for health-care providers*. Washington, DC: Consortium for Spinal Cord Medicine.

RESNA (Rehabilitation Engineering and Assistive Technology Society of North America). 2016a. *ATP statistics*. http://www.resna.org/get-certified/atp-statistics (accessed September 1, 2016).

RESNA. 2016b. *About*. http://www.resna.org/about (accessed August 1, 2016).

RESNA. 2016c. *Certification*. http://www.resna.org/certification (accessed February 3, 2017).

Routhier, F., C. Vincent, J. Desrosiers, and S. Nadeau. 2003. Mobility of wheelchair users: A proposed performance assessment framework. *Disability and Rehabilitation* 25(1):19-34.

Salminen, A. L., A. Brandt, K. Samuelsson, O. Töytäri, and A. Malmivaara. 2009. Mobility devices to promote activity and participation: A systematic review. *Journal of Rehabilitation Medicine* 41(9):697-706.

Scherer, M. J. 2002. *Assistive technology: Matching device and consumer for successful rehabilitation*. Washington, DC: American Psychological Association.

Schofield, R., A. Porter-Armstrong, and M. Stinson. 2013. Reviewing the literature on the effectiveness of pressure relieving movements. *Nursing Research and Practice* 2013.

Smith, E. M., E. M. Giesbrecht, W. B. Mortenson, and W. C. Miller. 2016. Prevalence of wheelchair and scooter use among community-dwelling Canadians. *Physical Therapy* 96(8):1135-1142.

Soydan, Y., S. Koksal, and O. Ciobanu. 2012. *Training of wheelchair users for maintenance*. Paper presented at 4th International Congress of Educational Research, Istanbul, May 4-7.

Sui Generis Seat. 2015. *Sui Generis Seat*. http://suigenerisseat.com (accessed April 6, 2017).

Toro, M. L., A. M. Koontz, and R. A. Cooper. 2013. The impact of transfer setup on the performance of independent wheelchair transfers. *Human Factors* 55(3):567-580.

Toro, M. L., C. Eke, and J. Pearlman. 2016. The impact of the World Health Organization 8-steps in wheelchair service provision in wheelchair users in a less resourced setting: A cohort study in Indonesia. *BMC Health Services Research* 16(1):26.

Trefler, E. M., S. G. P. Fitzgerald, D. A. P. Hobson, T. M. S. Bursick, and R. M. S. Joseph. 2004. Outcomes of wheelchair systems intervention with residents of long-term care facilities. *Assistive Technology* 16(1):18-27.

U.S. Census Bureau. 2016. *Survey of income and program participation: 2008 panel wave 06*. https://www.census.gov/programs-surveys/sipp/data/2008-panel/wave-6.html (accessed August 12, 2016).

van Roosmalen, L., G. E. Bertocci, D. A. Hobson, and P. Karg. 2002. Preliminary evaluation of wheelchair occupant restraint system usage in motor vehicles. *Journal of Rehabilitation Research & Development* 39(1):83-93.

Wang, H., H.-Y. Liu, J. Pearlman, R. Cooper, A. Jefferds, S. Connor, and R. A. Cooper. 2010. Relationship between wheelchair durability and wheelchair type and years of test. *Disability and Rehabilitation: Assistive Technology* 5(5):318-322.

WinterGreen Research. 2012. *Manual wheelchair market shares, strategies, and forecasts, worldwide, 2012 to 2018*. http://www.marketresearchstore.com/report/manual-wheelchair-market-shares-strategies-and-forecasts-worldwide-2394 (accessed August 11, 2016).

WHO (World Health Organization). 2008. *Guidelines on the provision of manual wheelchairs in less resourced settings*. http://apps.who.int/iris/bitstream/10665/43960/1/9789241547482_eng.pdf (accessed February 24, 2017).

Worobey, L. 2016. *Wheelchair breakdown: What is failing and what to do about it—Implications for users and clinicians and a potential intervention*. http://asia-mmg.societyhq.com/2016annual/guide/protected/syllabus/lectures/2016-PA-1461334033-3953.pdf (accessed February 1, 2017).

Worobey, L., M. Oyster, G. Nemunaitis, R. Cooper, and M. L. Boninger. 2012. Increases in wheelchair breakdowns, repairs, and adverse consequences for people with traumatic spinal cord injury. *American Journal of Physical Medicine & Rehabilitation/Association of Academic Physiatrists* 91(6):463.

Worobey, L., J. Pearlman, T. Dyson-Hudson, and M. Boninger. 2016. Clinician competency with wheelchair maintenance and the efficacy of a wheelchair maintenance training program. *Archives of Physical Medicine and Rehabilitation* 97(10):e55.

Young, J. B., P. W. Belfield, B. H. Mascie-Taylor, and G. P. Mulley. 1985. The neglected hospital wheelchair. *British Medical Journal* 291(6506):1388-1389.

CHAPTER 3 ANNEX TABLES BEGIN ON THE NEXT PAGE

ANNEX TABLE 3-1
Taxonomy of Wheeled and Seated Mobility Devices[a]

Device	Cost Range	Population	Intended Use	Requirements for Use
Manual Wheelchairs				
Standard (K0001), Hemi (K0002), and Lightweight (K0003)	$300–$600	Primarily elderly	Limited use for short time periods; may be used by individuals who can stand and walk to some degree	Upper-extremity function intact; good endurance in chair
High-Strength Lightweight (K0004)	$900–$2,000	Primarily for transport of individuals who have physical impairment and obesity	May be used by individuals who can stand and walk to some degree; users spend at least 2 hours/day in the wheelchair	Upper-extremity function intact; able to self-propel the wheelchair
Ultra-lightweight (K0005), Custom Manual (K0008), and Other (K0009)	$1,800–$4,000	Almost all ages (e.g., 18 months to 100 years)	Used as primary or sole mode of mobility	Able to self-propel the wheelchair; motivation
Heavy-Duty (K0006) and Extra-Heavy Duty (K0007)	$500–$2,000	Primarily for transport of individuals who have physical impairment and obesity	For individuals who weigh more than 250 pounds (K0006) or more than 350 pounds (K0007)	Weight more than 250 or 350 pounds

	Need for Training and Adaption	Benefits of Device	Limitations of Device	Life Span of Device (Years)	Maintenance	Other Considerations
	Minimal	Inexpensive and readily available	Heavy; difficult to propel; limited customiz-ability	1-3 years	Minimal	For temporary use or transport of people within a health care facility
	Minimal		Heavy; difficult to propel; difficult to transport	1-3 years	Minimal	Limited seating options, do not accommodate specialized seating needs
	Moderate training for advanced wheelchair skills	Offers customized fit and configurability; easier to lift; easier to propel, essential for those with limited endurance or strength, such as patients with tetraplegia	Expense and difficulty of getting approval for funding	3-5 years	Moderate; requires experienced technicians	Must be prescribed by a licensed/certified medical professional
	Minimal	Can be used by people with weight above 250 or 350 pounds	Heavy; difficult to propel	3-5 years	Moderate because of weight of user	Often better served with a powered wheelchair

continued

ANNEX TABLE 3-1
Continued

Device	Cost Range	Population	Intended Use	Requirements for Use
Powered Wheelchairs				
Scooter/Power Operated Vehicle	$1,000–$6,000	Primarily elderly or people with early onset of progressive conditions (e.g., multiple sclerosis)	Supplemental form of mobility for those who can stand and ambulate to some degree	Cognitive ability to operate; arm and hand function intact
Group 1 Powered Wheelchair	$3,000–$8,000	Primarily elderly, temporary use, or back-up	Primarily indoor use	Cognitive ability to operate; arm and some hand function intact; ability to perform independent weight shift and transfers
Group 2 Powered Wheelchair	$3,000–$20,000		Long-term use for individuals who can still independently weight shift or transfer	Cognitive ability to operate; arm and some hand function intact
Group 3 Powered Wheelchair	$8,000–$35,000	Long-term wheelchair users without effective ability to propel a manual wheelchair, perform an independent weight shift, or propel in the community	Long-term use for individuals who cannot independently weight shift or transfer	Cognitive ability to operate; arm and some hand function intact or ability to use hands-free interface
Group 4 Powered Wheelchair	$10,000–$40,000	Active indoor/outdoor long-term wheelchair users without effective ability to propel a manual wheelchair, perform an independent weight shift, or propel in the community	Long-term use for individuals who cannot independently weight shift or transfer; better designed for use outside of the home; ideal for active users	Cognitive ability to operate; arm and some hand function intact or ability to use hands-free interface

[a]Wheeled and seated mobility devices are medical devices with wheels that are intended to provide mobility to persons with restricted or no ability to ambulate without assistance from technology.

	Need for Training and Adaption	Benefits of Device	Limitations of Device	Life Span of Device (Years)	Maintenance	Other Considerations
	Minimal	Intuitive to use	Poor seating for support and pressure reduction; instability and tipping; large turning radius	1–5 years	Moderate; requires regular tire and battery maintenance	Requires additional equipment to transfer; difficult to use in-home, or when made for in-home presents safety risk in community
	Minimal	Relative ease of use; lightweight compared with other powered wheelchairs; can be portable	Short range of only 3–5 miles; few advanced features, such as tilt or recline	1–3 years	Frequent tire, battery, and hardware maintenance	Not durable for regular users of a powered wheelchair
	Moderate; need for an experienced licensed/certified medical professional	Limited seat functions and customi-zability	Not as durable as Group 3; limited seat functions and customi-zability	3–5 years	Minimal to moderate	
	Moderate; need for an experienced licensed/certified medical professional	Intermediate range and speed	Designed for use in the home	3–5 years	Requires skilled technicians	
	Moderate; need for an experienced licensed/certified medical professional	Longest range and highest speed; most customizable and greatest number of options; greatest durability	Expense	3–5 years	Requires skilled technicians	Limited funding available

ANNEX TABLE 3-2
Functionality of Wheeled and Seated Mobility Devices

Device	Standing: 1-Fixed seat height 2-Manual seat elevation 3-Powered seat elevation 4-Manual standing 5-Powered standing	Balancing - Seated or Standing: 1-Supports basic linear seated balance 2-Provides for adjustable seated balance 3-Provides for custom seated balance 4-Support for standing balance	Climbing: 1-Ramps 2-Curb-cuts 3-Thresholds 4-Curbs 5-Steps 6-Stairs	Balancing - Seating and Positioning: 1-Fixed 2-Adjustable Manual Seating Functions 3-Powered Seating Functions	Mobility Indoors: 1-Firm, stable flooring (wood, tile, cement) 2-Compliant flooring (carpet, artificial turf) 3-Ramps 4-Turning space 5-Size (width, length)
Manual wheelchairs					
Standard (K0001), Hemi (K0002), and Lightweight (K0003)	1	1	1, 2, 3	1	1
High-Strength Lightweight (K0004)	1	1	1, 2, 3	1	1
Ultra-lightweight (K0005), Custom Manual (K0008), and Other (K0009)	1	2	1, 2, 3, 4	1, 2	1, 2, 3, 4, 5

	Mobility Outdoors: 1-Americans with Disabilities Act (ADA) surfaces 2-Non-ADA pedestrian surfaces 3-Natural terrain	Reaching: 1-Provides floor level support 2-Provides chair-level support 3-Provides variable seat elevation above chair level 4-Provides standing	Carrying: 1-Unable to carry items without impacting mobility or function 2-Able to carry 10 lb without impacting mobility or function 3-Able to carry 25 lb without impacting mobility or function	Dexterous Movements: 1-Requires gross motor function 2-Requires fine motor function	Lifting: 1-Does not extend range of lifting 2-Extends range of lifting 6-12 inches 3-Extends range of lifting greater than 12 inches	Communication: 1-Does not support use of communication device; 2-Accommodates mechanical connection of communication device; 3-Provides mechanical and electronic (e.g., charging) connection of communication device
	1	2	1	1	1	1
	1	2	2	1	1	1
	1, 2	2	2	1	1	1

continued

ANNEX TABLE 3-2
Continued

Device	Standing: 1-Fixed seat height 2-Manual seat elevation 3-Powered seat elevation 4-Manual standing 5-Powered standing	Balancing - Seated or Standing: 1-Supports basic linear seated balance 2-Provides for adjustable seated balance 3-Provides for custom seated balance 4-Support for standing balance	Climbing: 1-Ramps 2-Curb-cuts 3-Thresholds 4-Curbs 5-Steps 6-Stairs	Balancing - Seating and Positioning: 1-Fixed 2-Adjustable Manual Seating Functions 3-Powered Seating Functions	Mobility Indoors: 1-Firm, stable flooring (wood, tile, cement) 2-Compliant flooring (carpet, artificial turf) 3-Ramps 4-Turning space 5-Size (width, length)
Heavy-Duty (K0006) and Extra-Heavy-Duty (K0007)	1	1	1, 2, 3	1	1
Powered Wheelchairs					
Scooter/ Power Operated Vehicle	1, 3	1	1, 2, 3	1	1, 2, 3
Group 1 Powered Wheelchair	1	1	1, 2, 3	1	1, 2, 3, 4, 5
Group 2 Powered Wheelchair	1, 3	2	1, 2, 3	3	1, 2, 3, 4, 5
Group 3 Powered Wheelchair	1, 3	2, 3	1, 2, 3	3	1, 2, 3, 4, 5
Group 4 Powered Wheelchair	1, 3, 5	2, 3, 4	1, 2, 3, 4, 5, 6	3	1, 2, 3, 4, 5

	Mobility Outdoors: 1-Americans with Disabilities Act (ADA) surfaces 2-Non-ADA pedestrian surfaces 3-Natural terrain	Reaching: 1-Provides floor level support 2-Provides chair-level support 3-Provides variable seat elevation above chair level 4-Provides standing	Carrying: 1-Unable to carry items without impacting mobility or function 2-Able to carry 10 lb without impacting mobility or function 3-Able to carry 25 lb without impacting mobility or function	Dexterous Movements: 1-Requires gross motor function 2-Requires fine motor function	Lifting: 1-Does not extend range of lifting 2-Extends range of lifting 6-12 inches 3-Extends range of lifting greater than 12 inches	Communication: 1-Does not support use of communication device; 2-Accommodates mechanical connection of communication device; 3-Provides mechanical and electronic (e.g., charging) connection of communication device
	1	2	1	1	1	1
	1, 2	2	2	1	1	2
	1	2	3	2	1	2
	1, 2	2, 3	3	2	2	2
	1, 2	2, 3	3	2	2	3
	1, 2, 3	1, 2, 3, 4	3	2	3	3

4

Upper-Extremity Prostheses

This chapter provides an overview of the various levels of amputation and congenital limb absence, their prevalence, and the types of prosthetic devices commercially available for each level. In addition, it reviews relevant clinical considerations pertaining to upper-extremity prostheses (UEPs), including their role in helping to mitigate the effects of impairments due to missing limbs. The evaluation and monitoring of individuals who need UEPs, the training and adaptation required to use such a device, and considerations of access and availability are addressed in turn. The chapter ends with findings and conclusions. Note that the discussion of prostheses and amputation, unless otherwise specified, applies to persons with congenital absence of a limb as well as to those with acquired amputation.

OVERVIEW OF CONDITIONS BENEFITING FROM UPPER-EXTREMITY PROSTHESES

Upper-extremity (upper-limb) amputations are defined by the level at which they occur (see Figure 4-1). Although congenital limb absence is properly defined with a slightly altered taxonomy, individuals are fit with prosthetic devices according to the corresponding amputation level regardless of whether the limb deficiency is congenital or acquired (Schuch and Pritham, 1994). The remaining part of the limb is often referred to as the "stump"; however, the more accepted term in the United States and the term used in this report is "residual limb."

Amputation of one limb is termed "unilateral amputation," while amputation of both the right and the left limb is termed "bilateral amputation."

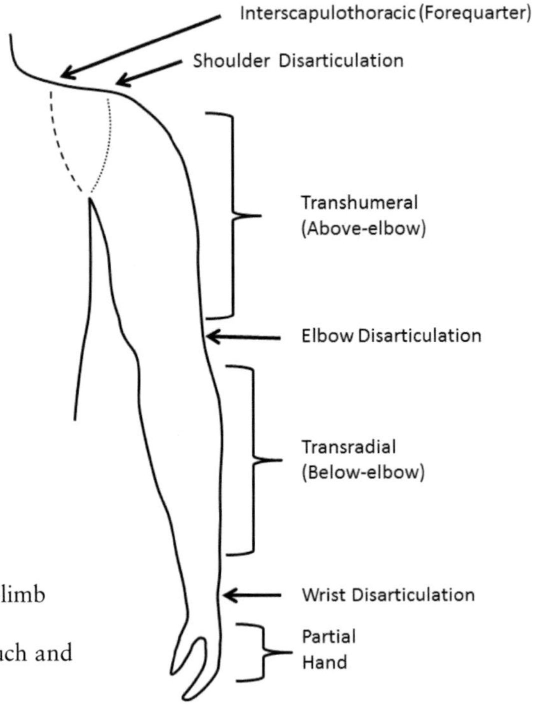

FIGURE 4-1 Levels of upper-limb amputation.
SOURCE: Adapted from Schuch and Pritham, 1994.

Given the added challenges in performing tasks with bilateral as opposed to unilateral amputations, prostheses used for bilateral amputations often have additional features. For example, wrist flexion units and a variety of components (e.g., two different hook styles) may increase the range of functional movement for people with these amputations and allow for improved performance of activities of daily living (Lehneis and Dickey, 1992; Uellendahl and Heckathorne, 1989).

A "transradial amputation" (or "below-elbow amputation") occurs through the long bones of the radius and ulna, while a "transhumeral amputation" (or "above-elbow amputation") occurs through the humerus. An amputation through a joint is called a "disarticulation." Therefore, an individual may have a wrist disarticulation amputation (between the carpals and radius and ulna), an elbow disarticulation (between the radius and ulna and humerus), or a shoulder disarticulation (between the humerus and scapula). Amputations proximal (closer to the center of the body) to the shoulder are termed "interscapulothoracic amputations" (sometimes called "forequarter amputations"). Partial hand amputations are amputations distal to the wrist joint, best described by the bones that are involved using the International Organization for Standardization terminology (ISO, n.d.): (phalangeal, metacarpo-phalangeal disarticulation, metacarpal, carpo-metacarpal disarticulation, and carpal).

In the United States in 2005, it is estimated that 41,000 people experienced upper-limb loss at levels at or above the wrist (Ziegler-Graham et al., 2008), with upper-limb amputations accounting for the majority of trauma-related amputations (68.6 percent) (Dillingham, 1998). According to data available for 2013, more than 10 times more lower- than upper-limb amputations were performed (O&P Almanac, 2016). During this year, 10,365 upper-limb amputations were performed. Of these, 5.2 percent occurred at the wrist disarticulation and transradial level, 6.1 percent were elbow disarticulation or transhumeral, and 2.3 percent were at the shoulder or higher. The majority (75.6 percent) were finger amputations (O&P Almanac, 2016). Similar percentages by level have been documented by the National Trauma Data Bank and by surveys of individuals with amputation (Inkellis et al., 2015).

The majority of all upper-limb amputations are the result of trauma (Raichle et al., 2008; Ziegler-Graham et al., 2008). Other common causes of upper-limb loss are vascular/infection, congenital absence, and cancer (Raichle et al., 2008). In general, the distribution across levels is the same for all causes, with the exception of cancer, which is more likely to result in a higher level of amputation (Dillingham, 1998). Partial hand amputations are the most common, accounting for 75 percent of all traumatic amputations (O&P Almanac, 2016). An estimated 500,000 people were affected by amputation of the hand or fingers in the United States in 2005 (Ziegler-Graham et al., 2008).

The function of the upper extremities is far more difficult to replace than that of the lower extremities. This is the case because the primary functions of the lower limbs are more limited and concern primarily maintenance and achievement of upright stance and various types of locomotion (e.g., walking, running, hopping, jumping, stair climbing). In contrast, the primary functions of the upper extremities include not only gross and fine motor activities but also more complex combinations of activities, such as self-care, interaction with the environment and others, and self-expression. An upper extremity is a high degree-of-freedom system, allowing for great mobility to move the hand into a range of positions around the body. The complexity of the human upper extremity is illustrated by the massive proportion of space within the motor and sensory areas of the brain (the motor and sensory homunculi) dedicated to the motor control and sensation of the hand and fingers. Thus, it is not surprising that persons with upper-limb amputation are generally less satisfied with the restoration of function provided by their prostheses relative to those with lower-limb amputation (Raichle et al., 2008).

TAXONOMY[1]

There are four main categories of prostheses, defined by the method used to control the device.

The most basic is the *passive prosthesis*. A passive prosthesis allows for no active movement of any of the joints. These are the lightest-weight devices because they contain no motors and few mechanical systems. Although these devices are often termed "cosmetic," they can provide function by assisting the intact hand/arm with bimanual tasks. For example, a passive prosthesis can be used to hold down papers when writing, to help carry items, or to stabilize objects held in the intact hand. They can also fill out and support clothing. Since they provide for no other controlled "function," however, these devices are not discussed in detail in the remainder of this chapter.

Next is the *body-powered prosthesis* (see Figure 4-2), so called because it is moved by the individual's remaining body. Typically, a harness with a strap that lies over the lower third of the scapula connects to a cable that operates the device. With biscapular abduction, the cable is pulled in the same way that pulling the handle on a bicycle break pulls on the cable that closes the brakes. The benefits of body-powered prostheses are that they are relatively lightweight and durable, can be made to be waterproof, and can provide feedback to the user based on the tension in the control cable. The disadvantages are that they require harnessing, and the user must have the strength and range of motion to pull the cable sufficiently to make the device work in all positions, particularly overhead.

Third is the *externally powered prosthesis* (see Figure 4-3). Whereas a body-powered system's power comes from the user's movements, an externally powered prosthesis is powered by batteries contained within the system. The device can be controlled with various inputs, including electromyographic (EMG) signals, force-sensing resistors, pull switches, and push switches (Esquenazi, 2015). Physical switches are a good complement to EMG signals for high-level amputees when multiple motors must be controlled or when the EMG signal is insufficient. Given that the most prevalent type of externally powered device is a myoelectric prosthesis, the following description focuses on those devices.

A typical myoelectric control scheme, direct control, uses EMG signals from two antagonist muscle contractions to operate two directions of movement. With a simple two-site direct control system, for example, wrist extensor EMG signals control opening of the hand, while wrist flexor EMG signals control closing of the hand. Thresholds are set for each muscle to

[1]The images in this section serve as examples of device categories only and should not be considered an endorsement of specific products or manufacturers.

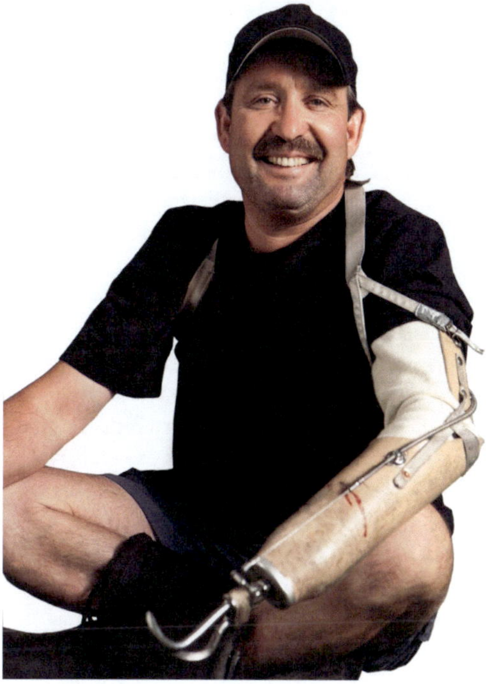

FIGURE 4-2 Body-powered prosthesis on a person with a transradial amputation. SOURCE: iStock.com/mikespics.

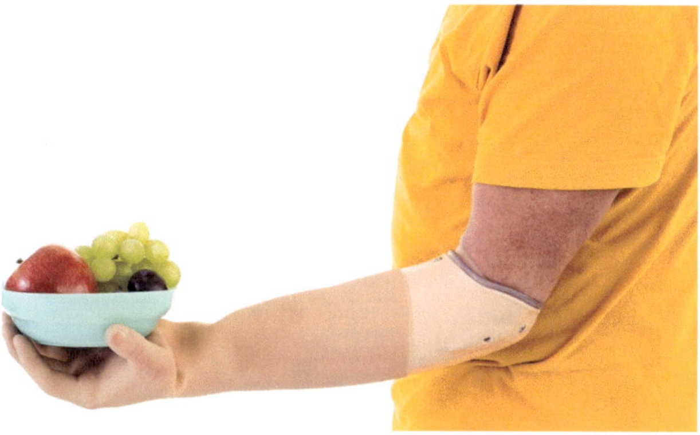

FIGURE 4-3 Myoelectric prosthesis on a person with a transradial amputation. SOURCE: iStock.com/Horsche.

allow some contraction without the occurrence of inadvertent movement. Most modern systems provide proportional control, in which the magnitude of the signal above the threshold is proportional to the speed of device movement and the generated grip force.

The benefits of myoelectric prostheses are that they typically use no harnessing or less harnessing than body-powered systems; they often can be operated in more planes of movement; the terminal devices (i.e., hands/hooks) can generate more force; and because there are no cables and straps on the outside of the device, they can appear more cosmetic. The disadvantages are that the batteries and motors make them heavier than body-powered systems; they can be water-resistant but not waterproof; they need to be charged daily; they require more maintenance than body-powered devices; and they are more expensive than those devices. Because of their complexity, they are also more prone to break and need repair (Biddiss and Chau, 2007b). In addition, myoelectric prostheses require that the electrode sensors that record signals from the muscles to control the device maintain contact with the skin. Thus, they require an intimate fit that may be uncomfortable or not tolerated by fragile skin or may be impeded or disrupted by scar tissue or excessive sweating. Contact with the electrodes also can be disrupted if the prosthesis is donned inappropriately or if changes occur in residual limb size or shape. Moreover, if more than two controlled motions (degrees of freedom) are available in the limb (e.g., elbow flexion and extension, as well as hand open and close), the same two antagonist muscles will be used for controlling each movement. In such cases, various strategies must be used to alternate control between the multiple movements in a sequential manner. The user must generate a trigger, such as co-contraction of both muscles or quick contraction of one muscle, to switch between the various movements, such as elbow and hand or various hand grip patterns. If the system is extremely complex (elbow, wrist rotation, various hand grasp patterns), the user may need to generate multiple types of triggers in a specific order to accomplish the various movements. Although there are many options for control with a trigger-controlled system, a user in a typical scenario would co-contract the wrist flexors and extensors to alternate control of wrist flexion between hand close and pronation or wrist extension between hand open and supination (Williams, 2004). When a multifunction hand is used, the various switching mechanisms, or triggers, such as co-contraction, impulse, and the like, can be used to alternate between the various hand grasps. These "Morse code" systems of control can be difficult to learn and cognitively burdensome to use.

A number of emerging technologies are being developed to overcome some of the above limitations of myoelectric prostheses. For grip selection there are devices that employ the use of gesture control by using imbedded accelerometers to switch grasp (Touch Bionics, n.d.-a). There are also passive radio frequency identification tags that can be placed in the environment, and when the device approaches these tags, it will automatically switch to the preconfigured grip needed in that location (Infinite Biomedical Technologies, n.d.; Touch Bionics, n.d.-b). With pattern recognition control, individuals do not use triggers to alternate the motors being controlled by the same two antagonist muscles (Chicoine et al., 2012; Englehart and Hudgins, 2003; Lock and Hargrove, 2014; Scheme and Englehart, 2011). Instead, numerous sensors are placed on the residual limb, and a microprocessor is "trained" to recognize the various patterns of movement, with the goal of making movements more intuitive and less mentally taxing (Deeny et al., 2014). For example, individuals with a transradial amputation can control wrist rotation and hand open/close by trying to contract the muscles in a way that feels more like they are performing those movements. Another emerging control option is inertial measurement unit (IMU) control, which will be available with the upcoming commercial release of the DEKA arm (anticipated in 2017) (see Figure 4-4) (Resnik et al., 2014b). With this technology, IMUs worn on the top of the shoes detect the speed and direction of foot movements, which can be programmed to control specific functions of the device, and the EMG sensors are implanted within the muscle tissue instead of being on the surface of the residential limb. Since a conventional myoelectric device requires that the sensors maintain contact with the skin in order to record accurate EMG signals to control

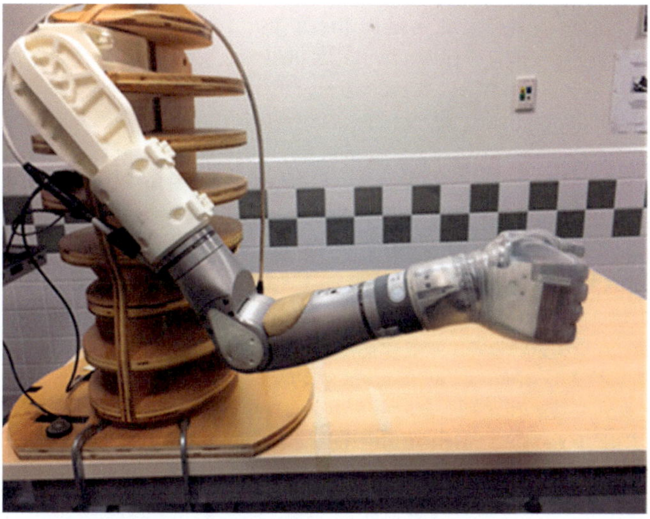

FIGURE 4-4 Transhumeral configuration of a DEKA arm.
SOURCE: Courtesy of the Providence VA Medical Center.

the device, a tight-fitting socket is necessary so that the sensors do not shift or pull away from the skin even as the user carries items, extends the arm in various planes, or perspires. Although not yet commercially available, methods such as IMUs worn on the feet (Resnik et al., 2014b) and EMG sensors implanted within the muscle tissue (Weir et al., 2003) avoid the use of surface EMG sensors and may allow a looser-fitting, and possibly more comfortable, socket fit.

The final category of devices is *hybrid prostheses*, which combine body-powered components and myoelectric/externally powered components in one device (see Figure 4-5). They are used for transhumeral and shoulder disarticulation prostheses and most commonly include a body-powered elbow and a myoelectric terminal device (hook or hand). This configuration allows both components to be operated simultaneously and provides the increased force of the powered hand for gripping, which is not required by the lightweight body-powered elbow. Annex Table 4-1 at the end of this chapter summarizes some of the features of body-powered, myoelectric, and hybrid prostheses for different levels of upper-limb amputation.

Prosthetic Components

For each missing joint, various options are available. For replacement shoulder function, there are only passive components, either friction or locking. Currently, no shoulder joints are commercially available that are motorized or body-powered; the same is true for replacement of humeral rotation. However, the commercial release of the DEKA arm will offer both powered shoulder movement and humeral rotation. At the elbow, there are motorized joints (myoelectric/externally powered) as well as body-powered joints. The motorized elbows have passive lift (how much can be carried) of approximately 50 pounds, which is comparable to body-powered elbows, although none of the motorized joints are able to flex actively with more than a few pounds held in the hand (Heckathorne, 1992). Available at the wrist are friction/locking and motorized wrist rotators; at this time, however, there are only friction/locking wrist flexion units.

Many varieties of terminal devices (hooks or hands) are available for both myoelectric and body-powered prostheses. There are body-powered hook options—called voluntary opening (VO) devices—in which pulling on the cable opens the device, and a spring or rubber bands cause it to close (see Figure 4-6). The hooks can be aluminum, titanium, or steel, depending on the durability needed, although the more durable ones are often heavier. One limitation of VO devices is that grip strength is limited by the rubber bands or springs used. To achieve a higher grip strength, the user must pull against this force every time the device is opened. Another variation is voluntary closing (VC) devices, in which pulling on the cable causes the

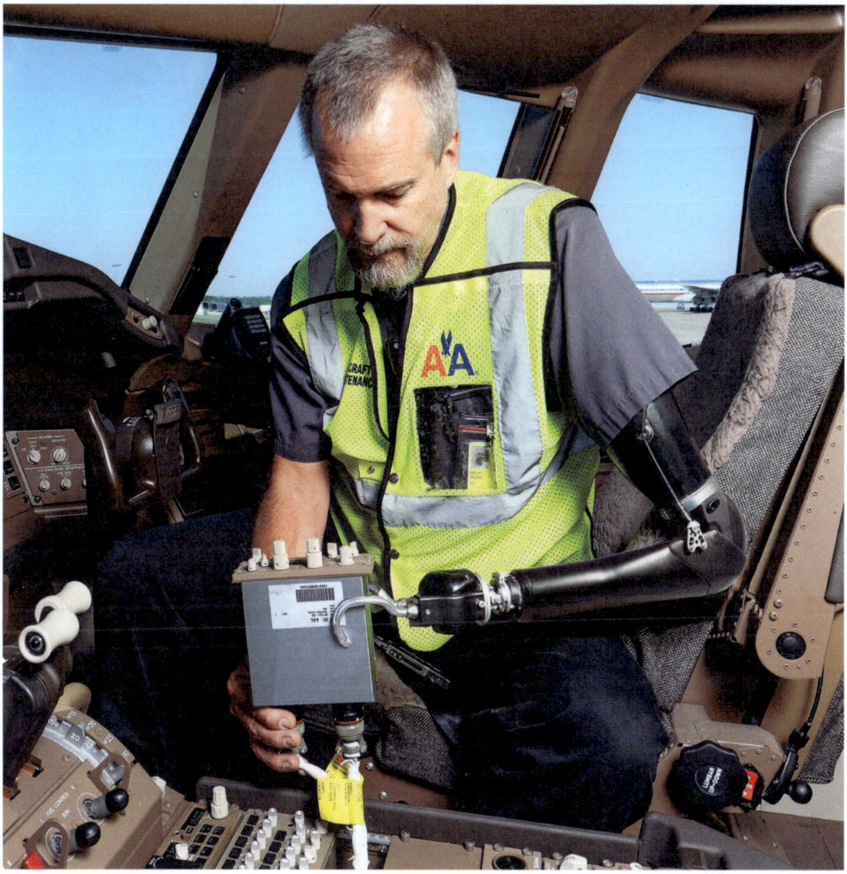

FIGURE 4-5 Example of a hybrid prosthesis.
SOURCE: Courtesy of Motion Control division of Fillauer.

device to close, and a lightweight spring causes it to open. The user can generate much higher grip forces with a VC than with a VO device, but unless using some kind of cleat or cable lock, must maintain tension on the harness to keep the device closed. The amount of force required varies across types of VC terminal devices (Smit and Plettenburg, 2010). Both VO and VC hands also exist. A body-powered prosthesis can be provided with a hook, a hand, or both to interchange in specific situations, most often for cosmesis or for use in social settings. Specialized work or recreation devices may also be interchanged on a body-powered system to maximize function during tasks when a traditional hook or hand device is not optimal (Texas Assistive Devices, 2016; TRS Prosthetics, 2016).

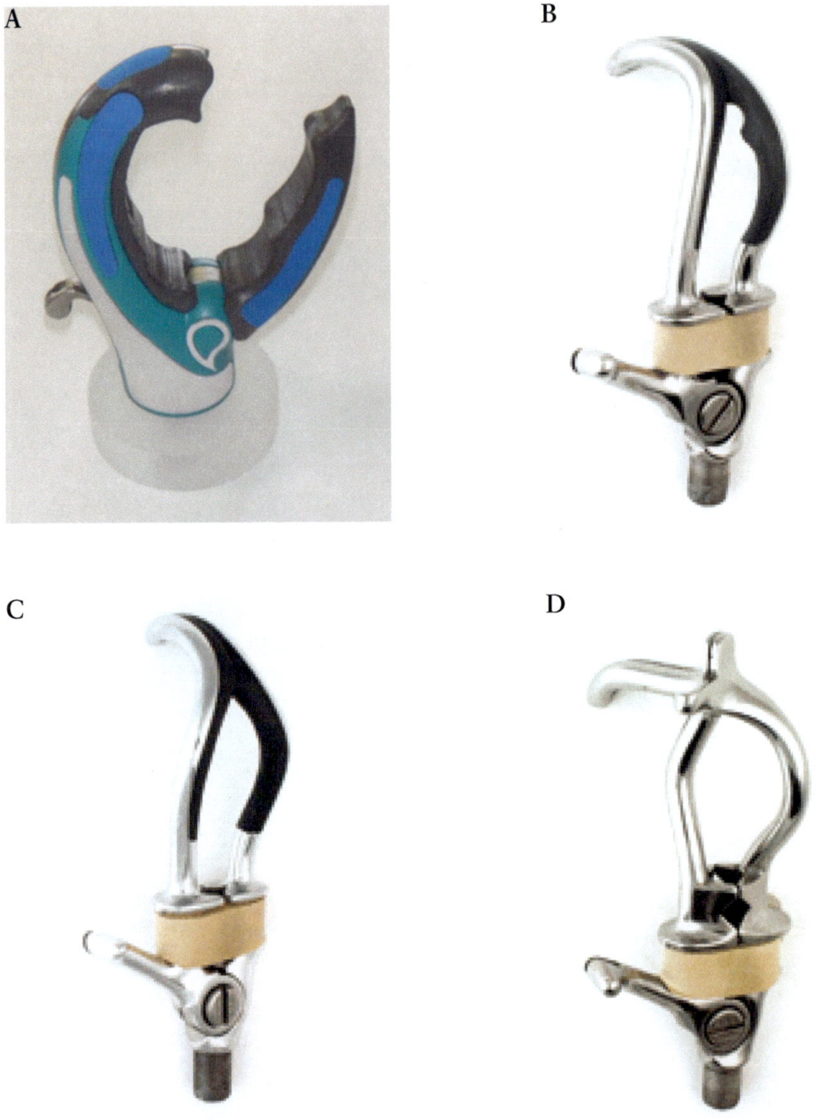

FIGURE 4-6 Examples of body-powered hooks.
NOTE: A. TRS GRIP 5, Voluntary Closing, Body-Powered Prehensor; B. Hosmer 5X Hook, canted-shape voluntary opening hook; C. Hosmer 555 Hook, lyre-shape voluntary opening; D. Hosmer 7 Work Hook, voluntary opening.
SOURCES: A. Courtesy of TRS Inc.; B-D. Photos for Hosmer Hooks provided by Fillauer LLC.

For body-powered systems, it is important that the individual have the range of motion and strength to operate the device. To fully open a standard VO hook, 2 inches of cable excursion is required. For a body-powered elbow, an additional 2.5 inches is required. To enable this full range of movement, the socket must fit well, and the harness must be properly fit to the user—a potentially time-consuming task. Proper fitting of the harness also often requires that it fit very tightly on the body, which can cause discomfort and lead to abandonment.

Motorized hooks and hands also are available (see Figures 4-7 and 4-8, respectively). They are much heavier (approximately 1-1.5 pounds) than the body-powered hooks (0.25-0.5 pound) and hands (0.75 pound) (Belter et al., 2013; Fillauer Companies, Inc., 2016; Hosmer, 2017; Steeper, 2016). The advantage of motorized hooks is that they are more durable than a motorized hand and can generate much more force than the frequently used VO hooks. Motorized hands can be divided into two categories: single-degree-of-freedom and multiarticulating. Single-degree-of-freedom hands have one motor and only open and close. They are the most durable type of myoelectric hand and can generate the most pinch force (Belter et al., 2013).

Multiarticulating hands have more than one motor to generate multiple grasp patterns (see Figure 4-9). The most complex have a motor in each digit. Because the motors are smaller, these hands cannot generate the same pinch force as a single-motor hand; by individually powering each digit, however, a more conforming grasp can be achieved.

A B

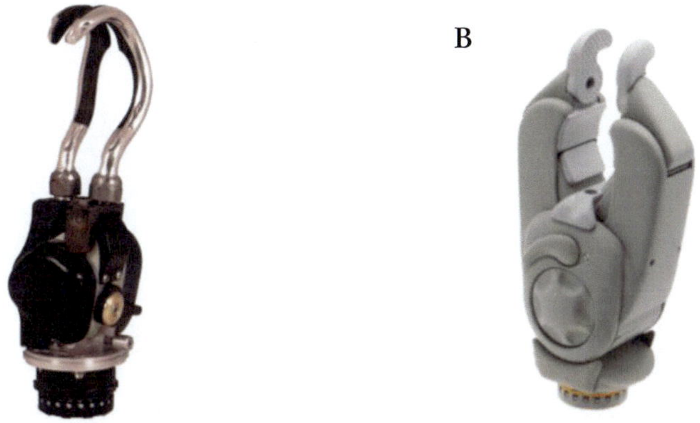

FIGURE 4-7 Examples of two powered hooks.
NOTE: A. Electronic Terminal Device (ETD) from Motion Control; B. Greifer from Ottobock.
SOURCES: A. Courtesy of Motion Control division of Fillauer; B. Courtesy of Ottobock.

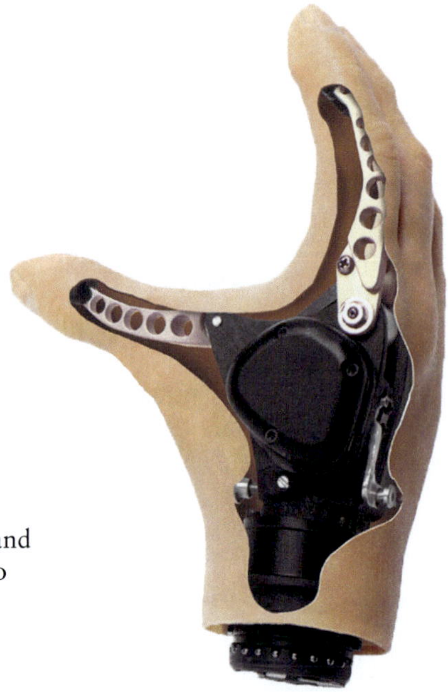

FIGURE 4-8 Single-degree-of-freedom hand showing cutout of glove and hand shell to display internal mechanism.
SOURCE: Courtesy of Motion Control division of Fillauer.

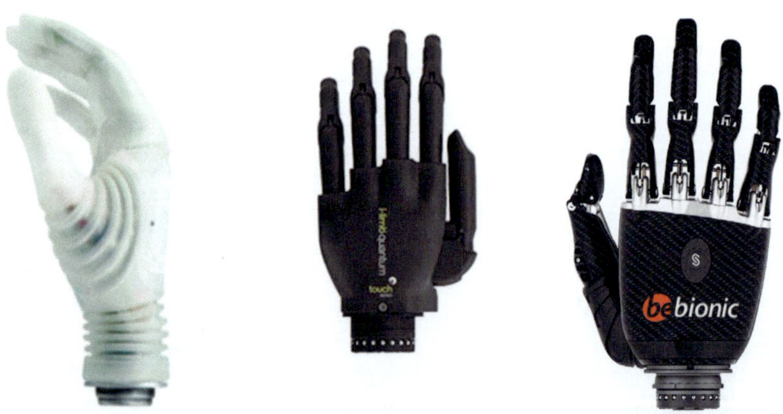

A B C

FIGURE 4-9 Examples of three multiarticular hands, all shown without a glove.
NOTE: A. Michelangelo hand; B. i-limb quantum XS; C. bebionic (small).
SOURCES: A. Ottobock, 2016a, courtesy of Ottobock; B. Courtesy of Touch Bionics by Össur; C. bebionic, courtesy of Steeper Group.

Prosthetic Sockets

Although component selection is important for prosthetic fitting, the aspect that most often impacts ultimate prosthesis use is the user interface, or socket. The socket is the framework that holds the device onto the remaining limb, and the comfort of the fitting, along with skin integrity, has a direct impact on acceptance of the device (Biddiss and Chau, 2007b,c; Schultz et al., 2007). During the initial fitting with a new device, an individual is typically fit first with a diagnostic or test socket. This type of socket often is made out of a clear material that allows the prosthetist to evaluate interface pressure and the presence of total contact and make adjustments as needed. Components often are connected to the check socket to confirm a comfortable and appropriate fit as the user operates the device in multiple planes. The check socket is then completed in the final materials, which may be of multiple types—for example, rigid laminations, flexible materials, and gel inserts. To improve socket comfort and therefore acceptance of the devices, prosthetists and engineers have continued to develop new materials, new socket designs, and designs that allow the user to customize the socket by tightening or loosening it for various functions and needs (Alley et al., 2011; Baschuk, 2016; Miguelez and Miguelez, 2003; Miguelez et al., 2016).

Obtaining a well-fitting socket can be challenging because the residual limb is often irregular in shape and density, with scarring, irregular soft tissue coverage, or the presence of bony projections. The prosthetic socket must optimize stability while controlling for movement such as slippage, translation, and rotation of the soft tissues and the socket itself (Resnik et al., 2014a). Even when the socket fits well, maintaining a consistent fit over time can be challenging because the shape and volume of the residual limb may change with changes in weight and fluid volume. Additionally, some people experience volume changes in their limb throughout the day, causing variability in socket fit and comfort even without long-term overall changes in body weight that may occur more slowly over time.

Osseointegration is an emerging surgical technique designed to bypass the impact of the socket on the success of the fitting. This technique, used clinically outside of the United States, was only recently approved by the U.S. Food and Drug Administration (FDA) for lower-limb applications (FDA, 2015) and has not yet been approved for upper-limb applications. The surgery entails connecting a metal rod to the remaining bone. The rod then protrudes through the skin (Aschoff et al., 2010; Branemark et al., 2001; Jönsson et al., 2011; Muderis et al., 2016; Palmquist et al., 2008; Pitkin, 2013), and the user can connect the prosthesis to the rod as desired. Although this technique does eliminate the need for a socket, challenges remain in interfacing with the residual limb to record EMG signals for a myoelectric prosthesis or to connect the control straps for a body-powered

BOX 4-1
Upper-Extremity Prostheses

Body-powered: The prosthesis is suspended from a harness that is fastened around the user's shoulder or upper torso. The user's upper-body movements control the utilization of the cable connections at the harness to the mechanical hand, hook, or elbow at the other end.

Myoelectric: The prosthesis is a battery-powered device activated by muscle electromyographic (EMG) signals in the residual limb. Signals are amplified and are applied to impulses needed to operate the hand, wrist, or elbow.

Hybrid: The prosthesis includes both electric and body-powered components, allowing the user to operate the elbow and hand simultaneously.

Terminal device: This is the distal portion of a prosthesis, often replacing hand function or appearance. Terminal devices provide the primary function of the ability to grip.

Prosthetic socket: The socket is the framework that holds the device onto the remaining limb. The comfort of the fitting has a direct impact on acceptance of the prosthesis by the user.

SOURCES: Biddiss and Chau, 2007b,c.

system. For myoelectric devices, research is ongoing to record EMG signals more directly through implanted myoelectric sensors (as discussed above) and through the osseointegration abutment (Ortiz-Catalan et al., 2012, 2014).

Box 4-1 provides a summary of definitions relevant to the taxonomy of UEPs.

CLINICAL CONSIDERATIONS

Mitigating the Effects of Impairment

Upper-limb amputation and limb deficiency are associated with self-reported disability and diminished functional performance (James et al., 2006; Lerman et al., 2005; Postema et al., 2012; Resnik et al., 2012; Tennent et al., 2014). These limitations and restrictions are greater with bilateral than with unilateral limb loss (Davidson, 2004). Disability also is typically greater with more proximal-level (transhumeral and shoulder-level) than with transradial-level amputation (Lerman et al., 2005; Resnik and Borgia, 2015), although people with partial hand amputation report greater disability than those with either transradial or transhumeral amputation (Davidson, 2004). Additionally, some evidence suggests that the impact on functional performance is greater for acquired than for congenital limb loss (James et al., 2006), although the evidence for this finding is mixed (Lerman et al., 2005).

Several small studies have found that persons with upper-limb amputation who use a prosthesis report less disability, as measured by the Disabilities of the Arm, Shoulder, and Hand (DASH) and QuickDASH questionnaires, relative to those who do not use such a device (Lifchez et al., 2005; Resnik and Borgia, 2015). However, as many as one-third of prosthesis users report that they do not find their device to be useful to them when performing daily activities or work functions (Datta et al., 2004). Prosthesis users report dissatisfaction with their ability to use their devices in such daily tasks as food preparation, eating, and self-care (Ritchie et al., 2011). And some research focused on pediatric congenital amputees has found no differences in functional performance between children who utilize a prosthesis and those who do not (James et al., 2006), suggesting that children adapt to limb deficiency at a young age and maximize function without the use of a prosthetic limb.

It is clear that currently available upper-limb prostheses cannot replace the complex functions of the missing upper limb because of limitations inherent in their control and design, their lack of sensory feedback, and the methods required to suspend them onto the residual limb. The human hand, wrist, elbow, and shoulder complex together comprises 32 bones, with dozens of movable joints and muscles, which together enable a wide field of active movement around the body, sometimes called the "functional envelope" (Harrtigan and Serrafin, 2004).

Although prosthesis use may in some instances partially mitigate the impact of upper-limb amputation on impairments in body functions and limitations in activity, the amount of mitigation provided by the prosthesis varies by the type of device used, as well as the level of amputation (see Annex Table 4-2) and, as discussed later in the chapter, of user training and ability. The findings in Annex Table 4-2 were determined through the consensus of committee members based on their expert knowledge, review of selected manufacturers' specifications, and review of the scientific literature. These findings are summarized below.

Body Image

The experience of acquired amputation is disruptive to one's body image and sense of self-esteem (Morris, 2008; Racey, 1992; Winchell, 1996). Body image includes physical, psychological, and social components. The upper extremities are an integral part of a person's self-identity, communication, and social interactions with others (Desteli et al., 2014), and acquired amputation, as well as congenital limb absence, can be associated with significant psychological distress, embarrassment, and shame due to perceived social stigma. Some persons with amputation may experience prejudice from others and a sense of injustice as a result of the visibility of their disability. For some people with limb loss, cosmetic restoration is highly valued, or even preferred over functional restoration, because of its mitigating effect on the disruption to body image. People with upper-limb loss in particular report high levels of distress about body image, and for them, the cosmetic aspects of the prosthesis are considered more important than is the case for people with lower-limb loss (Desteli et al., 2014). Thus, some people with limb loss may prefer terminal devices that resemble more closely the shape of the hand than a hook because they appear more like an unimpaired hand, and so may draw less attention to the prosthesis (Flannery and Faria, 1999; Hanson, 2003). Indeed, concerns about body image and the desire to improve cosmesis with prosthetic devices can result in rejection of prosthetic devices that may be more functional and may impact the choice of prosthetic devices, particularly for activities, such as work, that involve interaction with others (Morris, 2008; Racey, 1992; Winchell, 1996). Completely passive prostheses provide the best mitigation of cosmetic impairment. Cosmetic coverings can approximate the skin tone of the lost limb, and custom coverings may provide high-definition, cosmetic restoration that fully mirrors skin coloring, as well as anatomical details such as freckles or even hair of the lost limb. As discussed later in the chapter, however, access to such custom coverings varies because of limitations in reimbursement and the availability of providers who can make them.

Sensation

Research is under way on means of providing sensory function to prosthesis users (Carlsen et al., 2014; Chaubey et al., 2014; Cipriani et al., 2011, 2012; Clippinger et al., 1974; Hebert et al., 2014, 2016; Marasco et al., 2009; Nghiem et al., 2015; Rager et al., 2013; Schiefer et al., 2016; Schofield et al., 2014; Tabot et al., 2013; Tan et al., 2015; Tyler, 2015; Witteveen et al., 2014, 2015). Some existing devices have crude sensors for grip pressure or other features intended to provide the user with information on touch or object slip. However, all currently available devices fall short of restoring the sense of touch or proprioception of the missing appendage. Limited proprioception is available because users can feel the weight of the socket on the residual limb as the device is positioned in space and the muscular energy associated with the body movements required to pull the cable (for body-powered devices) or contraction of the musculature required to operate the myoelectric controls (for myoelectric devices). Loss of sensation makes control of grip force problematic, as prosthesis users cannot tell how hard they are gripping objects; thus, they are susceptible to dropping items because of too little or improper grip or to crushing fragile items by using a stronger grip than intended (Schiefer et al., 2016). To ensure that an object is held firmly, the user may be able to listen for the sound of the motors stalling or just hold a contraction after contacting an object so a large grip force is generated. For the most part, however, the user must rely on vision to modulate grip force and object placement (Sobuh et al., 2014), and so may avoid handling delicate, fragile, or slippery objects with the prosthesis. Lack of sensation also impairs the performance of fine motor activity.

Passive Range of Motion

No currently available upper-limb prosthesis can execute all of the passive movements of the human upper extremity. Although some advances have been achieved in improving the movements of multiarticulating prosthetic hands, even the most advanced of these devices, which may allow passive movement of the thumb or other digits, do not possess all of the passive range of motion of the human hand. The most commonly used terminal devices—body-powered and myoelectric hooks—have only a single degree of freedom, meaning that they can be moved only in two opposing directions—open and closed. Other myoelectric devices, such as the i-limb and Michelangelo hands, have a movable thumb and compliance in the digits that enable some degree of passive movement to conform to grasped objects.

Some existing prosthetic wrists allow passive wrist pronation and supination. However, prosthetic wrists lack full passive flexion/extension and radial/ulnar deviation, although there are some compliant wrists that allow a small amount of passive wrist movement in these directions. In contrast, most prosthetic elbows possess good passive flexion and extension movement, although some myoelectric elbows can be positioned only by motor action. Some shoulder-level prostheses have a fixed shoulder joint that does not move at all, while others can be manually positioned and then locked in a limited set of positions or held in place with friction.

Active Range of Motion

Active control of the movements of upper-limb prostheses is limited by both hardware constraints and currently available prosthetic control options. Even when passive range of motion is available (as described above), the user may not have active range of motion or control of that range. This may be because the device lacks the actuators and motors to move the joint. Some hand designs, for example, are under actuated, meaning that joints are linked together so they can be powered by a single motor or action. As another example, certain multiarticulating hands that have passive thumb movement require the user to position the thumb manually to change the thumb alignment. Further, no currently available devices allow active control over wrist flexion and extension or radial and ulnar deviation, humeral rotation, or powered shoulder movement in any direction.

Limitations in the active range of motion of any joint negatively impact the size of the functional envelope and are considered a contributing factor in the compensatory movements of the trunk observed in kinematic studies of upper-limb prosthesis users (Carey et al., 2008). This abnormal movement may, in turn, be associated with overreliance and overuse injuries of the sound side that have been reported (for people with unilateral amputation) and the more proximal joints and/or the neck and back (Burger and Vidmar, 2016; Østlie et al., 2011; Postema et al., 2012, 2016a).

The current standard for controlling prostheses is direct control, meaning that the user directly operates a specific control to activate a single intended movement, such as wrist extension to control hand opening (Phillips et al., 2013). In most cases, each intended prosthesis movement must be activated by the user in a sequential fashion, and it is difficult, if not impossible, to engage available powered movements simultaneously. Users of traditional two-site EMG myoelectric devices who may have powered elbow flexion/extension, wrist pronation/supination, and terminal device open/close cannot operate any of these movements simultaneously. Instead, they must use an alternate signal (frequently a muscular co-contraction) to switch control between joints (also termed switch modes). Another challenge for users of myoelectric prostheses is that active range of movement may not always function reliably. It is well known that myoelectric controls may function erratically if the surface electrode contact is disrupted. As discussed earlier, this can sometimes happen if the socket fit changes as a result of changes in residual limb volume or if the residuum becomes excessively sweaty.

Activities

Grasp, fine motor use, dexterous activities, and handling objects The human hand has more than 30 distinct grasp (grip) patterns (Cutosky, 1989), which are sometimes grouped into 6 or more major categories based on the shape of the grasping hand. Commercially available prostheses have between 1 and 14 (Ottobock, 2016b; Steeper, 2016; Touch Bionics, 2016). However, the most commonly used single-degree-of-freedom terminal device, the split hook, has a single grasp, although there are various styles of hooks. Grip strength and speed vary widely across these devices and type of grip (Belter et al., 2014; van der Niet et al., 2013).

Studies reporting the overall functionality of commercially available devices compared with limbs of intact subjects, as measured by the overall index-of-function score of the Southampton Hand Assessment Procedure (SHAP), show wide variation in mitigation of impairments of grasp. To date, no terminal device tested has been shown to restore function completely to all major grasp patterns. Body-powered terminal devices may be VO or VC, with some evidence that VC devices are associated with faster task performance as measured by the SHAP (Berning et al., 2014). SHAP index-of-function scores for several two-joint, single-degree-of-freedom terminal devices have been reported to be about 74 percent and 43-84 percent, respectively, compared with the functionality typical of an intact hand (Dalley et al., 2012; Luchetti et al., 2015; van der Niet et al., 2013).[2] The SHAP index-of-function scores for several commercially available multi-articulating hands have been reported in multiple studies: 52-76 percent for the i-limb Hand (Dalley et al., 2012; van der Niet et al., 2013), 87-88 percent for the i-limb Pulse (van der Niet et al., 2013), and 75-89 percent for the Michelangelo hand (Luchetti et al., 2015). Other research has found that myoelectric prosthesis users had average index-of-function scores of 43-50 percent compared with an intact hand (Bouwsema et al., 2012).

Few studies have directly compared the dexterity of myoelectric and body-powered terminal devices or multiarticulating and conventional myoelectric terminal devices. In one study, the functionality of a myoelectrically controlled single-degree-of-freedom terminal device was reported to be lower than that of a single-degree-of-freedom body-powered device as measured by the SHAP (Kyberd, 2011). Another study, comparing the performance of six transradial amputees using both a multiarticulating (Michelangelo) hand and a standard myoelectric hand, found better dexterity (box and blocks test and SHAP tests) using the multiarticulating hand (Luchetti et al., 2015).

---

[2]The index of functionality is the percent of function compared with an index hand as measured by the SHAP test.

Partial hand amputations range from single-digit amputations to those that involve multiple digits or part of the hand itself. Although single-digit amputations typically do not result in significant functional deficits, partial hand amputations that involve multiple digits and/or the thumb, compromising prehension force and sensation, can result in significant disability. Many people with partial hand amputations lose the opposition of digits necessary for an effective grasp, particularly if the amputation involves the thumb. Restoration of grasp to persons who have lost part but not all of their hand has been particularly challenging, with little research having been conducted in this area. A single study of 10 people with partial hand amputations showed that prosthesis use improved the strength of some but not all grips and also improved self-reported difficulty in the performance of specific activities (Lifchez et al., 2005).

Several studies have found substantially lower dexterity in users of upper-limb prostheses of all amputation levels compared with age-matched norms (Resnik and Borgia, 2012), as well as slower time to complete movements and activities (Bouwsema et al., 2010b; Cowley et al., 2016). Slower speeds are attributable, in part, to the fact that prosthesis users must perform more discrete submovements to perform basic tasks (Doeringer and Hogan, 1995; Fraser and Wing, 1981). In addition, grasping is uncoupled from reaching when one is using a prosthesis, which makes reaching for and grasping an object take longer (Blough et al., 2010; Bouwsema et al., 2012; Cowley et al., 2016).

Lifting, carrying, and reaching overhead Lifting and carrying objects with a prosthesis can be limited by the design restrictions of the prosthetic components, the method used to attach the prosthesis to the socket, or the socket and its suspension system. Lifting and carrying can be limited if the prosthesis hardware will not support the weight of the object, if the device detaches from the socket, or if the socket slips from the residuum. The functional envelope, or the space around the body in which the prosthesis can be used reliably, is often limited. Even when individuals with amputation have use of their own shoulder joint for reaching activities, they may be unable to use their prosthesis when reaching overhead because of the constraints of the harnessing that operates the cable. Users of myoelectric devices may also have difficulty operating their device in a full range of body positions because involuntary co-contraction of residual limb muscles that often occurs when stabilizing the limb against gravity can interfere with voluntary control of residual musculature.

Effects of Multiple Impairments on Impairment Mitigation

Acquired upper-limb amputations and congenital limb deficiencies are often associated with other impairments and comorbidities that affect overall function and can impact the use of prosthetic devices to mitigate impairment. The function of the upper extremities is complex and requires coordinated movements of multiple joints, visual feedback, sensation, and proprioception to accomplish even simple tasks.

Persons with amputation often have comorbid injuries, such as burns, nerve damage, or muscular loss, that interfere with the skin integrity, range of motion, strength, and/or sensation of the residual limb. Weakness of the proximal arm or trunk musculature and/or pain in the proximal joints, neck, or back can make it difficult to lift the weight of the prosthetic limb or to tolerate wearing a prosthesis for long periods. Thus, even those who wish to wear an upper-limb prosthesis may be unable to do so to the extent that they desire. Comorbid injuries and conditions that affect vision, cognitive ability, or the upper extremity/trunk proximal to the limb deficiency will make using a prosthesis more challenging and will limit the impairment mitigation effects of a prosthetic device. In addition, comorbid conditions that cause limb volume fluctuations, such as diabetes or renal or cardiovascular disease, can impact a person's ability to fit comfortably and consistently in a prosthetic device.

As noted earlier, beyond the physical conditions that often accompany upper-limb deficiency, the impact of limb loss or deficiency on body image, social role, and psychological health is substantial (Gallagher et al., 2007). In addition to the body image issues discussed above, it is estimated that at least 27 percent of people with limb loss experience symptoms of depression and that the risk for developing depression is greater for people with comorbid conditions (Desmond, 2007; McKechnie and John, 2014; Perkins et al., 2012). People with traumatic amputations are also at increased risk of developing posttraumatic stress disorder (PTSD), with prevalence rates estimated at 17-77 percent (Copuroglu et al., 2010; Tennent et al., 2014; Vincent et al., 2015).

In addition to psychological distress, upper-limb loss is frequently associated with chronic pain (Hanley et al., 2009; Kooijman et al., 2000). Several studies have found that people with upper-limb amputation report more postamputation pain relative to people with lower-limb amputation (Bosmans et al., 2010; Davidson et al., 2010). It is important to consider this high prevalence of postamputation pain, including phantom limb pain, when examining the use of prosthetic devices, as pain is a common reason why people with limb loss are not able to wear prosthetic devices successfully or restrict their use of the devices (Desmond et al., 2012).

Effects of User's Age on Prosthesis Use

Little is known about the association between age and use of upper-extremity prosthetic devices, particularly as children transition to adulthood and enter the workforce. A number of studies have examined factors that affect the use of prosthetic devices in children with either congenital limb deficiencies or acquired amputation. In general, these studies have found that young children with acquired amputation are more likely to become users of upper-extremity prosthetic devices if they begin using them at a younger age (Dabaghi-Richerand et al., 2015; Meurs et al., 2006). One study of 218 children aged 2-20 years in the Netherlands found that the majority preferred the use of unaffected parts of the body to accomplish tasks (>60 percent) over adaptive devices (<48 percent) and prostheses (<9 percent) (Vasluian et al., 2013). In this study, 27 percent of children reported having difficulties with work (the majority of these were children aged 13-20, and work for them was defined as any part-time, summer, or full-time job), yet none of these children reported using adaptive or prosthetic devices for their work. The children in this study who used both adaptive devices and prostheses reported higher satisfaction with the use of adaptive devices for specific activities compared with prosthetic devices because of the former devices' dimensions, weight, adjustability, and ease of use.

Another survey conducted in Sweden (Sjoberg et al., 2014) found that a majority of adults with congenital limb deficiencies (68 percent) used assistive devices, including prosthetic devices, but there were gender differences in the types of devices used: those using body-powered prostheses were exclusively men, and women were more likely to use cosmetic prostheses. Among those with upper-limb deficiencies, the vast majority were either working or in school (93/108); however, 24 percent of people reported that their self-assessed work capacity was reduced because of their upper-limb deficiency.

A qualitative focus group study of children and adolescents (aged 8-20 years) with unilateral transradial congenital limb deficiencies found that the limitations they experienced were typically environmental—related to attitudes or lack of accommodations—rather than being due to the limb deficiency itself (de Jong et al., 2012). Study participants transitioning to adulthood and thus more dependent on adults reported that they were more limited in their function relative to those who had already transitioned to independence. This finding suggests that the transition period itself is challenging for adolescents with limb deficiency, a phenomenon that has been recognized in other populations of people with disabilities (Donkervoort et al., 2009). This qualitative study also highlights that children and adolescents with upper-limb deficiency use many different and creative strategies to accomplish activities that do not necessarily rely on adaptive or prosthetic devices.

Prosthesis Use and Prognosis for Occupational/Educational Success

As noted earlier, congenital limb absence and acquired upper-limb amputation can significantly affect a person's ability to work. Although a number of studies have reported return-to-work rates of 50-75 percent following lower-limb amputation (Dajpratham et al., 2008; Fisher et al., 2003; Schoppen et al., 2001a,b), the committee found limited data, particularly from the United States, documenting work reintegration following acquired upper-limb amputation. Several studies specifically examining return to work after upper-limb amputation have found employment rates of approximately 57-85 percent; however, none of these studies were conducted in the United States (Datta et al., 2004; Fernandez et al., 2000; Jones and Davidson, 1995; Millstein et al., 1986; Postema et al., 2016b). One of the studies found that a majority of people who returned to work changed their employment because of limitations associated with their amputation (Datta et al., 2004). Another study, conducted in the Netherlands, found that individuals with amputation were employed at lower rates (57 percent for acquired amputation, 74 percent for congenital limb absence) than their age- and sex-matched peers (82 percent) but reported similar work productivity. This study also found that prosthesis use was a predictor of employment (Postema et al., 2016b). Other studies similarly found a positive association between prosthesis use and return to work following amputation (Fernandez et al., 2000; Millstein et al., 1985, 1986). The precise relationship between prosthesis use and return to work is unclear (Fernandez et al, 2000), although some have speculated that positive attitude and motivation may contribute to both (Millstein et al., 1985).

A study of people with partial hand amputation found that fewer than half were able to return to the same job, and most found prosthetic devices insufficient to meet the demands of their work, although cosmetic prostheses were important to their work success (Burger et al., 2007). While a limited sample, a recent survey of people with major limb amputation in Ireland found that 92 percent (n = 11/12) of those with upper-limb amputation experienced difficulty with employment or job seeking, even more so than people with lower-limb amputation (69 percent, n = 96) (Gallagher et al., 2011). Another European study found that 38 percent of people with upper-limb amputation required modifications to their job duties but that people with amputation reported job satisfaction similar to that of age- and gender-matched controls (van der Sluis et al., 2009). One small case series found that of 13 civilians with upper-limb amputation in the United States, 4 were able to return to work in any capacity, although none were able to return to their specific preinjury employment (Livingston et al., 1994). These findings are consistent with those of international studies, which found that upper-limb amputees typically returned to work in jobs that had fewer physical demands but required greater intellectual skills (e.g., clerical, service, managerial work) (Millstein et al., 1985). Similar findings also emerged from a study showing higher rates of return to work following upper-limb amputation in the building industry than in agriculture, presumably because agriculture offers fewer job opportunities compatible with a missing upper limb (Fernandez et al., 2000). Higher levels of employment for people with upper-limb amputation in more skilled jobs may explain the positive association found between postinjury employment and higher levels of education (Postema et al., 2016b), as well as receipt of vocational services (Millstein et al., 1985). Younger age at amputation and male sex also have been positively associated with return to work (Postema et al., 2016b).

In the United States, most of the studies examining the relationship between upper-extremity amputation and work duties were conducted in military populations. Although return-to-duty rates remain low for both upper- and lower-limb amputations, return to active duty is particularly challenging for people with upper-limb amputation (Belisle et al., 2013; Hurley et al., 2015). Roughly 75 percent of combat amputees from the global wars on terror were retired because of the amputation (Belisle et al., 2013). A recent study of all U.S. military amputations from 2001 to 2011 identified 153 people with upper-extremity loss (Tennent et al., 2014). In this population, no upper-extremity amputees were found to be fit for full duty, although 12 percent were allowed to continue on active duty (Tennent et al., 2014). Earlier studies had found higher return-to-duty rates for upper-limb amputees (17-22 percent), only slightly lower than the rates for lower-limb amputees (18-25 percent) (Stinner et al., 2010). Although military amputees are a unique population, and these findings may not be applicable to the general civilian population with upper-extremity amputation, they highlight the difficulties associated with return to work following upper-extremity loss. Further, upper-extremity amputees were more likely than lower-extremity amputees to experience PTSD and comorbid nerve injuries that impacted function (Tennent et al., 2014).

There are many reasons why employment may be difficult after upper-limb amputation, including limited ability to perform tasks repetitively (either with or without a prosthesis). One study found that bilateral amputees were less successful in returning to work relative to unilateral amputees (Millstein et al., 1985). Associated musculoskeletal complaints, including overuse injuries of the remaining limb, and pain also are negatively associated with return to work (Millstein et al, 1985; Postema et al., 2016b), and the impact of limb loss on psychological health, body image, and social role may negatively affect return to work as well (Saradjian et al., 2008). Depending on the type of work, each of these issues may impact one's ability to perform repetitive tasks involving the upper extremities and consequently, the quality of work and work productivity (Postema et al., 2016b). In addition, professions in which interactions with the public or social interactions are integral to job function may be more challenging for people who experience perceived social stigma or public self-consciousness due to their upper-limb loss (Saradjian et al., 2008).

Employment has been associated with decreased rejection rates of upper-limb prosthetics (Postema et al., 2016b), although this association depends in part on the level of amputation. Studies suggest greater employment among individuals with transradial relative to transhumeral amputations (Fernandez et al., 2000; Millstein et al., 1985), presumably because retention of one's elbow helps with carrying out work-related tasks (Fernandez et al., 2000). Some studies suggest that people with more proximal amputations use prostheses primarily for cosmesis while at work, whereas people with transradial amputations use prostheses for functional activities, and people with partial hand amputations more frequently choose not to use such devices at all (Burger et al., 2007; Postema et al., 2016b).

In summary, although research in the United States is lacking, international studies suggest that male sex, younger age, medium or high level of education, prosthesis use, good general health (fewer comorbidities), and positive attitude are predictors of work participation among upper-limb amputees (Fernandez et al., 2000; Millstein et al., 1985; 1986; Postema et al., 2016b; Raichle et al., 2008). Importantly, issues of prosthesis reliability and the need for repair also impact device use in the work environment and may contribute to work interruptions.

Prosthesis Wear-Time

Few statistics on prosthesis wear-time are available. Unlike a lower-limb prosthesis that is often required for ambulation, an upper-limb prosthesis can be donned and used when necessary, either for a small portion of the day or for the entire day. However, a few studies do report on the number of individuals studied who use an upper-limb prosthesis daily. An Israeli study of 42 people with upper-limb amputation fit with a combination of body-powered, myoelectric, and passive devices found that 21 (50 percent) used the prosthesis daily, 9 (21.43 percent) used it intermittently, and 12 (28.57 percent) did not use it at all (Dudkiewicz et al., 2004). Millstein and colleagues (1986) found higher daily usage results: 89 percent of below-elbow amputees, 76 percent of above-elbow amputees, and only 60 percent of higher-level amputees. Raichle and colleagues (2008) surveyed 107 people with upper-limb amputation and found that having a proximal amputation was related to greater use in terms of hours per day, while having a distal amputation was associated with greater use in terms of days per month.

Prosthesis Acceptance and Rejection

In addition to issues of comfort and body image discussed earlier, the prevalence of prosthesis use is associated with the level of amputation, loss of the dominant versus nondominant hand, bilateral versus unilateral amputation, and time since amputation. The term *rejection* is used in this chapter because it encompasses but is broader than *abandonment*. In some cases, amputees reject use of a certain type of prosthesis from the start, which is different from abandonment of a device later. Primary rejection rates (rejecting any use of a prosthesis) appear to be related to the level of amputation, age at the time of amputation, gender, and discrepancies between perceived needs and the availability of prosthetic devices that will meet those needs (Burger and Marinček, 1994; Dougherty et al., 2010; McFarland et al., 2010; Østlie et al., 2012a). Additionally, a large proportion of people who use upper-limb prostheses use a combination of devices (body-powered, myoelectric, and cosmetic), depending on their activities and goals (Crandall and Tomhave, 2002). And as noted earlier, even when functional devices are provided, many individuals may still choose to wear a device only for cosmetic purposes (Burger and Marinček, 1994).

Amputation Level

Rates of rejection of prosthesis use for people with upper-limb amputation range from 30 to 80 percent, with the rates typically being lowest for those with transradial amputations (Tintle et al., 2010; Wright et al., 1995) and highest for those with transhumeral or shoulder-level amputations as well as partial hand amputations (Burger and Marinček, 1994; Kruger and Fishman, 1993; Østlie et al., 2012a; Silcox et al., 1993). Research by Biddiss and Chau (2007a,b) supports the finding that individuals with a more proximal level of amputation compared with those with a more distal level of amputation are more likely to reject use of a prosthetic device. Rejection of prosthesis use in people with shoulder- or transhumeral-level amputations likely reflects the increased weight of the device, increased energy expenditure necessary to control the device, and more limited ability to improve function compared with prosthetic devices for transradial-level amputations (Østlie et al., 2012a). Higher rejection rates in people with partial hand amputations likely reflect the limited ability of partial hand prostheses to restore grasp ability adequately or to improve function compared with use of the limb without a device (Burger and Marinček, 1994; Burger et al., 2007).

Loss of Dominant Versus Nondominant Hand and Bilateral Versus Unilateral Amputation

Findings are mixed with respect to loss of the dominant or nondominant hand. Some studies have found increased wear-time when the dominant hand has been amputated (Burger and Marinček, 1994; Dudkiewicz et al., 2004; Hacking et al., 1997), while others have found little correlation been loss of the dominant hand and prosthetic use (Gaine et al., 1997).

The most thorough report of bilateral usage is a survey of 242 individuals, 15 percent of whom had bilateral amputations. Overall, those with unilateral and bilateral acquired amputation had similar rejection rates. However, those with congenital bilateral limb absence had significantly higher rejection rates (75 percent) than those with congenital unilateral absence (28 percent) ($p = 0.004$) (Biddiss and Chau, 2007a).

Time Since Amputation

Multiple studies have found that early prosthetic fitting and rehabilitation positively impacted prosthesis success (Biddiss and Chau, 2007b, 2008; Gaine et al., 1997; Kejlaa, 1993; Malone et al., 1984; Roeschlein and Domholdt, 1989). And in a clinical review of 23 cases involving traumatic amputation, none who were fit after 12 weeks returned to gainful employment (Gaine et al., 1997).

Age

Some studies have found that age is not a factor in prosthesis success (Burger and Marinček, 1994; Hacking et al., 1997; Roeschlein and Domholdt, 1989; Wright et al., 1995). Conversely, others have found an increased risk of rejection among the elderly (Biddiss and Chau, 2007a,b; Østlie et al., 2012a) and at certain life stages (adolescence and early adulthood) (Biddiss and Chau, 2007a).

Gender

Surveys generally have found an association between increased prosthesis rejection rates and gender, with women more likely to reject the devices (Kyberd and Hill, 2011; Østlie et al., 2012a), although other research has not found this relationship (Raichle et al., 2008). Secondary rejection of prosthetic devices (rejection after trial use) is associated with female gender and proximal upper-extremity amputation.

Level of Education

Level of education has not been associated with prosthesis use among individuals with upper-limb amputation (Raichle et al., 2008).

Perceived Needs

Individuals who wear their prostheses generally express satisfaction with their devices, while those who reject their devices express dissatisfaction (Biddiss et al., 2007). Addressing user desires therefore has the potential to reduce rejection rates. The most important aspects of prosthetic design that users consistently desire are comfort and reduced weight (Atkins et al., 1996; Biddiss and Chau, 2007c; Biddiss et al., 2007; Kyberd and Hill, 2011). Yet, while most users desire a device that is lighter-weight, that desire often is in conflict with the desire for more function (see the discussion of device taxonomy earlier in this chapter).

Various surveys of prosthesis users reveal similar user desires but no single design factor that would address the functional needs of all users (Kyberd and Hill, 2011). In general, body-powered prosthesis users desire additional wrist movement and better control mechanisms, as well as better cables and harness comfort (Atkins et al., 1996). Users of myoelectric devices desire components that have additional degrees of freedom (e.g., powered wrist movement, additional grips) and that are more durable, quieter, lighter-weight, and more cosmetic, with an improved control system and longer-lasting batteries (Atkins et al., 1996; Kyberd and Hill, 2011). Users also identify glove durability, improved sensory feedback, and increased dexterity as design priorities for myoelectric devices (Biddiss et al., 2007).

Overall, given the advantages and disadvantages of the various prosthetic devices, trade-offs are entailed in the prescription and fitting of the devices. Therefore, a key component of acceptance of a prosthetic device will be careful consideration of the individual's needs and goals and whether the device meets the expectations of the user (Burger and Marinček, 1994; Østlie et al., 2012a).

EVALUATION AND MONITORING

The need for a multidisciplinary team approach is acknowledged in the first evidence-based clinical practice guidelines for the rehabilitation of persons with upper-limb amputation, released in 2014 (Management of Upper Extremity Amputation Rehabilitation Working Group, 2014). Nonetheless, there are still no clear universally accepted guidelines for prosthesis prescription or prosthetic training. Given the myriad factors that influence the type of device prescribed and the type and amount of prosthetic training received, a comprehensive clinical assessment by a trained (multidisciplinary) clinical team (including physician(s), occupational and physical therapists, experts in prosthetics and orthotics) can help in assessing the appropriateness and readiness for use of an upper-limb prosthesis, and it can guide the prescription of an appropriate device or (devices) and a training program to meet an individual's needs. It is important to remember that the team centers around the individual, his or her capacity and needs. Therefore, this comprehensive assessment, performed in the outpatient setting during the preprosthetic phase, ideally will incorporate the following components that can impact prosthesis use and outcomes: current health status, current function and future functional goals and preferences, pain, social and cultural context, residual limb assessment, contralateral limb and trunk assessment, neurologic assessment, behavioral and cognitive assessment, lifestyle and occupational demands, and insurance status. Such an assessment, however, is frequently not available (Management of Upper Extremity Amputation Rehabilitation Working Group, 2014).

Lifelong Care

A person with an upper-limb amputation requires lifelong care, including at least annual rechecks with the clinical team to ensure both that his or her needs are being met by the rehabilitation process and the device and that functional abilities have been optimized (Management of Upper Extremity Amputation Rehabilitation Working Group, 2014). That said, there are no data on the prevalence of this practice pattern, and it is not clear that persons with amputation have access to regular annual amputation care. Studies on the frequency of upper-limb prosthetic replacements suggest that persons with upper-limb amputation receive a replacement device every 1 to 5 years (Blough et al., 2010; Dudkiewicz et al., 2004; Etter et al., 2014). A single study showed that provision of a new prosthesis was associated with an immediate decline in function (likely due to the acclimation required to become familiar with a new device), which could be remedied by prosthetic training (Dromerick et al., 2008). Indeed, it is widely recognized that prosthetic training needs to occur whenever a person with amputation, even an experienced prosthesis user, receives a new type of device (Management of Upper Extremity Amputation Rehabilitation Working Group, 2014). However, experienced prosthesis users may require fewer training sessions than inexperienced users to learn to use a new type of device (Management of Upper Extremity Amputation Rehabilitation Working Group, 2014).

Considerations for Prescription of Body-Powered and Myoelectric Devices

A recent systematic review of the literature (Carey et al., 2015) found that evidence was insufficient to determine the functional superiority of myoelectric versus body-powered prostheses. Each type of device has its merits and drawbacks. Body-powered devices are generally more robust and reliable, can be used in wet or dirty environments, and may require shorter training periods. In contrast, research suggests that myoelectric devices provide better cosmesis, improve phantom-limb pain, and are more accepted for light-intensity work (Carey et al., 2015). However, myoelectric devices require more training to use, are more prone to breakage, may become unreliable in hot and humid environments and in cases of weight fluctuation, and cannot be used in a wet environment. In a long-term follow-up study of pediatric patients fit at one center, a majority of the patients were provided with both myoelectric and body-powered devices, as well as a passive cosmetic prosthesis. A passive cosmetic hand was the prosthesis of choice for 44 percent of the individuals, and only 15 percent chose the myoelectric device (Crandall and Tomhave, 2002). In this study, 41 percent of those who used a prosthesis used multiple types of devices on a daily basis. Likewise, a survey of 50 service members from the Operation Enduring Freedom/Operation Iraqi Freedom era with unilateral upper-limb amputation, all of whom were provided with three types of devices (passive, body-powered, and myoelectric) within 1 year of their amputation, found that many used more than one type of device (McFarland et al., 2010).

TRAINING AND ADAPTATION

Therapy services and a team approach to amputation care are necessary throughout all phases of prosthetic rehabilitation (Atkins, 2004; Bowers, 2004; MaGuire, 2008; Management of Upper Extremity Amputation Rehabilitation Working Group, 2014; Resnik et al., 2012). Prosthetic training can improve skill in prosthesis use and help those with upper-limb amputation make better functional use of their prostheses (Atkins, 2004; Management of Upper Extremity Amputation Rehabilitation Working Group, 2014; Silcox et al., 1993). Multiple studies have found an association between long-term prosthetic use and receipt of prosthetic training (Biddiss and Chau, 2007a; Davids et al., 2006; Egermann et al., 2009), in particular, individualized and "sufficient" prosthetic training (Østlie et al., 2012a,b). In contrast, other studies have found that the quality or amount of prosthetic training was not strongly associated with prosthesis use (Biddiss and Chau, 2007b; Burger and Marinček, 1994; Hacking et al., 1997; Silcox et al., 1993). This finding is consistent with that of prior research showing that lack of technical skill in using a myoelectric prosthesis in and of itself is not predictive of prosthesis rejection (Herberts et al., 1980). It is likely that other factors, such as the comfort and fit of the device, are more influential than skill in use in determining device adoption.

The source of most evidence on the recommended type and amount of training in use of upper-limb prostheses is expert opinion (Management of Upper Extremity Amputation Rehabilitation Working Group, 2014), with training protocols being published largely in seminal textbooks (Atkins, 2004; Dillingham, 1998) and a handful of peer-reviewed papers (Johnson and Mansfield, 2014; Smurr et al., 2008) and available through prosthetic device manufacturers. Several recent papers focus on training for new special segments of the population, including those who have undergone targeted muscle reinnervation (Stubblefield et al., 2009), those using EMG pattern recognition control (Powell and Thakor, 2013; Powell et al., 2014; Scheme and Englehart, 2011; Simon et al., 2012), and those using the newly FDA-approved DEKA arm (Resnik et al., 2014b). Although training in prosthesis use is widely recognized as a key component of amputation rehabilitation, the relative value of intensive training or of specific training protocols for users of body-powered or myoelectric devices has not been well established (Davids et al., 2006).

The recently published comprehensive evidence-based clinical care guidelines for amputation rehabilitation (Management of Upper Extremity Amputation Rehabilitation Working Group, 2014) describe four phases of rehabilitation for the upper-limb amputee: perioperative care, preprosthetic training, prosthetic training, and lifelong care (Management of Upper Extremity Amputation Rehabilitation Working Group, 2014). Lifelong care was discussed above; the following sections focus on two other phases that are particularly pertinent to this report—preprosthetic and prosthetic training.

Preprosthetic Training

The preprosthetic training phase begins after acute wound healing, but it may begin even prior to amputation, once the decision to amputate has been made. This phase focuses on the skills needed to be independent in basic self-care activities, without a prosthesis. One-handed skills training also includes techniques to minimize overuse injuries of the intact limb and to prevent changes in posture that may occur as a result of upper-limb loss. If the dominant hand has been lost, training to alter hand dominance, including handwriting training, may also occur, since the prosthesis will only act as an assist. Additionally, preprosthetic training typically involves training in care of the residual limb (e.g., hygiene, shaping, desensitization, scar management) and development of an exercise program to maintain normal range of movement and to increase muscle strength that may be needed for operation of a prosthesis. If myoelectric controls are anticipated, myosite training may begin in this phase.

Prosthetic Training

The average amount of time needed to train patients with upper-limb amputation varies by level of amputation, type of device, and such other factors as the presence of comorbid conditions. The optimal frequency of training visits, the intensity and duration of training, and the time needed to acclimate fully to a new prosthesis have not been studied. Some have suggested that persons with transradial amputation require, on average, 3-5 weeks of training (Dakpa and Heger, 1997); others have suggested that 5 hours of training is sufficient for people with transradial amputation, 10 hours for those with transhumeral amputation, and 12-20 hours for those with bilateral amputation (Atkins, 2004); and still others have suggested that gaining proficiency can require from a few days to several months (Johnson and Mansfield, 2014). Although the committee suspects that skills in prosthesis use may improve over time, with greater experience, no studies evaluating the length of time required to become a fully proficient, "expert" prosthesis user could be found. Although some detailed protocols are available in the professional and scientific literature (Atkins, 2004; Resnik et al., 2014c; Smurr et al., 2008), few studies have examined the effectiveness of specific approaches to prosthetic training. Given the small numbers of upper-limb amputees, most of these studies were conducted with able-bodied participants instead (Bouwsema et al., 2008, 2010a, 2014; Clingman and Pidcoe, 2014; Lake, 1997). One such study demonstrated that those with 8 hours of training on a prosthesis simulator had better performance than those who were not trained (Lake, 1997).

The current evidence-based guidelines state that prosthetic training should include the following components: education, controls training, and functional training (Management of Upper Extremity Amputation Rehabilitation Working Group, 2014). Education includes instruction in putting on and taking off the prosthesis, caring for the residual limb, caring for and understanding the components of the prosthesis, and safely using the device. Generally speaking, most people require an adjustment period to acclimate to wearing a prosthesis and to learn to use it before they can wear the device full-time or for extended periods. Users need to acclimate to wearing a prosthesis through a graduated wear schedule (Management of Upper Extremity Amputation Rehabilitation Working Group, 2014), and the fit and function of the device must be reassessed periodically during prosthetic training. Prosthetic fit (i.e., the socket and harnessing) may need to be modified by the prosthetist to address such issues as pain in the residuum, skin breakdown, or changes in socket fit and comfort.

Controls training teaches the patient how to operate each aspect of the prosthesis while avoiding unnecessary compensatory movements and using good body mechanics. Users of body-powered devices must learn the movements needed to operate the harness and to position any movable joints (e.g., wrist rotators, elbow) manually, while users of myoelectric devices must learn to isolate and control specific muscles and, in some instances, switch between modes of control. Several studies of able-bodied subjects have examined the content of prosthetic controls training and found that use of a myoelectric trainer improved myoelectric signal control (Clingman and Pidcoe, 2014). However, a recent study of able-bodied subjects found no differences in skill acquisition among three approaches to myoelectric controls training: use of a prosthesis simulator, a virtual prosthesis on a computer screen, or an isolated prosthetic hand (Bouwsema et al., 2010a). Nevertheless, use of a virtual trainer has become a widely accepted method of myoelectric controls training (Johnson and Mansfield, 2014).

Controls training typically includes repetitive drills to enable the user to practice specific prosthesis actions and commonly used movements, such as grasp and release of objects. Preliminary evidence gathered on able-bodied subjects suggests that the structure of the training approach (blocked practice versus random practice of skills) does not impact the rate of acquisition of prosthetic skills (Bouwsema et al., 2008). A study of four approaches to grasp training for users of myoelectric prostheses recommends that training programs begin with indirect grasping tasks but ultimately emphasize fine motor tasks (Bouwsema et al., 2014).

Functional skills training is designed to help individuals integrate use of their prostheses into their everyday tasks and to teach them strategies for maximizing their functional abilities. Because most prostheses lack movable wrists and have limited grasp positions, functional training often focuses on teaching prepositioning of the device in a functional position prior to utilization. Functional training typically progresses from using the prosthesis in unilateral activities to engaging it during bimanual activities. Ultimately, training should advance to engagement in community activities to increase the user's confidence in utilizing the device in public and in real-world situations (Johnson and Mansfield, 2014).

ACCESS AND AVAILABILITY

Access to and Availability of Devices

Data are scarce on the prevalence of use or incidence of prescription of upper-limb prostheses across the United States, largely because no single nationally representative source of data contains this information. Thus, most studies on the prevalence of use of these devices, as well as the rates of prosthetic prescription and repair, have used self-report surveys. Results of such surveys suggest that persons with major upper-limb amputation receive a new device every 1-5 years (Blough et al., 2010; MacKenzie et al., 2007).

A recent, large study on prosthesis prescription patterns in the Veterans Health Administration (VHA) used 10 years of data from the VHA's National Prosthetic Patient Database to calculate annual prescription and repair rates by level of amputation and type of device (Etter et al., 2014). The rate of prescription of upper-limb prostheses was 0.20/year for persons with shoulder-level amputation, 0.27/year for those with transhumeral amputation, and 0.26/year for those with transradial amputation (Etter et al., 2014). These data suggest that overall, veterans with major upper-limb amputation received a new prosthesis once every 3.6 years. The prescription rate for myoelectric devices, however, was 0.38/year compared with 0.23/year for body-powered devices, indicating that the former devices were being prescribed or replaced more frequently than the latter. Repair rates varied by level of amputation, with the least frequent repairs provided for persons with shoulder-level amputation (0.02/year) and more frequent repairs for those with transhumeral and transradial amputations (0.26/year and 0.21/year, respectively). Furthermore, compared with veterans over age 65, those under age 65 had higher incidence rates of both prescription of new devices and repair of existing devices. The results of this study are limited to the prescription and repair patterns within the VHA and likely are not generalizable beyond that system of care.

It should be noted that issues with the reliability of a prosthesis may impact vocational use. Particularly with myoelectric devices, which need more frequent repairs/replacement, not having a back-up device can be a barrier to successful participation at work.

As described in Appendix C and Chapter 3, the committee examined data for a 5 percent random sample of beneficiaries from the Medicare Durable Medical Equipment (DME) files for the years 2013-2014 to gain information on the frequency with which UEPs were prescribed within the 20- to 67-year-old population of beneficiaries. Although the population represented in the Medicare data is not necessarily representative of the overall population using UEPs, these data were available to the committee. The 5 percent sample is commonly used in research as the 100 percent dataset is so large that its use for research purposes is not feasible. Because of the underrepresentation of the 20- to 67-year-old cohort in Medicare claims data and the relatively low frequency of UEP claims, the 5 percent sample yielded a small study sample, which limited the presentation of granular information based on individual-level characteristics. Use of a 20 percent random sample and/or more years of data would improve future analyses. The Medicare DME data were linked to data from the Master Beneficiary files to obtain information on the demographic and clinical characteristics of device recipients. (See Appendix C for a detailed description of methods.) The committee identified all upper-limb prostheses provided by Medicare to persons aged 20-67 and then categorized the types of devices provided, as well as the characteristics of device recipients. Given the small sample size (fewer than 150 persons) and the Centers for Medicare & Medicaid Services' (CMS's) restrictions on reporting values for categories of 20 or fewer persons, the analyses reported here show proportions rather than absolute values.

Of the prosthetic components and devices provided to the 5 percent random sample of Medicare beneficiaries aged 20 to 67 in 2013, 43 percent were classified as body-powered, 27.6 percent as myoelectric, and the remainder as other (see Table 4-1). Table 4-2 shows the demographic characteristics of those Medicare recipients who received a device, including age, sex, and race/ethnicity. Most recipients were under age 65, suggesting that these were individuals with long-term disability. The majority of recipients were male (58.2 percent) and white (68.4 percent). Table 4-3 shows the distribution of amputation diagnoses among this sample. More than half (54.3 percent) had amputation at the transradial level; 23.9 percent had amputation at the transhumeral level; almost 20 percent had unspecified amputation diagnoses; and only 2.2 percent had partial hand amputation.

Medicare and most state Medicaid agencies and private insurance companies utilize the CMS DME, Prosthetics/Orthotics, and Supplies fee schedules for all procedure codes. In contrast with most medical care, time typically is not billed separately. Instead, the billing of a code (L–code in the case of prosthetic devices) is assumed to include the time needed to evaluate, fit, deliver, and follow up on the given device. Later modifications, adjustments, and repairs past the warranty period may be billed

TABLE 4-1
Upper-Limb Prostheses Provided to Beneficiaries by Type

Type of Device	Percentage	Cumulative Percentage[a]
Body-Powered	42.9	42.9
Myoelectric	27.6	70.4
Other	29.6	100.0

NOTE: Information from 5 percent random sample of 2013–2014 Durable Medical Equipment (DME) Medicare beneficiaries aged 20–67.

[a]Percentages may not total because of rounding.

SOURCE: DME Research Identifiable File, Centers for Medicare & Medicaid Services.

TABLE 4-2
Demographic Characteristics of Recipients of Upper-Limb Prostheses

Category	Percentage	Cumulative Percentage[a]
Age		
20–45	20.4	20.4
46–55	25.5	45.9
56–64	26.5	72.4
65–67	27.6	100.0
Sex		
Male	58.2	58.2
Female	41.8	100.0
Race/Ethnicity		
White	68.4	68.4
Black	18.4	86.7
Hispanic	8.2	94.9
Other	5.1	100.0

NOTE: Information from 5 percent random sample of 2013–2014 Durable Medical Equipment (DME) Medicare beneficiaries aged 20–67.

[a]Percentages may not total because of rounding.

SOURCE: DME Research Identifiable File, Centers for Medicare & Medicaid Services.

TABLE 4-3
Estimated Percentage of Upper-Limb Prosthetic Devices by Amputation Category

Amputation Category	Percentage	Cumulative Percentage[a]
Transradial/wrist disarticulation	54.3	54.3
Transhumeral	23.9	78.3
Level/side unspecified	19.6	97.8
Partial hand	2.2	100.0

NOTE: Information from 5 percent random sample of 2013–2014 Durable Medical Equipment (DME) Medicare beneficiaries aged 20–67.

[a]Percentages may not total because of rounding.

SOURCE: DME Research Identifiable File, Centers for Medicare & Medicaid Services.

as repair time and parts. When devices and components are provided for patients through private payment or workers' compensation insurance, payment can vary widely based on the selected codes and provider customary fee schedules, which may or may not cover the cost of the components. Medicare fee schedules are shown in Annex Table 4-1; however, they may not be representative of practice outside of Medicare. The existence of a device-specific code does not guarantee coverage, which, depending on the source of coverage, may require preauthorization or predetermination prior to delivery. Additionally, some recommended items may be noncoded, noncovered items to which no specific fee has been assigned.

Medicare does not provide preauthorization and instead may later request documentation to justify medical necessity. If the claim of medical necessity is not met, a claim will not be paid to a provider. In some situations, the provider anticipates that a device may be determined not medically necessary and therefore may be denied, and so they may ask a patient to sign an advance beneficiary notice (ABN). The ABN allows the patient to make an informed decision about whether to receive an item or service that may be determined noncoverable by Medicare and to accept financial responsibility should that be the case. An example is a device or parts "not otherwise specified" (code L7499), which includes any new technology. The challenge in these cases is that the new technology may be very expensive (>$10,000). A clinical facility, especially a smaller one that is less able to absorb the cost of an unpaid device or less confident in the justification for a complex upper-limb device, may be very concerned about assuming the risk of purchasing and delivering such an item for which payment is not assured. Likewise, a patient may be very hesitant to accept financial responsibility in case Medicare does not. In addition, Medicare, as well as other insurance providers, requires a copayment for service, which may represent a significant financial burden for individuals without secondary insurance coverage.

The committee recognizes that limited or lack of evidence about the impact of upper-limb loss, prosthesis use, and amputation rehabilitation on activity and participation may affect decisions by funding sources about which devices and services to cover. Such information on outcomes could contribute to studies on the effectiveness or cost-effectiveness of different types of prostheses and help inform the development of rational resource utilization, including use by insurers and other funding sources to inform their coverage decisions.

Distribution of Experienced and Knowledgeable Clinicians

It is widely recognized among those who work frequently with individuals with upper-limb amputation that this population is best served by knowledgeable, trained clinical providers who work together as a team to provide amputation care. Yet, while limited data are available on utilization of rehabilitation services in the U.S. population, one study examining practice patterns found that only 27 percent of the people who had a unilateral amputation and used a prosthesis had received training from an occupational or a physical therapist, and only 22 percent had received more than 10 hours of training from either a therapist or a prosthetist (Kestner, 2006).

Requirements for becoming a certified prosthetist/orthotist have evolved to an entry-level master's degree from a school accredited by the Commission on Accreditation of Allied Health Education Programs. Students receive training in upper- and lower-limb prosthetic fittings. To achieve certification for each discipline, all students must also complete a 1-year residency (per discipline) working under a certified clinician at an American Board for Certification in Orthotics, Prosthetics and Pedorthics (ABC)-accredited residency location, followed by written and practical qualifying exams. The experience the student receives in upper-limb fittings will depend on the patients seen at the residency facility. Only 15 states have licensure for prosthetics and orthotics (ABC, 2017b). Those that do typically rely on the ABC certification examination as a requirement. There are approximately 14,000 ABC-certified clinicians (prosthetists, orthotists, and pedorthists) (ABC, 2017a).

Prosthesis users receive training from occupational or physical therapists, depending on the clinical environment and team. Both occupational and physical therapy training programs require training in upper-limb prosthetics as part of the accreditation process. However, there are no mandates regarding the extent or content of this training.

Given the relative rarity and geographic dispersion of persons with upper-limb amputation in the United States, it is difficult for physicians, prosthetists, and therapists to acquire expertise in working with this population. Although limited data on the workforce are available, a recent survey of ABC members found that only 150 of 1,145 prosthetist members (13 percent) would consider fitting a patient with a UEP (Stark, 2016). Nearly 72 percent of respondents to a survey of upper-limb practitioners categorized themselves as novices in upper-extremity prosthetics and indicated that they treated an average of three such patients per year. The 26.2 percent who considered themselves experts in the field treated an average of 25 such patients per year. Many prosthetists endorsed the idea that the fitting process for patients with upper-limb amputation is particularly complex and that few prosthetists are being educated in this practice specialty. The areas of greatest challenge in upper-limb prosthetics were identified as knowledge of componentry, patient training, patient variation, and functional adjustment.

Given the scarcity of clinicians, including physicians, prosthetists, and occupational therapists, who are specialists in caring for persons with upper-limb amputation, a skilled team approach to care may not be widely available across the United States. Because the typical clinician has minimal education specific to upper-limb amputation and may see very few of these patients over the course of his or her career (Alley, 2004), most have little opportunity to develop expertise with this patient population (Stark, 2016). In addition to having limited experience in prosthetic fitting, clinicians would also have limited experience in justifying the need for and benefits of certain devices to insurers, which also could negatively impact delivery and outcomes. Because of their lack of expertise, many prosthetists rely on consultations with upper-limb experts to treat their patients. Some clinicians and patients must travel long distances to deliver or receive care. This necessity may delay care and negatively impact outcomes (Stark, 2016).

In 2007, the VHA launched an Amputation System of Care (ASoC) to improve access to expertise and specialized training for veterans with amputation (VA, 2016). Seven geographically dispersed VHA medical centers were designated as Regional Amputation Care Centers (RACs). RACs provide interdisciplinary care and prosthetic fabrication facilities, and they serve as resources to other VHA medical centers by offering telerehabilitation, consultation, and education. In addition, 18 VHA sites were designated Polytrauma/Amputation Network Sites (PANS), which offer inpatient and outpatient amputation rehabilitation services and have prosthetic labs. The remaining VHA medical centers were designated Amputation Care Centers. These centers have interdisciplinary amputation care teams but may lack the resources of RACs or PANS; or they may be designated amputation points of contact for assessment and refer patients to sites with requisite resources. The goal of the ASoC is to offer a coordinated system of high-quality, multidisciplinary, lifelong care that can provide the "most advanced and appropriate prosthetic components to Veterans across the system of care regardless of geographic location" (VA, 2012).

FINDINGS AND CONCLUSIONS

Findings

Overview, Taxonomy, Prosthetic Components, Prosthetic Sockets

4-1. A variety of different types of upper-extremity prostheses (UEPs) are available, the major categories being cosmetic, body-powered, hybrid, and myoelectric devices. There also exist a range of socket interfaces, suspension methods, terminal devices, and other components for each of these categories.

4-2. Regardless of the type of prosthetic device used, a well-fitting and comfortable socket is essential to successful use of a prosthesis.

4-3. For some people with limb loss, cosmetic restoration is highly valued or even preferred over functional restoration because of its mitigating effect on the disruption to body image.

4-4. The complex function of an upper extremity is far more difficult to replace with a prosthesis relative to the function of a lower extremity.

Impairment Mitigation

4-5. Upper-extremity limb loss or deficiency results in a wide range of significant impairments to body functions and resulting limitations on activities and participation.

4-6. Currently available UEPs cannot replace the complex functions of the missing limb because of limitations inherent in their control and design, their lack of sensory feedback, and the methods required to suspend them onto the residual limb.

4-7. The extent of impairment mitigation provided by a prosthesis varies by the type of device, the level of amputation, and the user's training in using the device.

4-8. Relative to the upper extremities, the primary functions of the lower limbs are more limited and concern primarily maintenance and achievement of upright stance and various types of locomotion (walking, running, hopping, jumping, stair climbing). In contrast, the primary functions of the upper extremities include self-care, interaction with the environment and others, self-expression, and fine and gross motor activities.

Acceptance/Rejection of Prostheses and Factors Affecting Device Use

4-9. The fit and function of the prosthesis and thus its impairment-mitigating effects may be impacted by environmental factors that may change over time, such as exposure to moisture, heat, and dirt. The consistency of impairment mitigation also depends on the condition and volume of the residual limb, which impact socket fit and comfort.

4-10. Skin integrity and a well-fitting prosthetic socket are key factors for successful use of a UEP.

4-11. People with transradial amputations are more likely to use prosthetic devices relative to those whose amputations are either more proximal (transhumeral or shoulder-level) or more distal (partial hand amputations).

4-12. Overall rejection rates of currently available types of UEPs are high. Understanding of all factors related to successful prosthesis adoption is limited, although primary rejection rates appear to be related to comfort of the prosthetic socket, level of amputation, age at the time of amputation, gender, and discrepancies between users' perceived needs and the availability of prosthetic devices to meet these needs.

4-13. Data on durability and repair rates for UEPs are limited, but clinical experience indicates that these devices require frequent maintenance and repair that can interfere with their consistent use.

Prognosis for Occupational Success

4-14. The extent of impairment mitigation provided by a prosthesis varies by the type of device and the level of amputation. In addition to design selection, impairment mitigation is dependent on socket fit, which may change in various environments and over time.

4-15. The only U.S. data available on vocational reintegration following upper-extremity amputation come from the military health care system. The committee could find no other studies examining the impact of prosthetic devices and rehabilitation strategies on work participation in the United States.

4-16. International studies and studies of U.S. military personnel demonstrate that a significant percentage of people with acquired limb loss have difficulty returning to work at all, and those who do usually require job modifications and adaptations to be successful.

4-17. International studies suggest that use of UEPs is a predictor of work participation and that employment is associated with decreased prosthesis rejection rates.

Access and Availability

4-18. Users need training to utilize UEPs effectively. Prosthetic training begins in the preprosthetic phase and continues upon device acquisition.

4-19. Persons with amputation require lifelong care with annual rechecks to ensure that their prosthetic needs are being met.

4-20. Recent evidence-based clinical practice guidelines (Management of Upper Extremity Amputation Rehabilitation Working Group, 2014) acknowledge the importance of taking a multidisciplinary team approach to the rehabilitation of people with upper-limb amputation.

4-21. There are no universally accepted guidelines for prescription of prosthetics and training in their use.

4-22. Data on the prevalence of use and prescription of UEPs are fragmented and limited.

4-23. Within the United States, people with limb loss or limb deficiency experience significant barriers to accessing and successfully using prosthetic devices.

4-24. Medicare and other insurers may reject payment for devices and components that are new technologies or that they do not consider "medically necessary" even if prescribed by a trained professional.

4-25. Evidence suggests that prosthesis users may not receive adequate training in using their devices.

4-26. Data do not exist on the location and distribution of expertise, such as centers of excellence, in the care of persons with upper-limb amputation across the United States. There is no standardization for UEP centers of excellence except in the Veterans Health Administration (VHA), where access to services is limited to veterans.

Conclusions

Overview, Taxonomy, Prosthetic Components, Prosthetic Sockets

4-1. The type of UEPs provided, including the choice of terminal device and socket design, needs to be customized to meet individual needs. [Findings 4-1, 4-2, 4-3]

Impairment Mitigation

4-2. Despite advances in prosthetic designs and research, currently available UEPs are limited in their ability to mitigate impairments related to limb loss. [Findings 4-4, 4-5, 4-6, 4-8]

4-3. Many individuals would benefit from more than one type of prosthetic device and/or terminal device to mitigate their impairments. [Findings 4-1, 4-4, 4-8]

4-4. In the future, emerging technology, if made available to people with limb loss, may improve the ability of UEPs to mitigate impairments. [Findings 4-6, 4-9]

Acceptance/Rejection of Prostheses and Factors Affecting Device Use

4-5. Even for people who are able to obtain UEPs, rejection rates are high, in part because of discomfort with wearing the devices, limited ability of the devices to meet their needs, a lack of training in their use, and limited durability. [Findings 4-2, 4-4, 4-6, 4-7, 4-9 through 4-14, 4-18, 4-19, 4-25]

Prognosis for Occupational Success

4-6. In selected cases, UEPs could significantly improve the ability to work, depending on the specific job requirements and environmental and personal factors. [Findings 4-9, 4-11, 414, 4-16 through 4-18]

4-7. Comprehensive efforts to study the impact of upper-limb loss, prosthesis use, and amputation rehabilitation on activity and participation, including work participation, are needed. Such research may not only enhance knowledge in these areas but also inform the development of rational resource utilization, including informing cost-benefit analyses and coverage for devices and related services. [Findings 4-13, 4-15, 4-16, 4-22, 4-26]

Access and Availability

4-8. It is important that UEP prescriptions be generated by qualified providers and customized to individuals' functional goals and clinical conditions. [Findings 4-1, 4-2, 4-7, 4-9, 4-10, 4-12, 414, 4-19, 4-20]

4-9. Reimbursement for UEPs and related rehabilitation services is highly variable, which creates unequal access, particularly for new technologies. [Finding 4-24]

4-10. The provision of UEPs is contingent largely on reimbursement policy rather than patient need. In many cases, a mismatch exists between the UEPs covered by Medicare and other insurers as medically necessary and the products or technologies that would best meet the needs of users to enhance their participation in life roles. [Finding 4-24]

4-11. There is a need for more qualified providers (including physicians, prosthetists, and therapists) and clinics with the knowledge, skill, and expertise to properly evaluate, prescribe, fit, and train people in the use of UEPs. [Findings 4-21, 4-25, 4-26]

4-12. Many civilian users of UEPs could benefit from the establishment of regional amputation centers of excellence incorporating a specialty multidisciplinary team rehabilitation approach, similar to those in the VHA amputation system of care. [Finding 4-26]

General Conclusion

4-13. At this time, it is difficult to quantify fully the impact of UEPs on impairment mitigation and employability because of a lack of research on contextual/environmental factors that impact device use and job function and a lack of data on occupational success. Even as UEPs have the potential to improve functional capacity in work participation, their impact is limited by unequal access to the devices and training in their use.

REFERENCES

ABC (American Board for Certification in Orthotics, Prosthetics and Pedorthics). 2017a. *Learn who we are*. https://www.abcop.org/WhoWeAre/Pages/default.aspx (accessed January 5, 2017).

ABC. 2017b. *State licensure*. https://www.abcop.org/State-Licensure/Pages/state-licensure.aspx (accessed January 18, 2017).

Alley, R. D. 2004. The prosthetist's evaluation and planning process with the upper extremity amputee. In *Functional restoration of adults and children with upper extremity amputation*. New York: Demos Medical Publishing, Inc. Pp. 125-132.

Alley, R. D., T. W. Williams, III, M. J. Albuquerque, and D. E. Altobelli. 2011. Prosthetic sockets stabilized by alternating areas of tissue compression and release. *Journal of Rehabilitation Research & Development* 48(6):679-696.

Aschoff, H. H., R. E. Kennon, J. M. Keggi, and L. E. Rubin. 2010. Transcutaneous, distal femoral, intramedullary attachment for above-the-knee prostheses: An endo-exo device. *Journal of Bone & Joint Surgery* 92(Suppl. 2):180-186.

Atkins, D. 2004. Prosthetic training. In *Atlas of amputations and limb deficiencies: Surgical, prosthetic, and rehabilitation principles*, edited by D. G. Smith and J. W. Michael. Rosemont, IL: American Academy of Orthopaedic Surgeons. Pp. 27-284.

Atkins, D. J., D. C. Y. Heard, and W. H. Donovan. 1996. Epidemiologic overview of individuals with upper-limb loss and their reported research priorities. *Journal of Prosthetics and Orthotics* 8(1):211.

Baschuk, C. 2016. Application of elevated vacuum suspension in upper-limb prosthetics. *The Academy TODAY* 12(3).

Belisle, J. G., J. C. Wenke, and C. A. Krueger. 2013. Return-to-duty rates among U.S. military combat-related amputees in the global war on terror: Job description matters. *Journal of Trauma Acute Care Surgery* 75(2):279-286.

Belter, J. T., J. L. Segil, A. M. Dollar, and R. F. Weir. 2013. Mechanical design and performance specifications of anthropomorphic prosthetic hands: A review. *Journal of Rehabilitation Research & Development* 50(5):599-618.

Belter, J. T., B. C. Reynolds, and A. M. Dollar. 2014. Grasp and force based taxonomy of split-hook prosthetic terminal devices. *Conference of the IEEE Engineering in Medicine and Biology Society* 2014:6613-6618.

Berning, K., S. Cohick, R. Johnson, L. A. Miller, and J. W. Sensinger. 2014. Comparison of body-powered voluntary opening and voluntary closing prehensor for activities of daily life. *Journal of Rehabilitation Research & Development* 51(2):253-261.

Biddiss, E., and T. Chau. 2007a. The roles of predisposing characteristics, established need, and enabling resources on upper extremity prosthesis use and abandonment. *Disability Rehabilitation Assistive Technology* 2(2):71-84.

Biddiss, E., and T. Chau. 2007b. Upper-limb prosthetics: Critical factors in device abandonment. *American Journal of Physical Medicine & Rehabilitation* 86(12):977-987.

Biddiss, E., and T. Chau. 2007c. Upper limb prosthesis use and abandonment: A survey of the last 25 years. *Prosthetics and Orthotics International* 31(3):236-257.

Biddiss, E., and T. Chau. 2008. Multivariate prediction of upper limb prosthesis acceptance or rejection. *Disability Rehabilitation: Assistive Technology* 3(4):181-192.

Biddiss, E., D. Beaton, and T. Chau. 2007. Consumer design priorities for upper limb prosthetics. *Disability Rehabilitation: Assistive Technology* 2(6):346-357.

Blough, D. K., S. Hubbard, L. V. McFarland, D. G. Smith, J. M. Gambel, and G. E. Reiber. 2010. Prosthetic cost projections for service members with major limb loss from Vietnam and OIF/OEF. *Journal of Rehabilitation Research & Development* 47(4):387-402.

Bosmans, J. C., J. H. Geertzen, W. J. Post, C. P. van der Schans, and P. U. Dijkstra. 2010. Factors associated with phantom limb pain: A 3 1/2-year prospective study. *Clinical Rehabilitation* 24(5):444-453.

Bouwsema, H., C. K. van der Sluis, and R. M. Bongers. 2008. The role of order of practice in learning to handle an upper-limb prosthesis. *Archives of Physical Medicine and Rehabilitation* 89(9):1759-1764.

Bouwsema, H., C. K. van der Sluis, and R. M. Bongers. 2010a. Learning to control opening and closing a myoelectric hand. *Archives of Physical Medicine and Rehabilitation* 91(9):1442-1446.

Bouwsema, H., C. K. van der Sluis, and R. M. Bongers. 2010b. Movement characteristics of upper extremity prostheses during basic goal-directed tasks. *Clinical Biomechanics (Bristol, Avon)* 25(6):523-529.

Bouwsema, H., P. J. Kyberd, W. Hill, C. K. van der Sluis, and R. M. Bongers. 2012. Determining skill level in myoelectric prosthesis use with multiple outcome measures. *Journal of Rehabilitation Research & Development* 49(9):1331-1348.

Bouwsema, H., C. K. van der Sluis, and R. M. Bongers. 2014. Changes in performance over time while learning to use a myoelectric prosthesis. *Journal of Neuroengineering and Rehabilitation* 11(1):16.

Bowers, R. 2004. The team approach to amputee rehabilitation. *Senior Step* 1.

Branemark, R., P. I. Branemark, B. Rydevik, and R. R. Myers. 2001. Osseointegration in skeletal reconstruction and rehabilitation: A review. *Journal of Rehabilitation Research & Development* 38(2):175-181.

Burger, H., and Č. Marinček. 1994. Upper limb prosthetic use in Slovenia. *Prosthetics and Orthotics International* 18(1):25-33.

Burger, H., and G. Vidmar. 2016. A survey of overuse problems in patients with acquired or congenital upper limb deficiency. *Prosthetics and Orthotics International* 40(4):497-502.

Burger, H., T. Maver, and Č. Marinček. 2007. Partial hand amputation and work. *Disability and Rehabilitation* 29(17):1317-1321.

Carey, S. L., M. Jason Highsmith, M. E. Maitland, and R. V. Dubey. 2008. Compensatory movements of transradial prosthesis users during common tasks. *Clinical Biomechanics (Bristol, Avon)* 23(9):1128-1135.

Carey, S. L., D. J. Lura, and M. J. Highsmith. 2015. Differences in myoelectric and body-powered upper-limb prostheses: Systematic literature review. *Journal of Rehabilitation Research & Development* 52(3):247-262.

Carlsen, B. T., P. Prigge, and J. Peterson. 2014. Upper extremity limb loss: Functional restoration from prosthesis and targeted reinnervation to transplantation. *Journal of Hand Therapy* 27(2):106-113.

Chaubey, P., T. Rosenbaum-Chou, W. Daly, and D. Boone. 2014. Closed-loop vibratory haptic feedback in upper-limb prosthetic users. *Journal of Prosthetics and Orthotics* 26(3):120-127.

Chicoine, C. L., A. M. Simon, and L. J. Hargrove. 2012. Prosthesis-guided training of pattern recognition-controlled myoelectric prosthesis. *Conference of the IEEE Engineering in Medicine and Biology Society* 2012:1876-1879.

Cipriani, C., M. Controzzi, and M. C. Carrozza. 2011. The smarthand transradial prosthesis. *Journal of Neuroengineering and Rehabilitation* 8:29.

Cipriani, C., M. D'Alonzo, and M. C. Carrozza. 2012. A miniature vibrotactile sensory substitution device for multifingered hand prosthetics. *IEEE Transactions on Biomedical Engineering* 59(2):400-408.

Clingman, R., and P. Pidcoe. 2014. A novel myoelectric training device for upper limb prostheses. *IEEE Transactions and Neural Systems Rehabilitation Engineering* 22(4):879-885.

Clippinger, F. W., R. Avery, and B. R. Titus. 1974. A sensory feedback system for an upper-limb amputation prosthesis. *Bulletin of Prosthetics Research* 247-258.

Copuroglu, C., M. Ozcan, B. Yilmaz, Y. Gorgulu, E. Abay, and E. Yalniz. 2010. Acute stress disorder and post-traumatic stress disorder following traumatic amputation. *Acta Orthopaedica Belgica* 76(1):90-93.

Cowley, J., L. Resnik, J. Wilken, L. Smurr Walters, and D. Gates. 2016. Movement quality of conventional prostheses and the DEKA Arm during everyday tasks. *Prosthetics and Orthotics International* 41(1):33-40.

Crandall, R. C., and W. Tomhave. 2002. Pediatric unilateral below-elbow amputees: Retrospective analysis of 34 patients given multiple prosthetic options. *Journal of Pediatric Orthopaedics* 22(3):380-383.

Cutosky, M. 1989. On grasp choice, grasp models, and the design of hand for manufacturing tasks. *IEEE Transactions on Robotics and Automation* 5(3):269-279.

Dabaghi-Richerand, A., F. Haces-Garcia, and R. Capdevila-Leonori. 2015. Prognostic factors of a satisfactory functional result in patients with unilateral amputations of the upper limb above the wrist that use an upper limb prosthesis. *Revista Espanola de Cirugia Ortopedica y Traumatologia* 59(5):343-347.

Dajpratham, P., S. Tantiniramai, P. Lukkapichonchut, and S. Kaewnaree. 2008. Factors associated with vocational reintegration among the Thai lower limb amputees. *Journal of the Medical Association of Thailand* 91(2):234-239.

Dakpa, R., and H. Heger. 1997. Prosthesis management and training of adult upper limb amputees. *Current Orthopaedics* 11(3):193-202.

Dalley, S. A., D. A. Bennett, and M. Goldfarb. 2012. Preliminary functional assessment of a multigrasp myoelectric prosthesis. *Conference Proceedings of the IEEE Engineering in Medicine and Biology Society* 2012:4172-4175.

Datta, D., K. Selvarajah, and N. Davey. 2004. Functional outcome of patients with proximal upper limb deficiency—acquired and congenital. *Clinical Rehabilitation* 18(2):172-177.

Davids, J. R., L. V. Wagner, L. C. Meyer, and D. W. Blackhurst. 2006. Prosthetic management of children with unilateral congenital below-elbow deficiency. *Journal of Bone and Joint Surgery: Series A* 88(6):1294-1300.

Davidson, J. 2004. A comparison of upper limb amputees and patients with upper limb injuries using the Disability of the Arm, Shoulder and Hand (DASH). *Disability and Rehabilitation* 26(14-15):917-923.

Davidson, J. H., K. E. Khor, and L. E. Jones. 2010. A cross-sectional study of post-amputation pain in upper and lower limb amputees, experience of a tertiary referral amputee clinic. *Disability and Rehabilitation* 32(22):1855-1862.

de Jong, I. G., H. A. Reinders-Messelink, K. Tates, W. G. Janssen, M. J. Poelma, I. van Wijk, and C. K. van der Sluis. 2012. Activity and participation of children and adolescents with unilateral congenital below elbow deficiency: An online focus group study. *Journal of Rehabilitation Medicine* 44(10):885-892.

Deeny, S., C. Chicoine, L. Hargrove, T. Parrish, and A. Jayaraman. 2014. A simple ERP method for quantitative analysis of cognitive workload in myoelectric prosthesis control and human-machine interaction. *PLOS One* 9(11):e112091.

Desmond, D. M. 2007. Coping, affective distress, and psychosocial adjustment among people with traumatic upper limb amputations. *Journal of Psychosomatic Research* 62(1):15-21.

Desmond, D. M., L. Coffey, P. Gallagher, M. MacLachlan, S. Wegener, and F. O'Keeffe. 2012. Limb amputation. In *The Oxford handbook of rehabilitation psychology*, 1st ed., edited by P. Kennedy. New York: Oxford University Press. Pp. 351-367.

Desteli, E. E., Y. Imren, M. Erdogan, G. Sarisoy, and S. Cosgun. 2014. Comparison of upper limb amputees and lower limb amputees: A psychosocial perspective. *European Journal of Trauma and Emergency Surgery* 40(6):735-739.

Dillingham, T. 1998. Rehabilitation of the upper limb amputee. In *Textbook of military medicine part IV surgical combat casualty care: Rehabilitation of the injured combatant.* Washington, DC: Office of the Surgeon General, U.S. Department of the Army. Pp. 33-77.

Doeringer, J. A., and N. Hogan. 1995. Performance of above elbow body-powered prostheses in visually guided unconstrained motion tasks. *IEEE Transactions on Biomedical Engineering* 42(6):621-631.

Donkervoort, M., D. J. Wiegerink, J. van Meeteren, H. J. Stam, and M. E. Roebroeck. 2009. Transition to adulthood: Validation of the Rotterdam Transition Profile for young adults with cerebral palsy and normal intelligence. *Developmental Medicine and Child Neurology* 51(1):53-62.

Dougherty, P. J., L. V. McFarland, D. G. Smith, A. Esquenazi, D. J. Blake, and G. E. Reiber. 2010. Multiple traumatic limb loss: A comparison of Vietnam veterans to OIF/OEF servicemembers. *Journal of Rehabilitation Research & Development* 47(4):333-348.

Dromerick, A. W., C. N. Schabowsky, R. J. Holley, B. Monroe, A. Markotic, and P. S. Lum. 2008. Effect of training on upper-extremity prosthetic performance and motor learning: A single-case study. *Archives of Physical Medicine and Rehabilitation* 89(6):1199-1204.

Dudkiewicz, I., R. Gabrielov, I. Seiv-Ner, G. Zelig, and M. Heim. 2004. Evaluation of prosthetic usage in upper limb amputees. *Disability and Rehabilitation* 26(1):60-63.

Egermann, M., P. Kasten, and M. Thomsen. 2009. Myoelectric hand prostheses in very young children. *International Orthopaedics* 33(4):1101-1105.

Englehart, K., and B. Hudgins. 2003. A robust, real-time control scheme for multifunction myoelectric control. *IEEE Transactions on Biomedical Engineering* 50(7):848-854.

Esquenazi, A. 2015. Upper limb amputation, rehabilitation & prosthetic restoration. In *Current diagnosis & treatment: Physical medicine & rehabilitation*, edited by I. B. Maitin and E. Cruz. New York: McGraw-Hill Education. Pp. 453-459.

Etter, K., M. Borgia, and L. Resnik. 2014. Prescription and repair rates of prosthetic limbs in the VA healthcare system: Implications for national prosthetic parity. *Disability and Rehabilitation: Assistive Technology* 10(6):1-8.

FDA (U.S. Food and Drug Administration). 2015. *FDA authorizes use of prosthesis for rehabilitation of above-the-knee amputations.* Silver Spring, MD: FDA.

Fernandez, A., I. Isusi, and M. Gomez. 2000. Factors conditioning the return to work of upper limb amputees in Asturias, Spain. *Prosthetics and Orthotics International* 24(2):143-147.

Fillauer Companies, Inc. 2016. *Fillauer Companies product catalog.* http://hosmer.com/products/PDFs/Fillauer%20Companies%20Catalog.zip (accessed January 24, 2017).

Fisher, K., R. S. Hanspal, and L. Marks. 2003. Return to work after lower limb amputation. *International Journal of Rehabilitation Research* 26(1):51-56.

Flannery, J. C., and S. H. Faria. 1999. Limb loss: Alterations in body image. *Journal of Vascular Nursing* 17(4):100-106.

Fraser, C., and A. W. Wing. 1981. A case study of reaching by a user of a manually-operated artificial hand. *Prosthetics and Orthotics International* 5(3):151-156.

Gaine, W. J., C. Smart, and M. Bransby-Zachary. 1997. Upper limb traumatic amputees: Review of prosthetic use. *Journal of Hand Surgery (British and European Volume)* 22(1):73-76.

Gallagher, P., O. Horgan, F. Franchignoni, A. Giordano, and M. MacLachlan. 2007. Body image in people with lower-limb amputation: A Rasch analysis of the amputee body image scale. *American Journal of Physical Medicine & Rehabilitation* 86(3):205-215.

Gallagher, P., M. A. O'Donovan, A. Doyle, and D. Desmond. 2011. Environmental barriers, activity limitations and participation restrictions experienced by people with major limb amputation. *Prosthetics and Orthotics International* 35(3):278-284.

Hacking, H. G. A., J.-P. van den Berg, K. T. Dahmen, and M. W. Post. 1997. Long-term outcome of upper limb prosthetic use in the Netherlands. *European Journal of Physical Medicine and Rehabilitation* 7(6):179-181.

Hanley, M. A., D. M. Ehde, M. Jensen, J. Czerniecki, D. G. Smith, and L. R. Robinson. 2009. Chronic pain associated with upper-limb loss. *American Journal of Physical Medicine & Rehabilitation* 88(9):742-751.

Hanson, W. 2003. Upper limb prosthetic components: Function vs. appearance. *In Motion* 13(6):29.

Harrtigan, B., and S. Serrafin. 2004. Kinesiology and functional characteristics of the upper limb. In *Atlas of amputations and limb deficiencies: Surgical, prosthetic, and rehabilitation principles*, 3rd ed., edited by D. G. Smith, J. W. Michael, and J. H. Bowker. Rosemont, IL: American Academy of Orthopaedic Surgeons. Pp. 101-116.

Hebert, J. S., J. L. Olson, M. J. Morhart, M. R. Dawson, P. D. Marasco, T. A. Kuiken, and K. M. Chan. 2014. Novel targeted sensory reinnervation technique to restore functional hand sensation after transhumeral amputation. *IEEE Transactions on Neural Systems and Rehabilitation Engineering* 22(4):765-773.

Hebert, J. S., K. M. Chan, and M. R. Dawson. 2016. Cutaneous sensory outcomes from three transhumeral targeted reinnervation cases. *Prosthetics and Orthotics International* 40(3):303-310.

Heckathorne, C. W. 1992. Upper-limb prosthetics: Components for adult externally powered systems. In *Atlas of limb prosthetics: Surgical, prosthetic, and rehabilitation principles*, 2nd ed., edited by J. H. Bowker and J. W. Michael. St. Louis, MO: Mosby-Year Book, Inc. Pp. 151-174.

Herberts, P., L. Korner, K. Caine, and L. Wensby. 1980. Rehabilitation of unilateral below-elbow amputees with myoelectric prostheses. *Scandinavian Journal of Rehabilitation Medicine* 12(3):123-128.

Hosmer. 2017. *Hosmer products*. http://hosmer.com/products (accessed January 5, 2017).

Hurley, R. K., Jr., J. C. Rivera, J. C. Wenke, and C. A. Krueger. 2015. Identifying obstacles to return to duty in severely injured combat-related servicemembers with amputation. *Journal of Rehabilitation Research & Development* 52(1):53-61.

Infinite Biomedical Technologies. n.d. *morph2*. http://www.i-biomed.com/morph2.html (accessed April 5, 2017).

Inkellis, E. R., E. E. Low, and S. Morshed. 2015. *Traumatic upper extremity amputations: An epidemiologic study using the National Trauma Data Bank*. Paper presented at American Academy of Orthotists & Prosthetists 41st Academy Annual Meeting & Scientific Symposium, New Orleans, LA, February 18-21. http://www.oandp.org/publications/jop/2015/2015-05.pdf (accessed January 21, 2017).

ISO (International Organization for Standardization). n.d. *Prosthetics and orthotics—vocabulary—part 4: Terms relating to limb amputation*. https://www.iso.org/obp/ui/#iso:std:iso:8549:-4:ed-1:v1:en (accessed January 18, 2017).

James, M. A., A. M. Bagley, K. Brasington, C. Lutz, S. McConnell, and F. Molitor. 2006. Impact of prostheses on function and quality of life for children with unilateral congenital below-the-elbow deficiency. *Journal of Bone & Joint Surgery: American Edition* 88(11):2356-2365.

Johnson, S. S., and E. Mansfield. 2014. Prosthetic training: Upper limb. *Physical Medicine and Rehabilitation Clinics of North America* 25(1):133-151.

Jones, L. E., and J. H. Davidson. 1995. The long-term outcome of upper limb amputees treated at a rehabilitation centre in Sydney, Australia. *Disability and Rehabilitation* 17(8):437-442.

Jönsson, S., K. Caine-Winterberger, and R. Brånemark. 2011. Osseointegration amputation prostheses on the upper limbs: Methods, prosthetics and rehabilitation. *Prosthetics and Orthotics International* 35(2):190-200.

Kejlaa, G. H. 1993. Consumer concerns and the functional value of prostheses to upper limb amputees. *Prosthetics and Orthotics International* 17(3):157-163.

Kestner, S. 2006. Defining the relationship between prosthetic wrist function and its use in performing work tasks and activities of daily living. *Journal of Prosthetics and Orthotics* 18(3):80-86.

Kooijman, C. M., P. U. Dijkstra, J. H. Geertzen, A. Elzinga, and C. P. van der Schans. 2000. Phantom pain and phantom sensations in upper limb amputees: An epidemiological study. *Pain* 87(1):33-41.

Kruger, L. M., and S. Fishman. 1993. Myoelectric and body-powered prostheses. *Journal of Pediatric Orthopaedics* 13(1):68-75.

Kyberd, P. J. 2011. The influence of control format and hand design in single axis myoelectric hands: Assessment of functionality of prosthetic hands using the Southampton hand assessment procedure. *Prosthetics and Orthotics International* 35(3):285-293.

Kyberd, P. J., and W. Hill. 2011. Survey of upper limb prosthesis users in Sweden, the United Kingdom and Canada. *Prosthetics and Orthotics International* 35(2):234-241.

Lake, C. 1997. Effects of prosthetic training on upper-extremity prosthesis use. *Journal of Prosthetics and Orthotics* 9(1):3-9.

Lehneis, H. R., and R. Dickey. 1992. Special considerations: Fitting and training the bilateral upper-limb amputee. In *Atlas of limb prosthetics: Surgical, prosthetic, and rehabilitation principles*, 2nd ed., edited by J. H. Bowker and J. W. Michael. St. Louis, MO: Mosby-Year Book, Inc. Pp. 311-324.

Lerman, J. A., E. Sullivan, D. A. Barnes, and R. J. Haynes. 2005. The Pediatric Outcomes Data Collection Instrument (PODCI) and functional assessment of patients with unilateral upper extremity deficiencies. *Journal of Pediatric Orthopaedics* 25(3):405-407.

Lifchez, S. D., J. Marchant-Hanson, H. S. Matloub, J. R. Sanger, W. W. Dzwierzynski, and H. H. Nguyen. 2005. Functional improvement with digital prosthesis use after multiple digit amputations. *American Society for Surgery of the Hand* 30(4):790-794.

Livingston, D. H., D. Keenan, D. Kim, J. Elcavage, and M. A. Malagnoni. 1994. Extent of disability following traumatic extremity amputation. *Journal of Trauma* 37(3):495-499.

Lock, B. A., and L. J. Hargrove. 2014. *Systems and methods for autoconfiguration of pattern-recognition controlled myoelectric prostheses* (application number 13/950,000). Washington, DC: U.S. Patent and Trademark Office. http://appft1.uspto.gov/netacgi/nph-Parser?Sect1=PTO1&Sect2=HITOFF&d=PG01&p=1&u=/netahtml/PTO/srchnum.html&r=1&f=G&l=50&s1=20140032462.PGNR (accessed January 24, 2017).

Luchetti, M., A. G. Cutti, G. Verni, R. Sacchetti, and N. Rossi. 2015. Impact of Michelangelo prosthetic hand: Findings from a crossover longitudinal study. *Journal of Rehabilitation Research & Development* 52(5):605-618.

MacKenzie, E. J., A. S. Jones, M. J. Bosse, R. C. Castillo, A. N. Pollak, L. X. Webb, M. F. Swiontkowski, J. F. Kellam, D. G. Smith, R. W. Sanders, A. L. Jones, A. J. Starr, M. P. McAndrew, B. M. Patterson, and A. R. Burgess. 2007. Health-care costs associated with amputation or reconstruction of a limb-threatening injury. *Journal of Bone & Joint Surgery American Edition* 89(8):1685-1692.

MaGuire, M. T. 2008. Empowering prosthetics: A team approach to prosthetics and limb loss. *REHAB Management*, December 1. http://www.rehabpub.com/2008/12/empowering-prosthetics (accessed January 21, 2017).

Malone, J. M., L. L. Fleming, J. Roberson, T. E. Whitesides, Jr., J. M. Leal, J. U. Poole, and R. S. Grodin. 1984. Immediate, early, and late postsurgical management of upper-limb amputation. *Journal of Rehabilitation Research & Development* 21(1):33-41.

Management of Upper Extremity Amputation Rehabilitation Working Group. 2014. *VA/DoD clinical practice guideline for the management of upper extremity amputation rehabilitation.* Washington, DC: VA, Department of Defense (DoD).

Marasco, P. D., A. E. Schultz, and T. A. Kuiken. 2009. Sensory capacity of reinnervated skin after redirection of amputated upper limb nerves to the chest. *Brain* 132(Pt. 6):1441-1448.

McFarland, L. V., S. Winkler, M. W. Jones, A. W. Heinemann, G. E. Reiber, and A. Esquenazi. 2010. Unilateral upper limb loss: Satisfaction and prosthetic device use in service members from Vietnam and OIF/OEF conflicts. *Journal of Rehabilitation Research & Development* 47(4):275-298.

McKechnie, P. S., and A. John. 2014. Anxiety and depression following traumatic limb amputation: A systematic review. *Injury* 45(12):1859-1866.

Meurs, M., C. G. Maathuis, C. Lucas, M. Hadders-Algra, and C. K. van der Sluis. 2006. Prescription of the first prosthesis and later use in children with congenital unilateral upper limb deficiency: A systematic review. *Prosthetics and Orthotics International* 30(2):165-173.

Miguelez, J. M., and M. D. Miguelez. 2003. The microframe: The next generation of interface design for glenohumeral disarticulation and associated levels of limb deficiency. *Journal of Prosthetics and Orthotics* 15(2):66-71.

Miguelez, J. M., M. Lang, R. Dodson, M. Cameron, and C. Hays. 2016. Building a better arm: Design and fabrication in upper-limb prosthetics. *O&P Edge*, July.

Millstein, S., D. Bain D, and G. A. Hunter. 1985. A review of employment patterns of industrial amputees—Factors influencing rehabilitation. *Prosthetics and Orthotics International* 9(2):69-78.

Millstein, S. G., H. Heger, and G. A. Hunter. 1986. Prosthetic use in adult upper limb amputees: A comparison of the body powered and electrically powered prostheses. *Prosthetics and Orthotics International* 10(1):27-34.

Morris, R. 2008. Focus on upper extremity: Therapeutic influences on the upper-limb amputee. *The Academy TODAY* 4(3).

Muderis, M. A., K. Tetsworth, A. Khemka, S. Wilmot, B. Bosley, S. J. Lord, and V. Glatt. 2016. The Osseointegration Group of Australia Accelerated Protocol (OGAAP-1) for two-stage osseointegrated reconstruction of amputated limbs. *The Bone & Joint Journal* 98-B(7):952-960.

Nghiem, B. T., I. C. Sando, R. B. Gillespie, B. L. McLaughlin, G. J. Gerling, N. B. Langhals, M. G. Urbanchek, and P. S. Cederna. 2015. Providing a sense of touch to prosthetic hands. *Plastic and Reconstructive Surgery* 135(6):1652-1663.

O&P Almanac. 2016. Amputation data from community hospitals. *O&P Almanac*, April, p. 8.

Ortiz-Catalan, M., R. Branemark, B. Hakansson, and J. Delbeke. 2012. On the viability of implantable electrodes for the natural control of artificial limbs: Review and discussion. *BioMedical Engineering OnLine* 11:33.

Ortiz-Catalan, M., B. Håkansson, and R. Brånemark. 2014. An osseointegrated human-machine gateway for long-term sensory feedback and motor control of artificial limbs. *Science Translational Medicine* 6(257):257re6.

Østlie, K., R. J. Franklin, O. H. Skjeldal, A. Skrondal, and P. Magnus. 2011. Musculoskeletal pain and overuse syndromes in adult acquired major upper-limb amputees. *Archives of Physical Medicine and Rehabilitation* 92(12):1967-1973.

Østlie, K., I. M. Lesjø, R. J. Franklin, B. Garfelt, O. H. Skjeldal, and P. Magnus. 2012a. Prosthesis rejection in acquired major upper-limb amputees: A population-based survey. *Disability and Rehabilitation: Assistive Technology* 7(4):294-303.

Østlie, K., I. M. Lesjø, R. J. Franklin, B. Garfelt, O. H. Skjeldal, and P. Magnus. 2012b. Prosthesis use in adult acquired major upper-limb amputees: Patterns of wear, prosthetic skills and the actual use of prostheses in activities of daily life. *Disability and Rehabilitation: Assistive Technology* 7(6):479-493.

Ottobock. 2016a. *Michelangelo hand.* https://professionals.ottobockus.com/Prosthetics/Upper-Limb-Prosthetics/Michelangelo-Axon-Bus-System/Michelangelo-Hand/c/2001 (accessed January 24, 2017).

Ottobock. 2016b. *Michelangelo prosthetic hand.* http://www.ottobockus.com/prosthetics/upper-limb-prosthetics/solution-overview/michelangelo-prosthetic-hand (accessed January 24, 2017).

Palmquist, A., T. Jarmar, L. Emanuelsson, R. Branemark, H. Engqvist, and P. Thomsen. 2008. Forearm bone-anchored amputation prosthesis: A case study on the osseointegration. *Acta Orthopaedica* 79(1):78-85.

Perkins, Z. B., H. D. De'Ath, G. Sharp, and N. R. Tai. 2012. Factors affecting outcome after traumatic limb amputation. *British Journal of Surgery Society* 99(Suppl. 1):75-86.

Phillips, S., L. Resnik, and G. Latlief. 2013. Endpoint control for a powered shoulder prosthesis. *Journal of Prosthetics and Orthotics* 25(4):193-200.

Pitkin, M. 2013. Design features of implants for direct skeletal attachment of limb prostheses. *Journal of BioMedical Materials Research: Part A* 101(11):3339-3348.

Postema, S. G., C. K. van der Sluis, K. Waldenlov, and L. M. Norling Hermansson. 2012. Body structures and physical complaints in upper limb reduction deficiency: A 24-year follow-up study. *PLOS One* 7(11):e49727.

Postema, S. G., R. M. Bongers, M. A. Brouwers, H. Burger, L. M. Norling-Hermansson, M. F. Reneman, P. U. Dijkstra, and C. K. van der Sluis. 2016a. Musculoskeletal complaints in transverse upper limb reduction deficiency and amputation in the Netherlands: Prevalence, predictors, and effect on health. *Archives of Physical Medicine and Rehabilitation* 97(7): 1137-1145.

Postema, S. G., R. M. Bongers, M. A. Brouwers, H. Burger, L. M. Norling-Hermansson, M. F. Reneman, P. U. Dijkstra, and C. K. van der Sluis. 2016b. Upper limb absence: Predictors of work participation and work productivity. *Archives of Physical Medicine and Rehabilitation* 97(6):892-899.

Powell, M. A., and N. V. Thakor. 2013. A training strategy for learning pattern recognition control for myoelectric prostheses. *Journal of Prosthetics and Orthotics* 25(1):30-41.

Powell, M. A., R. R. Kaliki, and N. V. Thakor. 2014. User training for pattern recognition-based myoelectric prostheses: Improving phantom limb movement consistency and distinguishability. *IEEE Transactions on Neural Systems and Rehabilitation Engineering* 22(3):522-532.

Racey, J. 1992. Psychological adaptation to amputation. In *Atlas of limb prosthetics: Surgical, prosthetic, and rehabilitation principles*, 2nd ed., edited by J. H. Bowker and J. W. Michael. St. Louis, MO: Mosby-Year Book, Inc. Pp. 707-716.

Rager, D. M., D. Alvares, I. Birznieks, S. J. Redmond, J. W. Morley, N. H. Lovell, and R. M. Vickery. 2013. Generating tactile afferent stimulation patterns for slip and touch feedback in neural prosthetics. *Annual International Conference of the IEEE Engineering in Medicine and Biology Society* 2013:5922-5925.

Raichle, K. A., M. A. Hanley, I. Molton, N. J. Kadel, K. Campbell, E. Phelps, D. Ehde, and D. G. Smith. 2008. Prosthesis use in persons with lower- and upper-limb amputation. *Journal of Rehabilitation Research & Development* 45(7):961-972.

Resnik, L., and M. Borgia. 2012. Reliability and validity of outcome measures for upper limb amputation. *Journal of Prosthetics and Orthotics* 24(4):192-212.

Resnik, L., and M. Borgia. 2015. Reliability, validity, and responsiveness of the quickdash in patients with upper limb amputation. *Archives of Physical Medicine and Rehabilitation* 96(9):1676-1683.

Resnik, L., M. R. Meucci, S. Lieberman-Klinger, C. Fantini, D. L. Kelty, R. Disla, and N. Sasson. 2012. Advanced upper limb prosthetic devices: Implications for upper limb prosthetic rehabilitation. *Archives of Physical Medicine and Rehabilitation* 93(4):710-717.

Resnik, L., T. Patel, S. G. Cooney, J. J. Crisco, and C. Fantini. 2014a. Comparison of transhumeral socket designs utilizing patient assessment and in vivo skeletal and socket motion tracking: A case study. *Disability and Rehabilitation: Assistive Technology* 11(5):423-432.

Resnik, L., S. L. Klinger, and K. Etter. 2014b. The DEKA Arm: Its features, functionality, and evolution during the Veterans Affairs study to optimize the DEKA arm. *Prosthetics and Orthotics International* 38(6):492-504.

Resnik, L., S. L. Klinger, K. Korp, and L. S. Walters. 2014c. Training protocol for a powered shoulder prosthesis. *Journal of Rehabilitation Research & Development* 51(8):vii-xvi.

Ritchie, S., S. Wiggins, and A. Sanford. 2011. Perceptions of cosmesis and function in adults with upper limb prostheses: A systematic literature review. *Prosthetics and Orthotics International* 35(4):332-341.

Roeschlein, R. A., and E. Domholdt. 1989. Factors related to successful upper extremity prosthetic use. *Prosthetics and Orthotics International* 13(1):14-18.

Saradjian, A., A. R. Thompson, and D. Datta. 2008. The experience of men using an upper limb prosthesis following amputation: positive coping and minimizing feeling different. *Disability and Rehabilitation* 30(11):871-883.

Scheme, E., and K. Englehart. 2011. Electromyogram pattern recognition for control of powered upper-limb prostheses: State of the art and challenges for clinical use. *Journal of Rehabilitation Research & Development* 48(6):643-659.

Schiefer, M., D. Tan, S. M. Sidek, and D. J. Tyler. 2016. Sensory feedback by peripheral nerve stimulation improves task performance in individuals with upper limb loss using a myoelectric prosthesis. *Journal of Neural Engineering* 13(1):016001.

Schofield, J. S., K. R. Evans, J. P. Carey, and J. S. Hebert. 2014. Applications of sensory feedback in motorized upper extremity prosthesis: A review. *Expert Review of Medical Devices* 11(5):499-511.

Schoppen, T., A. Boonstra, J. W. Groothoff, J. de Vries, L. N. Goeken, and W. H. Eisma. 2001a. Employment status, job characteristics, and work-related health experience of people with a lower limb amputation in the Netherlands. *Archives of Physical Medicine and Rehabilitation* 82(2):239-245.

Schoppen, T., A. Boonstra, J. W. Groothoff, E. van Sonderen, L. N. Goeken, and W. H. Eisma. 2001b. Factors related to successful job reintegration of people with a lower limb amputation. *Archives of Physical Medicine and Rehabilitation* 82(10):1425-1431.

Schuch, C. M., and C. H. Pritham. 1994. International standards organization terminology: Application to prosthetics and orthotics. *Journal of Prosthetics and Orthotics* 6(1):29-33.

Schultz, A., S. Baade, and T. Kuiken. 2007. Expert opinions on success factors for upper-limb prostheses. *Journal of Rehabilitation Research & Development* 44(4):483-490.

Silcox, D. H., III, M. D. Rooks, R. R. Vogel, and L. L. Fleming. 1993. Myoelectric prostheses. A long-term follow-up and a study of the use of alternate prostheses. *Journal of Bone & Joint Surgery: American Edition* 75(12):1781-1789.

Simon, A. M., B. A. Lock, and K. A. Stubblefield. 2012. Patient training for functional use of pattern recognition-controlled prostheses. *Journal of Prosthetics and Orthotics* 24(2):56-64.

Sjoberg, L., Y. Nilsagard, and C. Fredriksson. 2014. Life situation of adults with congenital limb reduction deficiency in Sweden. *Disability and Rehabilitation* 36(18):1562-1571.

Smit, G., and D. H. Plettenburg. 2010. Efficiency of voluntary closing hand and hook prostheses. *Prosthetics and Orthotics International* 34(4):411-427.

Smurr, L. M., K. Gulick, K. Yancosek, and O. Ganz. 2008. Managing the upper extremity amputee: A protocol for success. *Journal of Hand Therapy* 21(2):160-176.

Sobuh, M. M., L. P. Kenney, A. J. Galpin, S. B. Thies, J. McLaughlin, J. Kulkarni, and P. Kyberd. 2014. Visuomotor behaviours when using a myoelectric prosthesis. *Journal of NeuroEngineering and Rehabilitation* 11:72.

Stark, G. 2016. *Competency, risk, and acceptance of upper limb prosthetic technology*. Presentation to the Committee on the Use of Selected Assistive Products and Technologies in Eliminating or Reducing the Effects of Impairments, Washington, DC, May 16.

Steeper. 2016. *Bebionic technical manual*. http://bebionic.com/uploads/files/RSLLIT317_-_Tech_Manual_Medium_Large_Hand_web1.pdf (accessed January 18, 2017).

Stinner, D. J., T. C. Burns, K. L. Kirk, and J. R. Ficke. 2010. Return to duty rate of amputee soldiers in the current conflicts in Afghanistan and Iraq. *Journal of Trauma and Acute Care Surgery* 68(6):1476-1479.

Stubblefield, K. A., L. A. Miller, R. D. Lipschutz, and T. A. Kuiken. 2009. Occupational therapy protocol for amputees with targeted muscle reinnervation. *Journal of Rehabilitation Research & Development* 46(4):481-488.

Tabot, G. A., J. F. Dammann, J. A. Berg, F. V. Tenore, J. L. Boback, R. J. Vogelstein, and S. J. Bensmaia. 2013. Restoring the sense of touch with a prosthetic hand through a brain interface. *Proceedings of the National Academy of Sciences of the United States of America* 110(45):18279-18284.

Tan, D. W., M. A. Schiefer, M. W. Keith, J. R. Anderson, and D. J. Tyler. 2015. Stability and selectivity of a chronic, multi-contact cuff electrode for sensory stimulation in human amputees. *Journal of Neural Engineering* 12(2):026002.

Tennent, D. J., J. C. Wenke, J. C. Rivera, and C. A. Krueger. 2014. Characterisation and outcomes of upper extremity amputations. *Injury* 45(6):965-969.

Texas Assistive Devices. 2016. *Manufacturers of upper extremity components for persons with hand dysfunction and amputation*. http://www.n-abler.org (accessed January 21, 2017).

Tintle, S. M., M. F. Baechler, G. P. Nanos, III, J. A. Forsberg, and B. K. Potter. 2010. Traumatic and trauma-related amputations: Part II: Upper extremity and future directions. *Journal of Bone & Joint Surgery: American Edition* 92(18):2934-2945.

Touch Bionics. 2016. *Touch Bionics i-limb ultra*. http://www.touchbionics.com/products/active-prostheses/i-limb-ultra (accessed January 21, 2017).

Touch Bionics. n.d.-a. *Touch bionics i-limb quantum*. http://www.touchbionics.com/products/active-prostheses/i-limb%E2%84%A2-quantum (accessed April 5, 2017).

Touch Bionics. n.d.-b. *Grip chips demo*. http://www.i-biomed.com/morph2.html (accessed April 5, 2017).

TRS Prosthetics. 2016. *Sports: Prosthetics for sports and activities*. http://www.trsprosthetics.com/shop-category/sports (accessed January 21, 2017).

Tyler, D. J. 2015. Neural interfaces for somatosensory feedback: Bringing life to a prosthesis. *Current Opinion in Neurology* 28(6):574-581.

Uellendahl, J., and C. W. Heckathorne. 1989. Creative prosthetic solutions for bilateral upper extremity amputation. In *Comprehensive management of the upper-limb amputee*, edited by D. J. Atkins and R. H. Meier. New York: Springer. Pp. 225-237.

VA (U.S. Department of Veterans Affairs). 2012. *VHA handbook 1172.03: Amputation system of care*. Washington, DC: VA.

VA. 2016. *Rehabilitation and prosthetic services: Amputation system of care*. http://www.prosthetics.va.gov/PROSTHETICS/asoc/index.asp (accessed January 18, 2017).

van der Niet, O., R. M. Bongers, and C. K. van der Sluis. 2013. Functionality of i-limb and i-limb pulse hands: Case report. *Journal of Rehabilitation Research & Development* 50(8):1123-1128.

van der Sluis, C. K., P. P. Hartman, T. Schoppen, and P. U. Dijkstra. 2009. Job adjustments, job satisfaction and health experience in upper and lower limb amputees. *Prosthetics and Orthotics International* 33(1):41-51.

Vasluian, E., I. G. de Jong, W. G. Janssen, M. J. Poelma, I. van Wijk, H. A. Reinders-Messelink, and C. K. van der Sluis. 2013. Opinions of youngsters with congenital below-elbow deficiency, and those of their parents and professionals concerning prosthetic use and rehabilitation treatment. *PLOS One* 8(6):e67101.

Vincent, H. K., M. Horodyski, K. R. Vincent, S. T. Brisbane, and K. K. Sadasivan. 2015. Psychological distress after orthopedic trauma: Prevalence in patients and implications for rehabilitation. *PM&R* 7(9):978-989.

Weir, R. F., P. R. Troyk, G. DeMichele, and T. Kuiken. 2003. *Implantable myoelectric sensors (IMES) for upper-extremity prosthesis control—preliminary work*. Paper presented at IEEE Engineering in Medicine and Biology Society, Cancun, Mexico, September 17-21.

Williams, T. W. 2004. Control of powered upper extremity prostheses. In *Functional restoration of adults and children with upper extremity amputation*, edited by R. H. Meier and D. J. Atkins. New York: Demos Medical Publishing, Inc. Pp. 207-224.

Winchell, E. 1996. Body image: Acceptance is step one. *In Motion* 6(4).

Witteveen, H. J., F. Luft, J. S. Rietman, and P. H. Veltink. 2014. Stiffness feedback for myoelectric forearm prostheses using vibrotactile stimulation. *IEEE Transactions on Neural Systems and Rehabilitation Engineering* 22(1):53-61.

Witteveen, H. J., H. S. Rietman, and P. H. Veltink. 2015. Vibrotactile grasping force and hand aperture feedback for myoelectric forearm prosthesis users. *Prosthetics and Orthotics International* 39(3):204-212.

Wright, T. W., A. D. Hagen, and M. B. Wood. 1995. Prosthetic usage in major upper extremity amputations. *The Journal of Hand Surgery* 20(4):619-622.

Ziegler-Graham, K., E. J. MacKenzie, P. L. Ephraim, T. G. Travison, and R. Brookmeyer. 2008. Estimating the prevalence of limb loss in the United States: 2005 to 2050. *Archives of Physical Medicine and Rehabilitation* 89(3):422-429.

CHAPTER 4 ANNEX TABLES BEGIN ON THE NEXT PAGE

ANNEX TABLE 4-1
Upper-Limb Prosthetic Device Taxonomy

Device	Estimated Cost[a]	Indications/Requirements for Use
Body-Powered		
Transradial	$4,400	• Skin integrity that allows socket wear and harness use • Adequate strength and range of motion (ROM) for biscapular abduction • Skilled prosthetist and occupational therapist (OT) needed to help patient learn to use effectively
Transhumeral	$6,000	
Shoulder disarticulation	$11,300	
Myoelectric		
Transradial	$15,100	• Skin integrity that allows an intimate socket fit to maintain electrode contact • Ability to contract isolated muscles voluntarily to activate myosites • Consistent access to electricity • Skilled prosthetist and OT needed to help patient learn to use effectively
Transhumeral	$56,200	
Shoulder disarticulation	$65,700	
Hybrid		
Transhumeral	$19,200	• Skin integrity that allows an intimate socket fit to maintain electrode contact • Ability to contract isolated muscles voluntarily to activate myosites • Consistent access to electricity • Skilled prosthetist and OT needed to help patient learn to use effectively
Shoulder disarticulation	$32,500	

	Relative Contraindications	Benefits of Device	Limitations of Device
	• Limited scapular ROM/ strength or shoulder pain may limit use of harness	• Lighter weight than myoelectric • More durable (better tolerates water/dirt) • Requires less maintenance • User can make some adjustments/self-repair • Less expensive option than myoelectric or hybrid	• Some transradial (TR) sockets may limit elbow ROM • Weight limitations—lifting and carrying activities depend on the positioning of the object in relation to the body • Socket style and harnessing may limit shoulder ROM in shoulder-level amputees • Terminal devices have only one grasp
	• Not recommended for driving and operating heavy equipment • Fluctuating limb volume can interfere with electrode contact, and make performance erratic	• Uses no harnessing or less harnessing compared with body-powered systems • Can be used for overhead activities/in more planes • Can be used with a wider range of terminal devices that can generate more force • Can have better cosmesis • Externally powered terminal devices typically provide greater grip force than body-powered hooks and hands	• Heavier than body-powered systems • Less resistant to water and dust exposure • Requires more maintenance, more prone to breakage • May function inconsistently as a result of excessive sweating, change in limb volume • Most users unable to control terminal device and any other movement simultaneously • Can be cognitively taxing to use
	• Limited shoulder ROM/ strength or shoulder pain may limit use of harness • Fluctuating limb volume (transhumeral) can interfere with electrode contact and make performance erratic	• Both elbow and hand can be operated simultaneously • Lighter than a full myoelectric system for higher levels • Externally powered terminal devices typically provide greater grip force than body-powered hooks and hands	• May function inconsistently as a result of excessive sweating, change in limb volume • Requires more maintenance than body-powered systems (battery charging, more prone to breakage) • Less resistant to water and dust exposure

continued

ANNEX TABLE 4-1
Continued

Device	Estimated Cost[a]	Indications/Requirements for Use	
Terminal Devices			
Passive hand	$500[b]	• Used to stabilize objects and for cosmesis	
Body-powered hook	$400–$1,420	• Use of body-powered system	
Single-degree-of-freedom (DOF), body-powered hand	$1,100–$1,500	• Use of body-powered system	
Single-DOF powered hand	$6,800	• Use of myoelectric system	
Multiarticulating hand powered hand	$32,000[b]	• Use of myoelectric system	

	Relative Contraindications	Benefits of Device	Limitations of Device
	• Not appropriate if need to grasp objects	• Provides the best cosmetic restoration • Requires no training to use • Can be interchanged with other terminal devices	• Unable to use functionally to grasp objects—very limited in function • Large variability in price between off-the-shelf and custom designs • PVC designs can stain easily, and silicone, while stain-resistant, can tear
		• Less expensive than powered systems • Can grasp small objects • Available in multiple materials and grip styles • Allows good visibility of object manipulation	• Nonanthropomorphic
		• Less expensive than powered systems	• More effort required to operate than a body-powered hook • Limited visibility of object manipulation • Limited to a single grasp position—limits use for specific activities that require different hand positions
		• Least expensive powered option	• Limited visibility of object manipulation; makes grasp of smaller objects more challenging • Limited to a single grasp position—limits use for specific activities that require different hand positions
	• Cannot get wet	• More grasp positions—may be used for a wider range of activities • More cosmetic than hook	• Less durable/more prone to breakage • Must be used with a myoelectric or hybrid prosthesis • More expensive • May require more extensive training to use effectively

continued

ANNEX TABLE 4-1
Continued

Device	Estimated Cost[a]	Indications/Requirements for Use
Specialized terminal device: work attachment	$600	• Need for specialized terminal device for specific activities (e.g., holding tools with a specific shape and size)

NOTES:

Transradial body-powered includes codes L6100, L6615, L6660, L6675, L6680, L6687, L7400, L7403, L8415, L8435, and L8485.

Transhumeral body-powered includes codes L6250, L6615, L6620, L6635, L6660, L6665, L6676, L6682, L6688, L7401, L7404, L8415, L8435, and L8485.

Shoulder disarticulation body-powered includes codes L6300, L6615, L6620, L6635, L6641, L6646, L6647, L6660, L6665, L6672, L6684, L6689, L7402, and L7405.

Transradial myoelectric includes codes L6680, L6687, L6686, L6935, L7259, L7368, L7400, and L7403.

Transhumeral myoelectric includes codes L6682, L6688, L6955, L7181, L7259, L7368, L7401, and L7404.

Shoulder disarticulation myoelectric includes codes L6646, L6648, L6684, L6689, L6965, L7181, L7259, L7368, L7402, and L7405.

Transhumeral hybrid includes codes L6638, L6693, L6655, L6675, L6682, L6688, L6955, L7368, L7401, and L7404.

Shoulder disarticulation hybrid includes codes L6638, L6646, L6648, L6693, L6655, L6675, L6684, L6689, L6965, L7259, L7368, L7402, and L7405.

Passive hand includes codes L6703 and L6890.

Body-powered hook includes codes L6706 (low) and L6707 (high).

Body-powered hand includes codes L6708 (low) and L6709 (high) and L6890.

Sports/recreation/work attachment device includes code L6704.

Myoelectric hand (low) includes codes L6629, L6890, L7007, and L6882.

Myoelectric hand (high) includes codes L6621, L6629, L6890, L6880, L6881, and L6882.

[a]Estimated costs for devices include the base code and associated codes to create an example full system, excluding the terminal device (hook or hand). Codes shown are meant to be representative of a general estimate of billing for the upper-limb prosthesis design types and are not meant to be specific billing recommendations. Prices are based on the January 2015 Centers for Medicare & Medicaid Services (CMS) fee schedule for Illinois. Prices in the table have been rounded to the nearest $100.

[b]Any unlisted codes that might be suggested for a product (for example, advanced myoelectric devices, custom silicone gloves) are not included in these estimates.

	Relative Contraindications	Benefits of Device	Limitations of Device
		• Tailored grasp positions for specific activities • Can be more durable than multiarticulating hands • Can be water-resistant	• Less cosmetic • Often needs to be interchanged with other terminal devices to accomplish the broad range of activities people need to do

ANNEX TABLE 4-2
Ability of Upper-Limb Prosthetic Devices to Mitigate the Effects of Impairment

	Body-Powered		
	TR	TH	Shoulder
Sensation			
Proprioception	No	No	No
Touch function	No	No	No
Passive Range of Motion			
Fingers	Partial	Partial	Partial
Thumb	No	No	No
Wrist ulnar/radial deviation	No	No	No
Wrist flexion/extension	Var/partial	Var/partial	Var/partial
Wrist pronation/supination	Variable	Variable	Variable
Elbow flexion/extension	NA	Variable	Variable
Shoulder flexion/extension	NA	NA	Var/partial
Shoulder abduction/adduction	NA	NA	Var/partial
Shoulder rotation	NA	NA	Variable
Shoulder horizontal ad/abduction	NA	NA	Var/partial
Active Range of Motion			
Fingers	Partial	Partial	Partial
Thumb	No	No	No
Wrist ulnar/radial deviation	No	No	No
Wrist flexion/extension	No	No	No
Wrist pronation/supination	Var/Yes	NA	NA
Elbow flexion/extension	NA	Variable	No
Shoulder flexion/extension	NA	NA	No
Shoulder abduction/adduction	NA	NA	No
Shoulder rotation	NA	NA	No
Shoulder horizontal ad/abduction	NA	NA	No

	Myoelectric				Hybrid	
	TR	TH	Shoulder		TH	Shoulder
	No	No	No		No	No
	No	No	No		No	No
	Var/partial	Var/partial	Var/partial		Var/partial	Var/partial
	Var/partial	Var/partial	Var/partial		Var/partial	Var/partial
	No	No	No		No	No
	Var/partial	Var/partial	Var/partial		Var/partial	Var/partial
	Variable	Variable	Variable		Variable	Variable
	NA	Partial	Variable		Variable	Variable
	NA	NA	Var/partial		NA	Variable
	NA	NA	Var/partial		NA	Variable
	NA	NA	Variable		NA	Variable
	NA	NA	Var/partial		NA	Var/partial
	No	No	No		No	No
	No	No	No		No	No
	Var/Yes	Var/Yes	Var/Yes		Var/Yes	Var/Yes
	NA	Yes	Yes		No	No
	NA	NA	No		NA	No
	NA	NA	No		NA	No
	NA	NA	No		NA	No
	NA	NA	No		NA	No

continued

ANNEX TABLE 4-2
Continued

	Body-Powered		
	TR	TH	Shoulder
Activities			
Grasp	Partial	Partial	Partial
Fine motor use	Partial	Partial	Partial
Dexterous activities	Partial	Partial	Partial
Handling objects	Partial	Partial	Partial
Lifting <20 pounds	Partial	Partial	Partial
Lifting >20 pounds	Partial	Partial	Partial
Carrying <20 pounds	Partial	Partial	Partial
Carrying >20 pounds	Partial	Partial	Partial
Reaching forward	Variable	Partial	Partial
Overhead reaching	Var/partial	Var/partial	Var/partial
Considerations			
Indications	• Skin integrity that allows socket wear and harness use		
Contraindications	• Limited shoulder range of motion/strength or shoulder pain may limit use of harness		
Clinical expertise/training	• Needs trained prosthetist and occupational therapist to help patient learn to use effectively		
Limitations	• Socket style for some transradial-level amputees may limit elbow range of motion • Socket style and harnessing may limit shoulder range of motion in shoulder level amputees. • Weight limitations—lifting and carrying activities depend on the positioning of the object in relation to the body		

NOTE: NA = not applicable; TH = transhumeral; TR = transradial; Var = Variable.

	Myoelectric				Hybrid	
	TR	TH	Shoulder		TH	Shoulder
	Partial	Partial	Partial		Partial	Partial
	Partial	Partial	Partial		Partial	Partial
	Partial	Partial	Partial		Partial	Partial
	Partial	Partial	Partial		Partial	Partial
	Partial	Partial	Partial		Partial	Partial
	Var/partial	Var/partial	Var/partial		No	No
	Partial	Partial	Partial		Partial	Partial
	Var/partial	Var/partial	Var/partial		Var/partial	Var/partial
	Partial	Partial	Partial		Partial	Partial
	Partial	Partial	Partial		Partial	No
	• Skin integrity that allows socket wear • Requires active myosites • Most unable to control terminal device and any other movement simultaneously				• Skin integrity that allows socket wear • Requires active myosites	
	• Cannot get wet				• Limited shoulder range of motion/strength or shoulder pain may limit use of harness • Cannot get wet	
	• Needs trained prosthetist and occupational therapist to help patient learn to use effectively				• Needs trained prosthetist and occupational therapist to help patient learn to use effectively	
	• May function inconsistently as a result of excessive sweating, change in limb volume • Must have consistent access to electricity				• May function inconsistently as a result of excessive sweating, change in limb volume	

5

Selected Hearing Technologies[1]

This chapter provides an overview of assistive products and technologies that mitigate the effects of hearing loss. After briefly reviewing the prevalence and severity of hearing loss and the extent of use of hearing aids, the chapter presents a taxonomy of assistive devices for hearing loss. It then turns to clinical considerations in addressing hearing loss. Issues of evaluation and monitoring, training and adaptation, and access to and availability of hearing products and technologies and related services are then examined in turn. The chapter ends with findings and conclusions.

Hearing loss can manifest at any time throughout life or be present from birth. It has two categories of causes: congenital and acquired. Congenital causes lead to hearing loss or deafness at birth or soon after. They include genetic syndromes; maternal rubella, syphilis, or certain other infections during pregnancy; low birth weight; lack of oxygen at birth; and severe jaundice in the neonatal period (birth to 1 month). Almost 50 to 60 percent of childhood hearing loss in developed countries is genetic (Morton and Nance, 2006). Acquired hearing loss can be caused by meningitis, measles and mumps, otosclerosis, chronic ear infections, fluid or infection in the ear (otitis media), tympanic membrane (ear drum) thickening or perforation, some head injuries and other traumas, excessive long-term exposure to noise, cerumen (wax) or foreign bodies blocking the ear canal, or aging (WHO, 2015).

Conditions such as otitis media, ear canal blockage, and some forms

[1]Sections of this chapter draw heavily on a recent report titled *Hearing Health Care for Adults* (NASEM, 2016).

of otosclerosis can result in conductive hearing loss, which affects the outer or middle ear and is often treated medically or surgically (HLAA, 2017). Other conditions result in sensorineural hearing loss, which affects the inner ear, the auditory nerve, and more central auditory pathways; it is permanent and progressive and typically is not medically or surgically treatable. Therefore, common interventions for sensorineural hearing loss amplify sound and, if possible, improve the audibility of speech and other sounds. These interventions include hearing aids, assistive listening devices, aural rehabilitation services, and training to improve communication and coping strategies.

Age-related hearing loss, or presbycusis, is characterized by increased hearing thresholds (i.e., poorer ability to detect low-level sounds); impaired suprathreshold processing of higher-level sounds (including reduced frequency and temporal resolution); and impaired ability to understand speech, especially in noisy or complex listening environments (Yamasoba et al., 2013). Although the primary pathology of the process is unknown, it involves both intrinsic and extrinsic factors such as genetic mutations, degeneration of cellular structures in the cochlear lateral wall, age-related loss of auditory nerve fibers, and a lifetime of environmental exposures (especially to noise and ototoxic drugs) (Yamasoba et al., 2013). These factors affect the "ability of the inner ear and higher neural centers to process acoustic signals and effectively separate the primary speech signal from interfering speech and noise" (NASEM, 2016, p. 22). The functional consequences, regardless of which auditory pathways are affected, can include inability to hear low-level sounds, particularly high-frequency sounds; inability to understand subtle differences in spoken words (e.g., "I'll see you Sunday" versus "I'll see you someday"), especially in noisy environments; poorer ability to process acoustic information quickly relative to younger individuals; and difficulty identifying sources of sound (Roth, 2015; Yamasoba et al., 2013). There is no single etiologic pathway for age-related hearing loss since various factors influence its age of onset and severity. Individuals usually have symmetrical loss that is more apparent with high-frequency sounds and commonly more severe in men than in women (van Eyken et al., 2007).

OVERVIEW OF PREVALENCE AND SEVERITY OF HEARING LOSS AND USE OF HEARING AIDS

Prevalence

According to data from the National Health and Nutrition Examination Survey (NHANES), hearing loss is highly prevalent with aging. As shown in Figure 5-1, the prevalence of hearing loss rises with age from 0.3 percent

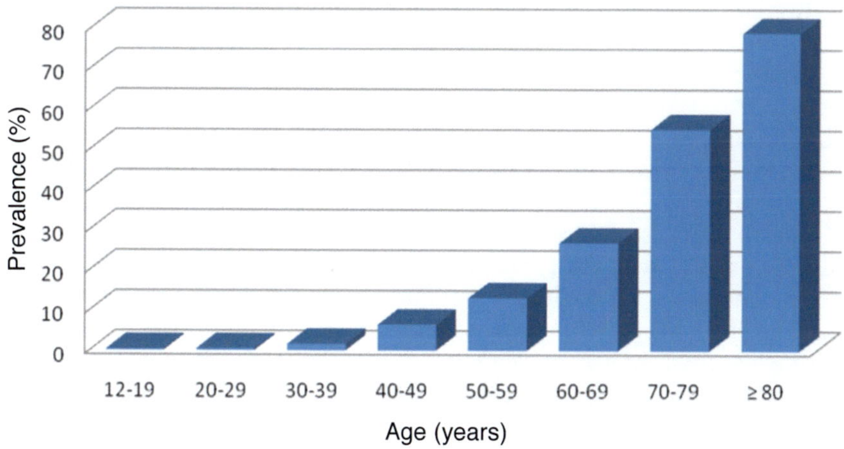

FIGURE 5-1 Prevalence of hearing loss in the United States by age, 2001-2008.
NOTE: Hearing loss is defined by a pure tone average (PTA) of 0.5-4 kHz thresholds in the better-hearing ear of greater than 25 dB.
SOURCE: Data from Lin et al., 2011d.

among those aged 12 to 19 to 79 percent among those aged 80 and older (Lin et al., 2011d). True population prevalence is likely underestimated because NHANES does not include data on individuals in assisted care facilities, group homes, or nursing homes or on individuals who were unable to come to the mobile examination center. NHANES data also show that 30 million individuals who are 12 and older have bilateral hearing loss, while 48 million have poor hearing in at least one ear (Lin et al., 2011d).

In the Epidemiology of Hearing Loss Study cohort, conductive hearing loss was present in 8 percent of participants; 0.2 percent had a history of otosclerosis (an uncommon but disabling form of hereditary hearing loss that can be aggravated by pregnancy, becomes disabling in midlife, and in older age is functionally complicated by presbycusis); and 1.9 percent reported the onset of the impairment before age 20 (Cruickshanks et al., 1998). Most participants with hearing loss had bilateral symmetrical loss, which is consistent with sensorineural hearing loss acquired in adulthood being the predominant type among adults.

Severity

Studies generally use a clinically significant cut point for defining hearing loss, which includes any hearing loss that is mild or greater (i.e., above

25 dB). However, the severity of the loss is a critical factor affecting the extent of its impact on communicative functioning and potential working capacity. Adults with a mild hearing loss, for example, may note only occasional communication problems in settings with background noise, while those with a severe to profound hearing loss may have trouble even in face-to-face conversation in a quiet room. The standardized prevalence of hearing loss by severity in individuals aged 12 and older is reported by Goman and Lin (2016) based on NHANES data from 2001 to 2010. Table 5-1 shows that most individuals with hearing loss had a mild loss, with moderate or greater losses becoming more prevalent with increasing age. The Blue Mountains Hearing Study also found that the severity of hearing loss increased with age (Mitchell et al., 2011), but again, the most common level of loss was mild, in this case until the oldest age group of 85 and above (Mitchell et al., 2011).

Extent of Hearing Aid Use

Compared with the prevalence of hearing loss in the United States, the prevalence of hearing aid use is low (see Table 5-2). In NHANES, 1999-2006, audiological testing was conducted in a sample of participants aged 50 to 69 from 1999 to 2004 and was conducted in all participants aged 70 and older in 2005. Using these data, Chien and Lin (2012) found that approximately 3.8 million, or 14.2 percent, of individuals in the United States who had hearing loss wore hearing aids (see Table 5-2). An earlier study (Lin et al., 2011c) found a strong relationship between hearing aid use and severity of hearing loss: 3 percent of those with mild loss, 40 percent of those with moderate loss, and 77 percent of those with severe loss wore a hearing aid regularly (Lin et al., 2011c). Other variables, such as college education and exposure to leisure noise, but not race/ethnicity, age, sex, or income, were significantly associated with hearing aid use (Lin et al., 2011c).

In the Epidemiology of Hearing Loss Study, current hearing aid use was 14.6 percent among individuals with hearing loss, while former use was 6 percent (Popelka et al., 1998). Current use was 33 percent among participants reporting significant communication problems and handicaps[2] and 32 percent among those with moderate to severe loss (Popelka et al., 1998). Hearing aid use was associated with factors that included severity of hearing loss, older age, college education, poor performance on word recognition tests, and self-reported hearing loss and handicap. Similar low use of hearing aids was seen in the adult children of participants in the

[2]Significant communication problems and handicaps refer to a Hearing Handicap Inventory for the Elderly (screening version) score greater than 8 (Popelka et al., 1998).

Epidemiology of Hearing Loss Study: 4 percent for those with mild loss and 23 percent for those with moderate to severe loss (Nash et al., 2013).

Although NHANES data demonstrate no differences in hearing aid use by race/ethnicity, this may be due to the low number of Hispanics/Latinos enrolled in the study (Nieman et al., 2016). Among those Hispanics/Latinos that were enrolled, hearing aid use was less than 10 percent (Lee et al., 1991). Even among individuals in the study with hearing loss more severe than mild (pure tone average greater than 40 dB), hearing aid use was low, at 5 percent among men and 11 percent among women.

TAXONOMY

Treatment for hearing loss includes hearing products and technologies (described below)[3] and auditory rehabilitation and counseling. The products and technologies differ based on various factors, including type of hearing loss, unique needs in daily life, personal preferences, and financial means.

Hearing Aids

Hearing aids are defined by the U.S. Food and Drug Administration (FDA) as "any wearable instrument or device designed for, offered for the purpose of, or represented as aiding persons with or compensating for, impaired hearing."[4] Components of hearing aids include the microphone, analog-to-digital converter, digital sound processor, output transducer, and battery. Unlike glasses that can correct vision loss, current hearing aids cannot correct or restore normal hearing. Instead, they improve the audibility of soft sounds such as speech or music and ensure that other audible sounds do not interfere by becoming too loud. Customizing hearing aids to suit users' needs is important. Greater satisfaction has routinely been documented in users whose hearing aids are fitted with real-ear probe microphone measurements and speech mapping as part of the fitting process (Cox and Alexander, 1999; Kochkin, 2009; Valente et al., 2006). Additionally, fewer postfitting adjustments are needed for patients whose fitting includes loudness scaling and speech-in-noise testing (Shi et al., 2007). Multiple studies have assessed the benefit of one versus two hearing aids and have found a preference for using two (Cox et al., 2011; Most et al., 2012; Noble and Gatehouse, 2006).

---

[3]Medical and surgical treatments (such as cochlear implants), as well as auditory rehabilitation and counseling, were not included in the statement of task for this study (see Box 1-1 in Chapter 1).

[4]21 CFR § 801.420.

TABLE 5-1
Prevalence of and Numbers of Individuals with Hearing Loss, by Age and Severity: National Health and Nutrition Examination Survey, United States, 2001–2010

Hearing Loss Category and Age, y	Prevalence, % (95% CI)					Number With Hearing Loss (Millions)				
	Mild	Moderate	Severe	Profound	Overall	Mild	Moderate	Severe	Profound	Overall
Bilateral[a]										
12–19 y	0.14 (0.04, 0.24)	0.03[b] (0.00, 0.06)	. . .[c]	0.00[b] (0.00, 0.01)	0.18 (0.07, 0.28)	0.05	0.01	. . .[c]	<0.01	0.06
20–29 y	0.34[b] (0.00, 0.88)	0.07[b] (0.00, 0.20)	. . .[c]	. . .[c]	0.42[b] (0.00, 0.97)	0.15	0.03	. . .[c]	. . .[c]	0.18
30–39 y	1.01[b] (0.18, 1.84)	0.55[b] (0.00, 1.21)	0.08[b] (0.00, 0.25)	. . .[c]	1.64 (0.23, 3.06)	0.41	0.23	0.03	. . .[c]	0.68
40–49 y	6.05 (3.71, 8.40)	0.48[b] (0.00, 1.01)	. . .[c]	. . .[c]	6.53 (4.19, 8.88)	2.46	0.20	. . .[c]	. . .[c]	2.65
50–59 y	10.48 (7.34, 13.62)	2.13 (0.79, 3.46)	0.35[b] (0.00, 0.78)	0.34[b] (0.00, 0.99)	13.29 (9.76, 16.81)	4.57	0.93	0.15	0.15	5.80
60–69 y	19.94 (15.03, 24.84)	5.85 (3.53, 8.17)	0.76[b] (0.00, 1.70)	0.25[b] (0.00, 0.75)	26.80 (22.25, 31.35)	6.92	2.03	0.27	0.09	9.31
70–79 y	35.62 (31.03, 40.22)	15.83 (13.63, 18.04)	2.86 (1.60, 4.12)	0.30[b] (0.02, 0.59)	54.62 (49.27, 59.97)	6.84	3.04	0.55	0.06	10.49
≥80 y	36.02 (32.03, 40.01)	37.92 (33.40, 42.44)	6.97 (4.94, 9.01)	0.56[b] (0.01, 1.10)	81.47 (78.12, 84.82)	3.98	4.19	0.77	0.06	9.01
Total						25.39	10.66	1.77	0.35	38.17
Loss in at least 1 ear (unilateral and bilateral)										
12–19 y	1.18 (0.77, 1.59)	0.46 (0.18, 0.74)	0.31 (0.11, 0.51)	0.01[b] (0.00, 0.03)	1.96 (1.39, 2.54)	0.39	0.15	0.10	< 0.01	0.65
20–29 y	2.32 (0.92, 3.72)	0.62[b] (0.00, 1.75)	0.02[b] (0.00, 0.05)	0.26[b] (0.00, 0.65)	3.22 (1.38, 5.07)	1.02	0.28	0.01	0.11	1.42
30–39 y	3.50 (1.91, 5.09)	1.38 (0.15, 2.62)	0.30[b] (0.00, 0.76)	0.25[b] (0.00, 0.63)	5.43 (3.28, 7.58)	1.44	0.57	0.12	0.10	2.23
40–49 y	10.02 (7.41, 12.64)	2.00 (1.01, 3.00)	0.86[b] (0.00, 1.88)	0.06[b] (0.00, 0.19)	12.95 (9.85, 16.04)	4.07	0.81	0.35	0.03	5.25
50–59 y	21.30 (16.57, 26.02)	5.49 (3.35, 7.63)	0.82[b] (0.06, 1.57)	1.08[b] (0.06, 2.10)	28.69 (23.63, 33.74)	9.30	2.40	0.36	0.47	12.52
60–69 y	29.38 (24.46, 34.29)	12.12[b] (8.62, 15.62)	2.06 (0.61, 3.51)	1.30[b] (0.29, 2.31)	44.86 (40.79, 48.92)	10.20	4.21	0.72	0.45	15.58
70–79 y	37.51 (33.10, 41.92)	21.14 (17.88, 24.40)	7.47 (5.75, 9.19)	2.04 (1.06, 3.01)	68.15 (62.78, 73.53)	7.21	4.06	1.43	0.39	13.09
≥80 y	31.42 (26.75, 36.08)	40.83 (36.42, 45.24)	13.80 (11.13, 16.47)	4.24 (2.49, 5.99)	90.29 (87.20, 93.39)	3.47	4.51	1.53	0.47	9.98
Total						37.10	16.99	4.61	2.03	60.73

Note. CI = confidence interval. Hearing loss was defined as a pure-tone average (at 0.5, 1, 2, and 4 kHz) of above 25 dB hearing level. The sample size was n = 9648.
[a]Severity of bilateral loss is based on the better ear.
[b]The unweighted number of individuals in the category is < 10.
[c]No individuals with this hearing loss severity level were observed in the sample.

SOURCE: Goman, A. M., and F. R. Lin. 2016. Prevalence of hearing loss by severity in the United States. *American Journal of Public Health* 106(10):1820-1822. American Public Health Association.

TABLE 5-2
Prevalence of Hearing Aid Use Among Adults with Hearing Loss[a] >25 dB (95% CI)[b]

	Sex		Hearing Loss Severity[c]		Total		
Age, years	Male	Female	Mild (>25–40 dB)	Moderate or Greater >40 dB	Overall Prevalence of Hearing Aid Use	Number with Hearing Aids, millions	Number with Hearing Loss[a] >25 dB, millions
50–59	4.3 (0–9.5)	4.5 (0–13.5)	2.7 (0–6.6)	11.8 (0–27.5)	4.3 (0–8.8)	0.20	4.5
60–69	7.3 (2.5–12.1)	7.2 (1.4–13.0)	2.6 (0–5.2)	23.9 (10.6–37.2)	7.3 (3.6–10.9)	0.44	6.1
70–79	21.1 (14.5–27.6)	12.7 (6.0–19.5)	3.4 (0.3–6.5)	47.8 (37.0–58.6)	17.0 (12.4–21.6)	1.5	8.8
80+	28.1 (20.3–35.9)	17.9 (11.2–24.7)	3.4 (0–7.7)	35.7 (28.7–42.7)	22.1 (18.5–25.8)	1.6	7.3
Estimated total number of individuals with hearing aids and with hearing loss, respectively, in millions					3.8[c]		26.7

NOTE: CI = confidence interval.

[a]Hearing loss defined as a speech-frequency pure tone average (PTA) of hearing thresholds at 0.5, 1, 2, and 4 kHz tones presented by air conduction in the better hearing ear of >25 dB.

[b]All values represent percent prevalence unless otherwise noted.

[c]Numbers do not sum to group total because of rounding.

SOURCE: Data from Chien and Lin, 2012.

Air-conduction hearing aids (discussed further below) capture sound vibrations through one or more microphones. The signal is treated, amplified, and played back through an earphone that is placed in the ear canal (Lorenzi and Chaix, 2016). These conventional hearing aids can be fitted behind the ear, in the ear, or in the ear canal. These various placements provide different levels of visibility and ease of control as well as different features (*Consumer Reports*, 2015; NIDCD, 2013).

Adults with mild to moderate sensorineural hearing loss typically have difficulty understanding speech, especially in noisy environments. When hearing loss is measured using a speech-in-noise task, the results may show that a more beneficial signal-to-noise ratio[5] is required to understand speech for individuals with loss relative to those with normal hearing. The signal-to-noise ratio may be improved when a hearing aid fits well (i.e., is properly programmed) and is capable of improving speech audibility at higher frequencies. In some cases, however, well-fit hearing aids may not improve the signal-to-noise ratio and therefore do not improve speech recognition in noisy environments. In addition to hearing aids, hearing assistive technologies (discussed below) and auditory rehabilitation may be useful for individuals with mild to moderate hearing loss.

Hearing Aid Telecoil and Induction Loop Technologies

Telecoils are small copper coils that are available for a majority of hearing aids but not for all types and models. However, most consumers are unaware of this feature or the fact that it can be added[6] (HLAA, 2016). Telecoils also can help in enhancing the performance of wired and wireless telephones.

Hearing induction loop technology[7] consists of a telecoil in a hearing aid or neck loop receiver and earphones connecting wirelessly to a room's sound system, which eliminates background noise and improves clarity of sound. The hearing loop, which is connected to the room's sound system, is wired around the perimeter of the room. The telecoil in the hearing aid or the receiver transmits electromagnetic signals from the sound system.

---

[5]Signal-to-noise ratio measures the signal strength relative to background noise (Rouse, 2016).

[6]According to the *Consumer's Guide to Hearing Aids* (HLAA, 2016), telecoils are available as a standard or an additional feature for a majority of hearing aids.

[7]Further discussion of hearing induction loop technology is not provided since this technology is beyond the scope of the committee's statement of task.

Hearing Assistive Technologies Beyond Hearing Aids

A variety of hearing assistive technologies beyond hearing aids can help individuals with hearing loss—particularly those whose loss is moderate to severe—connect to or receive information from communication channels such as a telephone or television or from sound systems in offices, classrooms, theaters, auditoriums, or other public spaces. These technologies range from products for personal and home use to systems made available in public spaces and for larger audiences to meet consumer needs, as well as to comply with requirements of antidiscrimination laws such as the Americans with Disabilities Act (ADA), which was revised in 2010 to include a number of requirements focused on individuals with hearing loss.

Personal Sound Amplification Products

Personal sound amplification products (PSAPs) include a wide range of devices currently classified by the FDA as designed to "amplify environmental sound for non-hearing impaired consumers" (FDA, 2013). Some PSAPs look very similar to hearing aids and may be a suitable amplification tool for those who cannot afford a hearing aid or are seeking a low-cost introduction to amplification. However, PSAPs are not meant to compensate for hearing impairment.

Wireless Connectivity in Hearing Aids

Wireless connectivity in hearing aids mitigates many communication issues through use of a remote microphone. When a speaker wears a remote microphone, background noise levels typically remain well below the signal of interest, the sources of reverberation are reduced, and the integrity of high-frequency speech sounds is maintained to a greater extent. Listening can thereby be enhanced in both quiet environments and those with background noise, in distance listening, and in listening to media (e.g., television, videos, music). Wireless connectivity systems are designed to work in conjunction with hearing aids. The systems are proprietary and require programming by an audiologist to ensure that they are recognized by hearing aids. They utilize a microphone and an auxiliary piece, often worn around the neck, to stream the sound from the external source to the user's hearing aid(s). Although not available from all hearing aid manufacturers at present, direct to hearing aid couplings are becoming more readily available.

Frequency-Modulated and Infrared Technologies

Radio signals are used to transmit sound from a speaker's microphone or other sound system in frequency modulated (FM) systems. FM may also be referred to as digital modulation (DM). Wireless FM transmissions can be processed by some hearing aids. In other cases, the user wears a receiver that is connected to earphones or a neck loop that converts the transmission to an electromagnetic signal that can be picked up by the telecoil in the user's hearing aid (ASHA, 2017b; Chisolm et al., 2007; Kim and Kim, 2014). FM/DM systems are beneficial in one-to-one communication in noisy environments. They are also used in large gathering places such as theaters, museums, and auditoriums and can be used to transmit sound from radio, television, and other sources (ASHA, 2017b). When radio signals penetrate the walls of a room, mixed signals can result unless different frequencies are used. Although performance varies among users, FM/DM systems can help with better hearing in an environment with background noise (Thibodeau, 2014).

Infrared technologies entail using infrared light waves that must be transmitted via line of sight. Like FM systems, they may transmit to either a receiver and headphones or a neck loop and hearing aid telecoil. While infrared systems can contain the signal in a room and are subject to less interference from other signals relative to FM systems, they have a drawback in that the light waves they transmit can compete with natural light (Holmes et al., 2000; Kim and Kim, 2014).

Hard-Wired Microphone Systems

Some very basic microphone systems whose components are tethered together limit the user to a range of about 4 to 6 feet from the speaker and provide limited amplification of a speaker's voice. These generic systems are not coupled to the user's hearing aid(s). Despite their limitations, they are low-cost and easy-to-use systems that can be purchased from a hearing health care provider or at a consumer electronic venue and can be a suitable solution for some listening situations.

Captioning

Captioning, which can be done either on-site or remotely, involves converting discussions or programming into text that is displayed on a screen. It is usually provided for live events, such as sports events in real time, and can be projected through television and other media, through a website, or directly onto a screen visible in the location of the event. In 1993, the ADA required closed captioning for the auditory portion of programs

BOX 5-1
Hearing Technologies

Hearing Aids: "Any wearable instrument or device designed for, offered for the purpose of, or represented as aiding persons with or compensating for, impaired hearing" (21 CFR § 801.420).

Hearing Assistive Technologies: "Encompasses a wide range of products—from traditional hearing aids regulated as medical devices to consumer-technology products and hearing assistive technologies—with the overall goal of enabling the user to hear and communicate better in their homes (e.g., television), in public spaces (e.g., movies and lectures), and through phones or other communications products and systems" (NASEM, 2016, p. 149).

Personal Sound Amplification Products: Personal sound amplification products include a wide range of devices currently classified by the FDA as designed to "amplify environmental sound for non-hearing impaired consumers" (FDA, 2013).

for all televisions 13 inches or larger (Holmes et al., 2000). Captioning also may be provided for telephones and may be used along with the Telecommunications Relay Service (TRS), discussed below.

Telecommunications Relay Service

The telecommunications relay service (TRS) is "a telephone service that allows persons with hearing or speech disabilities to place and receive telephone calls"[8] (FCC, 2016). The Federal Communications Commission manages the program. The service uses operators, called communication assistants, who facilitate calls for individuals with hearing and speech impairments. To initiate a TRS call, an individual with such an impairment dials 711 using a teletypewriter or other text input device and then gives the communication assistant the number of the individual being called. The communication assistant acts as a link between the two parties by converting text to voice and voice to text. This service also allows individuals with hearing loss to speak directly to the people being called and hear their voice. Captioning in conjunction with TRS may be preferred by users who have some hearing capacity and can use their own voices, whereas people who employ sign language to communicate may prefer video relay technology used along with sign language interpreters.

[8]There is no cost to the user for TRS.

Box 5-1 provides definitions of selected hearing technologies. More detailed information on the features and functionality of these devices is provided in Annex Tables 5-1 and 5-2, respectively, at the end of this chapter.

CLINICAL CONSIDERATIONS

Clinical considerations in addressing hearing loss include the functioning of affected individuals, particularly, in the present context, their functioning at work; the effectiveness of hearing aids and other assistive devices; and factors affecting the success of treatment.

Functioning

The World Health Organization has identified participation in work as one of the major areas of life (WHO, 2001). As the U.S. government increases the age at which an individual becomes eligible for Medicare, a larger number of adults will continue to work at later ages, which in turn will lead to a higher prevalence of hearing impairment in the workplace in the near future. Occupations today rely increasingly on communication skills, which places a greater burden on those suffering from hearing loss. Such issues as unemployment, underemployment, sick leave (due to stress), lower earning potential, and early retirement often are more pervasive among workers with hearing loss relative to their normal-hearing peers.

The U.S. Census Bureau reported an employment rate of 41.1 percent among adults of working age (21-64) with disabilities, compared with 79.1 percent of this age group without disabilities (Brault, 2012). Employment is also low among those who suffer from hearing difficulties (1,837) (Brault, 2012). One study found that hard-of-hearing professionals reported a sense of having lost their competitive edge and having been passed over for promotion or having missed job advancement opportunities as a result of their hearing loss (Tye-Murray et al., 2009). Nachtegaal and colleagues (2012) found a significant association between hearing loss and experiencing limitations in the kind or amount of work that can be performed, with the odds of experiencing such limitations increasing significantly with increases in the decibels of hearing loss. Another study found that sick leave was significantly higher (77 percent) among those with hearing loss relative to those with normal hearing (55 percent) because of "fatigue, strain and burnout" (Kramer et al., 2006). And according to Kochkin (2005), people with severe hearing loss earn $12,000 less per year than those with mild hearing loss.

Jennings and Shaw (2008) argue that the specific implications of hearing loss in the workplace are not fully understood because of the lack of research in this area. They note that the most pertinent experiences of workers with hearing loss on the job are mental distress, fatigue, need for recovery after work, and lack of knowledge and job control. The authors suggest further that, aside from equipment and environmental management (appropriate hearing assistive technology), hard-of-hearing workers would benefit from a more favorable signal-to-noise ratio. Additionally, they assert, it is important for hard-of-hearing workers to gain knowledge of how to disclose their hearing loss, how to educate their coworkers to be supportive, how to become better advocates for themselves, and how to better understand their rights to accommodation under the law.

The workplace is a complex environment. Thus, for a hard-of-hearing employee's abilities and limitations to be assessed and addressed adequately, a multilevel, multidisciplinary, and integrated approach is necessary. With such an approach, functioning and disability are seen as outcomes of interactions between a person's health condition (hearing loss) and contextual factors. As described in Chapter 2, contextual factors are both environmental (room acoustics, noise levels, colleagues, tasks, schedules) and personal (age, cognitive capacity, coping styles, education). In using the *International Classification of Functioning, Disability and Health* (ICF) to determine the goals of a rehabilitation program for someone with hearing loss, it is essential to involve that person, who is the one most qualified to identify the activity limitations and/or participation restrictions to be addressed. In addition, the rehabilitation program, its goals, and the technology to be used to achieve those goals need to be formulated in functional terms specific to the client (Southall et al., 2010).

Studies have examined the links between hearing loss and falls or declines in physical functioning and hospitalization, although more research, particularly longitudinal studies, is needed in this area. Severe hearing loss was found to be associated with increased risk of falls in a study of retired workers (Girard et al., 2014); in cross-sectional data from NHANES (Lin and Ferrucci, 2012); and in observational data from the Health ABC study, which also showed increased risk of frailty (Kamil et al., 2016). Further, in a study examining hospitalization of participants in the Health ABC study, a higher incidence of hospitalization and annual rate of hospitalization were found among those older adults with hearing loss (Genther et al., 2015). Higher rates of decline in physical functioning also were seen in the Health ABC study among participants with hearing loss (Chen et al., 2015).

The longitudinal Blue Mountains Health Study evaluated the effect of hearing impairment on independence and use of support services. At the baseline hearing test visit, a total of 1,457 participants reported no use of community support services, no use of nonspouse family or friend support, or an inability to go out alone. The 5-year incidence analysis showed that all three of these factors increased with age. Nonetheless, the results showed that baseline hearing loss was not significantly associated with the 5-year incidence of these factors. Results also showed, however, that, relative to people with normal hearing, those with moderate to severe hearing loss had a 2.7-fold increased risk of needing help from family and friends, indicating that individuals with these levels of hearing loss may have a greater need for support services relative to those without hearing loss.

Both the Wisconsin Longitudinal Study and the Medical Expenditure Panel Survey examined the impact of hearing on health care using self-reported hearing loss. In the Wisconsin Longitudinal Study, reports of difficulties and delays in accessing health care in the previous year were 1.85 times higher among individuals reporting than among those not reporting hearing loss (Pandhi et al., 2011). Results of the Medical Expenditure Panel Survey showed that individuals with hearing loss had better access to health care relative to those with other disabilities who experienced higher unmet needs due to environmental barriers (Horner-Johnson et al., 2014). Although several studies have reported longitudinal associations between hearing and mortality risk (Contrera et al., 2015; Fischer et al., 2014; Genther et al., 2015; Gopinath et al., 2013; Wahl et al., 2013), most have shown no association after controlling for confounding factors (Contrera et al., 2015; Genther et al., 2015; Wahl et al., 2013).

Effectiveness of Hearing Aids and Other Assistive Devices

More peer-reviewed studies have focused on the impact of hearing aid use among children relative to adults with hearing loss. As noted by Mäki-Torkko and colleagues (2001, p. 8), "only a few studies on hearing aid outcomes meet strict scientific criteria and even fewer studies correlate rehabilitation outcome with the degree of hearing impairment disability or handicap." Although studies have examined the use of hearing aids and owners' satisfaction with and barriers to their use, outcome measures used to assess the efficacy and effectiveness of hearing aids vary widely.

Studies of the effectiveness of hearing aids are primarily experimental studies examining the impact of specific technical aspects or components of the device using small numbers of study subjects; many have been focused on the technical rather than on the clinical or functional outcomes associated with hearing loss (Humes and Krull, 2012). There has been only one true randomized controlled trial of hearing loss treatment examining outcomes beyond measures of speech perception (Mulrow et al., 1990). This trial, which was conducted more than two decades ago, randomized 192 veterans into two groups: one with treatment (provision of a single monaural analog hearing aid) and one without. The results showed improved social and emotional function, communicative abilities, and cognitive function among the treatment group (Mulrow et al., 1990). These results, however, were not confirmed in a trial with a larger representative cohort that used more current hearing rehabilitative strategies (e.g., digital hearing aids) and evaluated cognitive and other functional outcomes comprehensively with longer follow-up periods.

Some observational epidemiological studies have examined the association of hearing aid use with functional outcomes, but the results of these studies are difficult to interpret. For example, most studies have demonstrated a trend toward a positive association between self-reported hearing aid use and cognitive functioning, yet these studies have not yielded data on other key variables (e.g., years of hearing aid use, adequacy of hearing aid fitting and rehabilitation) that would affect the success of hearing loss treatment, as well as any observed associations (Amieva et al., 2015; Dawes et al., 2015; Lin, 2011; Lin et al., 2011a,b, 2013). It is important, moreover, to interpret results of observational studies with caution because individuals who use a hearing aid differ significantly from those who do not with respect to both measured and unmeasured factors. Therefore, a randomized controlled trial would help determine whether hearing rehabilitative strategies can affect functional outcomes.

Most prior studies of the efficacy/effectiveness of hearing aids have focused on speech or other audiologic outcomes and have compared the results for different hearing aids rather than hearing aids versus placebo or no treatment. These studies often have compared different versions of a technology, such as directional and omnidirectional microphones (e.g., Gnewikow et al., 2009; Hawkins and Yacullo, 1984; Keidser et al., 2013; Wu et al., 2013), multimemory and volume controls (e.g., Banerjee, 2011), noise reduction technologies (e.g., Oeding and Valente, 2013), and various types of circuits and compression options (e.g., Hawkins and Naidoo, 1993; Kokx-Ryan et al., 2015; Moore et al., 2001; Shanks et al., 2002).

Only a few studies of hearing aids have used control groups or randomized methods. As noted by van Vliet (2005, p. 416), "Peer-reviewed publications describing performance of various techniques and hearing aid circuits are available, but high-quality evidence about what works for patients in the form of randomized, blinded studies designed to answer critical questions about candidacy for hearing aids, hearing aid selection, fitting, and rehabilitation are rare." A clinical trial conducted by the U.S. Department of Veterans Affairs (VA) and the National Institute on Deafness and Other Communication Disorders examined the benefits of hearing aids among 360 participants with sensorineural hearing loss. The participants were randomized to examine three hearing aid circuits that made up 70 percent of the U.S. hearing aid market at the time of the study (Larson et al., 2000; Noffsinger et al., 2002; Shanks et al., 2002). Each circuit was used for 3 months, and in this double-blinded study using six sequences of circuits, the major outcomes examined were loudness, noise interference, and overall quality. Some outcome measures included speech recognition tests, perceived sound quality, and self-reported assessment of benefit.

Participants using all three circuits reported considerable benefits and only "small differences" in loudness and distortion of sounds.

In a study by Yueh and colleagues (2001), 30 veterans with service-related hearing loss who were eligible to receive a hearing aid were randomly assigned to receive either a programmable hearing aid with a directional microphone or a nonprogrammable aid. Hearing-related quality of life was measured among these veterans as well as among 30 veterans with non-service-connected hearing loss who either did not have a hearing aid or received an assistive listening device. Results showed highest scores on measures of hearing-related quality of life among individuals using the programmable hearing aid, followed by the nonprogrammable aid, the assistive listening device, and finally no hearing device.

In a randomized crossover trial, Cox and colleagues (2014) examined speech understanding among 25 participants (with bilateral mild to moderate sensorineural hearing loss) who used four types of hearing aids (two basic and two premium level). Participants, who included both new and experienced hearing aid users, used each type of hearing aid for 1 month and then completed laboratory speech understanding tests, responded to standardized questionnaires, and recorded journal entries on their experiences with the hearing aids during the month. The study results showed benefits associated with all four types of hearing aids, with experienced users reporting greater benefits (Cox et al., 2014). No statistically significant differences in speech understanding were found between the premium and the basic hearing aids.

Some studies have examined hearing aid use longitudinally (Humes and Wilson, 2003; Humes et al., 2002; Turner et al., 1996). Contrary to what might be expected, these studies have produced no consistent evidence that users of hearing aids grow used to them over time and come to better understand amplified speech.

Factors Affecting the Success of Treatment

Myriad factors affect the success of hearing rehabilitative treatment in enhancing the functional capabilities of individuals with hearing loss. Among these factors are the extent of hearing loss; the type of hearing loss (sensorineural, conductive, or mixed); and the individual's word recognition abilities, processing speed, and ability to process speech in more complex listening environments (such as those that are noisy) (Gatehouse et al., 2003). These factors likely are best understood within the context of the ICF model. For example, the severity and duration of an individual's hearing loss (characterized by the structure/function of the cochlea and peripheral auditory system) and his or her intrinsic cognitive resources and auditory processing abilities will affect that person's hearing and communicative abilities (Gatehouse et al., 2003; Humes et al., 2006). Similarly, a person's functional abilities will be affected by environmental factors such as the listening environment at work/home, the communicative behaviors of other people, and the type of hearing aid or other assistive listening devices the individual is using. Finally, personal factors, such as an individual's willingness to utilize hearing rehabilitative strategies, also will greatly affect the benefit of any type of treatment and the person's resulting functional abilities. Therefore, assessment of an individual's lifestyle/job functions in conjunction with objective and subjective testing can help in determining which devices(s) will yield the greatest benefit for that person.

There are many reasons why people may not wear their hearing aids successfully after being fitted with them. First, users may have issues with the devices related to wearing or handling them and to their effectiveness. Moreover, a significant reason people do not use their hearing aids relates to their value for understanding speech (McCormack and Fortnum, 2013). The success of assistive listening technology varies with the listening situation. In almost all instances, users will benefit from some type of assistive technology in one-on-one communication in a quiet environment. Hearing aids, remote microphone technology, and PSAPs generally are used most successfully when the listener is in close proximity to the speaker, has no other auditory distractions, and can utilize speech reading (Mueller et al., 2006; Nilsson et al., 1992). Thus, small-group discussions in quiet environments utilizing properly programmed hearing aids will likely be beneficial for most users, and the more distance and background noise that are introduced, the less likely the user will have a favorable listening experience.

EVALUATION AND MONITORING

Given that hearing loss can make communication difficult, effective communication is especially important in health care settings to ensure patient safety and enable a person-centered approach (Middleton et al., 2010). Since performing hearing tests usually is not routine during primary care visits, the individual or family is responsible for recognizing symptoms of hearing loss and seeking treatment. Efforts to improve hearing health literacy are ongoing.

Individuals may seek audiological services and a hearing evaluation for several reasons: because of their own concerns, referral resulting from a medical evaluation that has revealed indicators of poor hearing, the advice of a family member or friend, or in the context of routine health care. An individual also may have congenital hearing loss that is stable or has progressed or may have incurred hearing loss due to injury or illness. Evaluations may vary based on the risk for ear disease. Regardless, any evaluation for hearing loss is focused on determining any impacts on overall functioning and the potential for treatment.

Patient History and Otoscopic Exam

The first step in an evaluation for hearing loss is to gather the person's medical and hearing history, including the duration and extent of the loss; salient past events and circumstances, such as ear infections or pain, a family history of hearing loss, and use of relevant prescription and over-the-counter medications; and any use of treatments for hearing loss. Further information may be gathered to assess the impact of hearing loss on the individual's daily life (see below). The second step is to perform an otoscopic examination "to evaluate the pinna (outer ear), external auditory canal, and tympanic membrane for any conditions that could be contributing to hearing loss or that may require further evaluation and treatment (e.g., cerumen impaction, an abnormality of the tympanic membrane, etc.)" (NASEM, 2016, p. 81). A patient may be referred to a physician for additional evaluation based on the results of these two steps.

Diagnostic Testing

Diagnostic testing for hearing loss includes pure tone, speech, and immittance audiometry.

Pure Tone Audiometry

Pure tone audiometry is a test that "measures the lowest intensity level at which an individual can detect calibrated pure tones at specific frequencies between 250–8,000 Hertz" (NASEM, 2016, p. 82). The "threshold" is defined as the intensity level at which the person can detect a calibrated pure tone 50 percent of the time. "Intensity levels are calibrated in decibels (dB) relative to average normal hearing (dB hearing level or dB HL) and can range from –10 dB HL to 120 dB HL" (NASEM, 2016, p. 82). Normal limits for pure tone thresholds are between –10 dB HL and 20 dB HL.

Pure tones can be delivered through headphones or delivered to the skull using a bone oscillator. When headphones are used, pure tones are delivered to each of the ears individually; the sound travels through each ear canal and middle ear to the cochlea within the inner ear (termed "air-conduction" hearing). When pure tones are delivered to the skull using a bone oscillator, the sound passes through the skull directly, stimulating the cochlea and bypassing the ear canal and middle ear ("bone-conduction" hearing). The practitioner conducting the test can draw conclusions about the nature of the hearing loss by looking at the patterns of air-conduction or bone-conduction thresholds, with the former thresholds being higher than the latter. A conductive hearing loss is the result of damage to or disease of the ear canal, eardrum, or middle ear, while a sensorineural hearing loss is identified when air-conduction and bone-conduction thresholds are similar but fall outside the limits of normal hearing.

Speech Audiometry

In a speech audiometry test, two-syllable words are transmitted to each ear individually through headphones to determine the speech recognition threshold—the lowest intensity level at which the person can repeat 50 percent of the words correctly. Some tests simulate quiet and/or noisy environments to help determine the individual's function needs and assess the potential benefits of amplification devices. If an individual shows disproportionately poor speech recognition relative to his or her thresholds for pure tones, changes to the function of the cochlea, auditory vestibular nerve, brainstem, or central processing may be suspected. While speech testing can guide a clinician in the development of a rehabilitation plan, there can be many variables that prevent speech testing from being an objective way of demonstrating the overall benefit that one can achieve from wearing hearing aids. These include variations in the measurement conditions (speech level, background noise level) as well as patient variability (hearing thresholds) and the available gain of the hearing aid at each frequency. Establishing objective measures of real-world communicative functioning is vital to promoting a better understanding of the effects of audiometric hearing function and hearing devices on real-world communicative function.

Immittance Audiometry

Immittance audiometry, also known as "acoustic impedance" or "admittance" testing, includes tympanometry and assessments of the acoustic reflex threshold. These tests are used to establish middle ear pressure and to estimate the transfer of acoustic energy through the middle ear system, which can help differentiate among different disorders.

Assessment of Communicative Function

During a functional communication assessment, an individual's hearing- and communication-related audiologic and nonaudiologic needs are defined, the impact of hearing loss on the individual and his or her communication partners (e.g., family) is established, and the services and technologies that can benefit the individual are determined (ASHA, 2017d; Valente et al., 2006). The use of technologies and/or rehabilitation to manage hearing difficulties may be beneficial and sufficient when a strong relationship exists between measured hearing impairment and reported hearing and communication difficulties. When such a relationship does not exist, on the other hand, other considerations come into play, such as the individual's environment, the people with whom the person interacts and how those people behave, as well as such personal factors as intellectual capacity and psychological state. These factors accord with the biopsychosocial model of the ICF as well as the framework of environmental facilitators described in Chapter 2.

In relation to the ICF framework, audiological testing identifies the impairment aspect of auditory function. Accordingly, it is important for audiologists to be aware of hearing difficulties that occur in situations that do not involve communication—for example, when attempting to locate sounds or recognizing the sound of a nearby event, such as a coin falling on the floor. It is also important to note that, because of variations in people's auditory environments, it can be difficult to evaluate an individual's ability to understand conversation in various settings and at various levels of intensity.

Finally, individuals with functional consequences from hearing loss usually have a chronic problem that is unlikely to improve spontaneously or through medical or surgical treatments. Thus, the goal of treatment is to maximize the capacity that remains to an individual.

Use of Results

The results of an audiological evaluation should be used to address the following:

- whether the individual's hearing loss is due to a medical condition that requires care
- whether the hearing loss is great enough to interfere with the individual's functioning and, if so, whether the person's complaints are traceable to the deficit
- whether psychosocial factors can explain any mismatch between the individual's complaints and his or her measured hearing loss and, if so, whether further evaluation or referral is necessary
- if there is no such mismatch, what treatment approach (e.g., technologies, rehabilitation) will best maximize the person's functioning
- if the person's hearing impairment is not of sufficient magnitude to indicate disease or compromise full functioning, whether there is a risk of that occurring in the future and, if so, whether there are ways to mitigate that risk

Such information can help drive the individualized audiological treatment plan. Some of these questions can be deferred to a referring physician after the audiological evaluation is performed. Although most of the traditional tests for auditory function focus on the diagnosis of disease, the same set of tests can be used to evaluate both the possibility of disease and the effects of hearing loss on function. Additional tests, such as otoacoustic emissions tests and tests for characterization of tinnitus, can be administered to distinguish among more complex forms of otologic disease or auditory dysfunction.

TRAINING AND ADAPTATION

As emphasized throughout this report with respect to all of the disabilities considered and as reflected in the ICF model, the impact of hearing loss depends on multiple factors, such as the individual's lifestyle, interactions with others, and environments. Therefore, two individuals with the same degree of hearing loss can report different difficulties. In addition, an individual's personality, coping style, resiliency, and duration of hearing loss may all play a role in how that person perceives his or her hearing abilities. Adaptation to hearing aid use also depends on many factors, such as degree of hearing loss, age and personality of the user, duration of the loss, and performance of the hearing aid (Brooks, 1996). These complex factors and interactions highlight the need for a personalized approach to treatment for hearing loss.

Selection, Fitting, Maintenance, and Use of Hearing Products and Technologies

Users of hearing products and technologies receive services that most commonly include the provision of and assistance with the use of hearing aids, consisting of device selection, fitting, verification, and validation, within the context of the functional communication assessment.[9,10] According to U.S. best practices in audiology, selection of a hearing aid is based on "an individual's needs and requirements for hearing aid gain, ear canal geometry, occlusion, special features (e.g., directional microphone, noise reduction circuit, feedback suppression, telecoil), ease of insertion and manipulating volume controls, and cosmetics" (NASEM, 2016, p. 85). Gain processing is initially determined by means of validated prescriptive

[9]Refer to ASHA (2017d) and Valente et al. (2006) for best practice guidelines for audiologic management of hearing loss in adults.

[10]Refer to Oh and Lee (2016) for a review of hearing aid fitting management across worldwide guidelines.

procedures, such as those developed by the National Acoustics Laboratories (Byrne and Dillon, 1986; Byrne et al., 2001; Johnson and Dillon, 2011; Mueller, 2005). Hearing aid evaluations also "include selection of output limiting and compression features, and consideration of the need for special technologies (e.g., bone-anchored hearing aids, contralateral routing of signal fittings, and middle-ear implants)" (NASEM, 2016, p. 85). The most reliable method for validating that prescriptive gain targets have been achieved is gain verification using a probe microphone ("real-ear" measures) (Abrams et al., 2012; Mueller, 2001).

Next, the provider discusses with the patient how best to operate, maintain, and use the selected device. With respect to the device, the focus is on insertion and removal, the schedule for use, features of the device, how to reduce feedback and change batteries, and maintenance. With respect to the patient, the focus is on establishing goals and expectations, adjusting to amplification, understanding communication strategies, and the possible need for supplementary treatment (e.g., training in speech reading or speech perception). The final step is to formulate a plan for assessing the benefits of the selected device, based on both subjective and objective measures (for examples, see Cox and Alexander, 1995; Cox et al., 2003; Dillon et al., 1997; Ventry and Weinstein, 1982). Follow-up visits also may be necessary to perform more adjustments; to provide further education on the correct operation, maintenance, and usage of the device (Desjardins and Doherty, 2009); and to ensure that the device provides optimal performance and that hearing is stable.

Although health care professionals who treat patients with hearing loss most commonly provide services and support for hearing aids, they may offer similar services for other hearing assistive technologies that they do not dispense. It is important for these professionals to be trained in the full range of such technologies so they can help patients determine which technology is most useful for meeting their needs.

A personalized approach to treatment for hearing loss is important to the user's experience. In a study by Abrams and Kihm (2015), 81 percent of hearing aid users reported satisfaction with their devices. The survey also showed the devices' positive impacts on relationships, work performance, ability to communicate, ability to participate in group activities, and overall quality of life (Abrams and Kihm, 2015). Factors that were barriers to hearing aid adoption included financial constraints, lack of perceived need, and being unaware of where to go to receive an evaluation (Abrams and Kihm, 2015).

User Training/Adaptation to Hearing Rehabilitation

Hearing aids cannot address all of the challenges of living with hearing loss, which include the loss itself, communication difficulties, changes in quality of life, and possible comorbidities. Rather, "hearing loss requires a holistic, individual-centered approach to care that blends both medical and non-medical solutions, such as auditory rehabilitation (also referred to as aural rehabilitation or audiological rehabilitation)" (NASEM, 2016, p. 86). Auditory rehabilitation is intended to help individuals with hearing loss learn how to live with that loss, to provide information on the use of hearing aids and other hearing assistive technologies, to teach strategies for better listening and communication, and in some cases to offer psychosocial support (ASHA, 2017a; Boothroyd, 2010; Sweetow and Palmer, 2005). Auditory rehabilitation programs can take many forms. They can be offered with a group in a community setting or on an individual basis in an audiology clinic; sessions may be led by an audiologist, a speech-language pathologist, or a trained volunteer; and individuals may take part in self-paced, multimedia rehabilitation programs from their homes (Bally and Bakke, 2007). Studies have consistently shown the benefits of group auditory rehabilitation (Hawkins, 2005; Laplante-Levesque et al., 2011; Northern and Beyer, 1999; Preminger, 2011).

ACCESS AND AVAILABILITY

The costs of hearing aids and other nonsurgical approaches to managing hearing loss, as well as related services, generally are not covered by health insurance, although coverage can vary from state to state depending on the insurer. Therefore, these costs most commonly are paid for out of pocket by consumers. The cost of a hearing aid or other assistive device is usually set according to a "bundled" pricing model that includes the cost of professional services in addition to that of the device itself. The price may also include fees for comprehensive assessment of hearing loss and hearing aid candidacy; assessment of communication needs; hearing aid fitting and programming; and other associated services, such as routine maintenance for a defined period of time and accessories. These services assist the user in achieving optimal fit and maximal benefit from the device and in learning strategies for maximizing the quality of communication. Alternatively, in an unbundled or itemized billing model, the prices of each test, device, and service are listed individually. In 2003, the average retail price for a pair of hearing aids was $4,700 (a bundled price including services) (range $3,300 to $6,000) (Strom, 2014). As a result, many adults with hearing loss and without sufficient financial resources or coverage of hearing devices and services do not receive care. While some emerging, less expensive hearing technologies (e.g., PSAPs) are available to consumers, these options vary substantially in quality and the ability to mitigate impairment effectively, and individuals may require additional assistance to utilize them optimally. Coverage of devices and services for individuals with hearing loss under various programs is reviewed below. Also described are the various types of hearing health care personnel.

Social Security Administration

Currently, U.S. Social Security Administration (SSA) disability benefits are available only for profound hearing loss or deafness, not for mild or moderate hearing loss. The loss must be diagnosed by an audiologist, an otolaryngologist, or a licensed physician. The criteria for qualifying for benefits include air-conduction results of 90 dB HL or worse in the better ear, with bone-conduction results of 60 dB HL or poorer in the better ear. Alternatively, one must receive a score poorer than 40 percent correct on word recognition testing. Such hearing loss is generally at a level at which conventional hearing aids cannot fully mitigate communication impairments. Therefore, the current criteria for hearing disability in SSA's *Listing of Impairments* generally reflect a level of hearing loss severity at which amplification with a hearing aid is insufficient to substantially mitigate impairments and restrictions on participation due to hearing loss. Currently, SSA's residual functional capacity assessment for hearing loss may include specific restrictions on the type of work an individual can do because of poor hearing, such as working near or operating hazardous machinery.

Medicare

Original Medicare (also referred to as Medicare Parts A and B) covers costs related to hospital stays and outpatient services and supplies considered medically necessary in diagnosing and treating a disease or condition. A hearing test is covered only if a physician or other health care provider orders the test to diagnose a hearing or balance disorder (CMS, 2016c). Audiologists who conduct this test also can be reimbursed. However, Medicare does not pay for other services they provide to beneficiaries, such as rehabilitation, despite its being within their scope of practice. The Social Security Amendments of 1965[11] specify that Medicare does not provide coverage of hearing aids. Section 1862(a)(7) of the act states, "Notwithstanding any other provision of this title, no payment may be made under part A or part B for any expenses incurred for items or services . . . where such expenses are for . . . hearing aids or examinations

[11]Social Security Amendments of 1965, Public Law 89-97 (July 30, 1965).

therefor." This policy is codified in the regulation at 42 CFR 411.15 (d), which states that hearing aids and examinations for the purpose of prescribing, fitting, or changing hearing aids are excluded from Medicare coverage.

Medicare Advantage

Under Medicare Advantage (also referred to as Medicare Part C), a person who is eligible for original Medicare (Parts A and B) can withdraw from that program and choose a private insurance plan instead. The federal government will then redirect money from what is paid into Medicare to the individual's Medicare Advantage program. Medicare Advantage allows beneficiaries to choose plans that meet their specific needs, such as coverage for hearing health care services and devices or the ability to purchase extra coverage for hearing health care. The number of beneficiaries enrolled in a Medicare Advantage plan has increased since 2004, with approximately 31 percent of Medicare beneficiaries joining such plans in 2015 (Kaiser Family Foundation, 2015).

Medicaid

As of early 2015, only 28 states covered purchases of hearing aids for adult Medicaid beneficiaries (HLAA, 2015). Medicaid coverage varies widely among states, in some cases being very limited. For individuals to be eligible for Medicaid coverage for hearing aids, they are required by states to have an established minimum hearing loss, and many states also require a medical exam in addition to an audiological evaluation to determine whether a hearing aid is medically necessary. However, some states have limitations on the types of hearing aids covered and on the number of aids and accessories that may be received in a given time period, and some impose annual caps on payment and even require prior approval from a physician. Another hurdle can be finding a provider who will accept Medicaid.

The Early and Periodic Screening, Diagnostic, and Treatment Program

The Early and Periodic Screening, Diagnostic, and Treatment (EPSDT) program provides health care services for children enrolled in Medicaid until they turn age 21 (CMS, 2016a). This program requires that each state provide minimum hearing health care services to its beneficiaries that include diagnosis, treatment, and hearing aids. When these beneficiaries turn 21, they transition to the Medicaid program for adults and receive hearing health care benefits provided by the state in which they reside, as described above. In states that do not provide hearing health care benefits to adults, the transition for children aging out of the EPSDT program is very challenging. Another challenge is that children covered under the Children's Health Insurance Program (CHIP)—a benefit program for uninsured individuals under age 19 whose family income is too high for them to enroll in Medicaid—may not be able to enroll in EPSDT since states are not required to extend this program to those covered by CHIP.

Patient Protection and Affordable Care Act

The Patient Protection and Affordable Care Act (ACA) requires individual state marketplace health insurance plans and expanded Medicaid programs to cover 10 "essential health benefits," including "rehabilitative and habilitative services and devices (services and devices to help people with injuries, disabilities, or chronic conditions gain or recover mental and physical skills)" (CMS, 2016b, p. 1). States vary in their interpretations of what constitutes the benefit. The benchmark insurance plans selected by states may not include hearing health care services or hearing aids for adults, and if this is the case, their expanded Medicaid program (if they have one) and the plans offered in their marketplace are not required to do so either. Only 7 of 50 states (Arizona, Hawaii, Nevada, New York, Rhode Island, Texas, and Wisconsin) and the District of Columbia chose benchmark plans that offer this coverage for adults, which varies by state.

Employer-Sponsored and Private Health Insurance

Few private insurance companies cover hearing health care for adults (Andrews, 2012; *Consumer Reports*, 2015). Employer-sponsored plans provide some coverage of hearing health care. Some cover diagnostic and evaluation services; others cover some or all costs of hearing aids; and some offer their employees the option of purchasing hearing health care insurance, similar to optional dental or vision insurance (ASHA, 2017c). By 2014, only three states—Arkansas, New Hampshire, and Rhode Island—mandated that health insurance plans include coverage for hearing aids for adults (ASHA, 2017e). However, self-insured plans are exempt from this mandate. This means that even in the states with mandated coverage, large self-insured companies with thousands of employees need not provide hearing health care coverage. Coverage for hearing aids and other services for adults with hearing loss is provided by some Federal Employee Health Benefits plans, fee-for-service plans, and health maintenance organizations (HMOs) (HLAA, 2008), but the comprehensiveness of the coverage varies among plans.

Benefits for Veterans

TRICARE is a health care program serving members of the military, military retirees, and their families that covers hearing aids and hearing aid services for beneficiaries with hearing loss that meets specific parameters (TRICARE, 2015). VA services and the Retiree At-Cost Hearing Aid Program also offer hearing services that military retirees may be able to access (MAA, 2016; TRICARE, 2015).

For U.S. military veterans, the most prevalent causes of service-related disability are hearing loss and tinnitus, which affect veterans of all ages; this makes audiology one of the most highly utilized services in the VA (Chandler, 2015; VA Office of the Inspector General, 2014). Veterans who are enrolled in the VA health care system receive diagnostic audiology services and hearing aids. Hearing aids provided through the VA cost qualified recipients very little or nothing; in most cases, however, veterans can qualify only if they have a predefined minimum hearing loss that resulted from active military service (Beck, 2015).[12] Veterans also may be eligible for service-connected disability compensation for hearing impairment based on results from unaided pure tone audiometry and unaided speech recognition scores. The amount of disability compensation varies according to the joint results on both of these tests according to the established VA Schedule for Rating Disabilities.[13]

Vocational Rehabilitation Programs

State vocational rehabilitation programs funded under the Rehabilitation Act of 1973[14] are focused on individuals who have a physical or an intellectual disability that prevents them from engaging in part- or full-time employment or postsecondary education. To qualify for the program requires a determination that vocational rehabilitation will help an individual with a disability gain employment or postsecondary education. Once this has been determined, eligible individuals work with a counselor to establish an Individualized Plan for Employment. The Workforce Innovation and Opportunity Act of 2014[15] amended the Rehabilitation Act of 1973 to require that all state agencies operating these programs allocate at least 15 percent of their federal funds to services for those transitioning from secondary education to postsecondary education or employment. An example

[12]38 CFR § 3.385.

[13]38 CFR § 4.87.

[14]Rehabilitation Act of 1973, Public Law 93-112, 93rd Cong. (September 26, 1973).

[15]Workforce Innovation and Opportunity Act, Public Law 113-128, 113th Cong. (July 22, 2014).

of such services is summer programs for students with hearing loss who are transitioning to college.

Vocational rehabilitation services for individuals with hearing loss or deafness include provision of hearing aids and other hearing health care services. These services are administered by the state and funded through the U.S. Department of Education's Rehabilitation Services Administration (U.S. Department of Education, 2016). State vocational rehabilitation agencies use a process termed "order of selection" for services in which the highest priority for benefits is given to clients with the most significant functional limitations, while those with less severe limitations may be placed on a waiting list to receive services. The state decides which functional limitations have the highest priority. People with hearing loss may not be accorded priority since their functional limitation may be seen as less significant than those of other consumers (University of Arkansas Rehabilitation Research and Training Center, 2008).

Hearing Health Care Personnel

There are a variety of providers with whom one can work to treat hearing loss. Insurance coverage for visits to these providers varies. Some insurance providers, for example, will cover an audiologist visit, but others require referral by a primary care physician before they will cover all or part of the cost of a hearing test. There are also some providers who may not be eligible to bill insurance. An overview of the various types of hearing health care personnel is presented below.

Hearing Instrument Specialists

Hearing instrument specialists, also known as hearing aid specialists, "identify individuals with hearing loss, assess their need for hearing aids, dispense hearing aids, and educate patients and their family members about their hearing loss" (NASEM, 2016, p. 76). By law, minimum qualifications for hearing instrument specialists in most states are a high school diploma, a 2-year apprenticeship, and a license to practice. Although licensure requirements vary from state to state, most states require completion of an annual application form and payment of a fee, and some states require certification by the business owner (offered through the National Board for Certification in Hearing Instrument Sciences). According to the U.S. Bureau of Labor Statistics, there are approximately 5,920 hearing instrument specialists in the United States; most are located in large cities (BLS, 2015b).

Audiologists

Audiologists offer services to identify patients with hearing difficulties, assess and diagnose their hearing needs, treat their needs through hearing aid dispensing and/or habilitation, and educate patients and caregivers about hearing loss prevention. Audiologists must obtain a doctor of audiology degree, which usually requires completion of a 4-year program in addition to a bachelor's degree from an accredited institution. Although state licensing requirements for audiologists vary, many states require an advanced degree, a qualifying examination, and supervised experience in a clinical fellowship, as well as ongoing continuing education. The United States currently has approximately 12,070 practicing audiologists; again, most are located in urban areas (BLS, 2015a).

Otolaryngologists

Otolaryngologists (i.e., ear, nose, and throat [ENT] physicians) are "physicians trained in the medical and surgical management and treatment of patients with diseases and disorders of the ear, nose, throat, and related structures of the head and neck" (NASEM, 2016, p. 76). They treat, medically and surgically, conditions of the ear that include hearing loss, ear infections, balance disorders, and tinnitus (American Academy of Otolaryngology-Head and Neck Surgery, 2015). Although there were approximately 10,000 otolaryngologists in the United States in 2009, the number of residents seeking board certification in this field has declined since 2006 (Neuwahl et al., 2012). There are various subspecialties in ENT medicine, not all of these physicians see patients with hearing loss.

Primary Care Providers

Primary care providers may often be the first to assess and diagnose patients with hearing loss, and they may even provide treatment to these patients without referring them to a hearing health care specialist. A primary care provider can treat outer or middle ear infections, identify and discontinue ototoxic medications, and conduct simple hearing screening tests and primary otologic examinations.

Availability of Hearing Health Care Personnel

These multiple entry points to accessing hearing health care and even the decline in otolaryngologists seeking board certification can create many challenges for adults with hearing loss. More qualified providers and clinics with the knowledge, skill, and expertise to properly evaluate, prescribe, and train people in the use of hearing devices are needed. Proper fitting and training are complex but necessary elements to maximize performance among hearing device users. Consumers who work with providers trained in the use of properly prescribed and fitted hearing devices can expect better results than those who use off-the-shelf products.

FINDINGS AND CONCLUSIONS

Findings

5-1. The distribution of providers and clinics with the knowledge, skill, and expertise to properly evaluate, prescribe, and train people in the use of hearing devices varies greatly throughout the United States.

5-2. Current SSA *Listing of Impairments* criteria for hearing disability generally reflect a level of hearing loss at which amplification with a hearing aid is insufficient to substantially mitigate impairments and restrictions on participation due to hearing loss.

5-3. There are no established objective measures of real-world communicative functioning.

5-4. Research investigating the impact of audiometric hearing function and/or hearing devices on real-world communicative functioning is extremely limited.

5-5. Audiologists cannot bill Medicare or insurance for audiological rehabilitation services.

5-6. Reimbursement for hearing aids is statutorily excluded by Medicare.

5-7. Compared with the prevalence of hearing loss, the prevalence of hearing aid use is low in the United States.

5-8. Access to hearing devices varies significantly across reimbursement and funding sources in the United States.

5-9. The vast majority of individuals do not have insurance that covers hearing aids or related services.

5-10. The cost for hearing aids is usually covered under a bundled model that includes the costs of the devices and of the professional services required to fit them properly and follow up for rehabilitation.

Conclusions

5-1. Qualified providers and clinics with the knowledge, skill, and expertise to properly evaluate, prescribe, and train people in the use of hearing devices are needed. [Finding 5-1]

5-2. Proper fitting and training are complex but necessary elements of maximizing performance among users of hearing devices. Consumers who work with providers trained in the use of properly prescribed and fitted hearing devices can expect better results than those who use off-the-shelf products. [Finding 5-1]

5-3. Even with advances in technology, hearing aids and other hearing assistive devices may help but do not fully mitigate impairments or restrictions on participation caused by hearing loss. Environmental and personal factors are as important in determining the overall communicative functioning of individuals with hearing loss. [Finding 5-2]

5-4. The establishment of objective measures of real-world communicative functioning is vital to promoting a better understanding of the effects on this functioning of audiometric hearing function and hearing devices. [Findings 5-3, 5-4]

5-5. The widespread lack of insurance coverage for hearing devices and related services is an impediment to optimizing communicative functioning and maintaining gainful employment among adults with hearing loss. [Findings 5-5, 5-6, 5-7, 5-8, 5-9]

REFERENCES

Abrams, H. B., and J. Kihm. 2015. *An introduction to MarkeTrak IX: A new baseline for the hearing aid market.* http://www.hearingreview.com/2015/05/introduction-marketrak-ix-new-baseline-hearing-aid-market (accessed February 6, 2017).

Abrams, H. B., T. H. Chisolm, M. McManus, and R. McArdle. 2012. Initial-fit approach versus verified prescription: Comparing self-perceived hearing aid benefit. *Journal of the American Academy of Audiology* 23(10):768-778.

American Academy of Otolaryngology-Head and Neck Surgery. 2015. *What is an otolaryngologist?* http://www.entnet.org/content/what-otolaryngologist (accessed January 13, 2017).

Amieva, H., C. Ouvrard, C. Giulioli, C. Meillon, L. Rullier, and J. F. Dartigues. 2015. Self-reported hearing loss, hearing aids, and cognitive decline in elderly adults: A 25-year study. *Journal of the American Geriatrics Society* 63(10):2099-2104.

Andrews, M. 2012. Unlike most insurers, United Healthcare is offering big discounts on hearing aids. *The Washington Post*, April 9. https://www.washingtonpost.com/national/health-science/unlike-most-insurers-unitedhealthcare-is-offering-big-discounts-on-hearing-aids/2012/04/09/gIQA8I0Z6S_story.html?utm_term=.41e62d96906d (accessed January 13, 2017).

ASHA (American Speech-Language-Hearing Association). 2017a. *Adult aural/audiologic rehabilitation.* http://www.asha.org/public/hearing/Adult-Aural-Rehabilitation (accessed January 13, 2017).

ASHA. 2017b. *FM systems.* http://www.asha.org/public/hearing/FM-Systems (accessed January 9, 2017).

ASHA. 2017c. *Health insurance coverage for hearing aids.* http://www.asha.org/public/hearing/Health-Insurance-Coverage-for-Hearing-Aids (accessed January 13, 2017).

ASHA. 2017d. *Hearing aids for adults.* http://www.asha.org/Practice-Portal/Professional-Issues/Hearing-Aids-for-Adults (accessed January 13, 2017).

ASHA. 2017e. *State insurance mandates for hearing aids.* http://www.asha.org/advocacy/state/issues/ha_reimbursement (accessed February 9, 2017).

Bally, S. J., and M. H. Bakke. 2007. A peer mentor training program for aural rehabilitation. *Trends in Amplification* 11(2):125-131.

Banerjee, S. 2011. Hearing aids in the real world: Use of multimemory and volume controls. *Journal of the American Academy of Audiology* 22(6):359-374.

Beck, L. 2015. *Perspective from Department of Veterans Affairs*. Presented at the Committee on Accessible and Affordable Hearing Health Care Meeting, Washington, DC, June 30.

Blackwell, D. L., J. W. Lucas, and T. C. Clarke. 2014. Summary health statistics for U.S. adults: National Health Interview Survey, 2012. *Vital and health statistics* 10(260):1-161.

BLS (U.S. Bureau of Labor Statistics). 2015a. *Occupational emloyment and wages, May 2015: 29-1181 Audiologists*. http://www.bls.gov/oes/current/oes291181.htm (accessed January 13, 2017).

BLS. 2015b. *Occupational employment and wages, May 2015: 29-2092 Hearing aid specialists*. https://www.bls.gov/oes/current/oes292092.htm (accessed January 13, 2017).

Boothroyd, A. 2010. Adapting to changed hearing: The potential role of formal training. *Journal of the American Academy of Audiology* 21(9):601-611.

Brault, M. W. 2012. Americans with disabilities: 2010. *Current Population Reports* 7:1-131.

Breitbart, D., J. Xu, J. Johnson, and R. Cox. 2014. *Is there a preference between hearing aids and personal sound amplification products (PSAPs)?* http://www.harlmemphis.org/files/2513/9628/6861/Breitbart2014.pdf (accessed February 6, 2017).

Brooks, D. N. 1996. The time course of adaptation to hearing aid use. *British Journal of Audiology* 30(1):55-62.

Byrne, D., and H. Dillon. 1986. The National Acoustic Laboratories' (NAL) new procedure for selecting the gain and frequency response of a hearing aid. *Ear and Hearing* 7(4):257-265.

Byrne, D., H. Dillon, T. Ching, R. Katsch, and G. Keidser. 2001. NAL-NL1 procedure for fitting nonlinear hearing aids: Characteristics and comparisons with other procedures. *Journal of the American Academy of Audiology* 12(1):37-51.

CDC (U.S. Centers for Disease Control and Prevention). 2011. *NHANES 2011-2012 questionnaire data*. https://wwwn.cdc.gov/Nchs/Nhanes/Search/DataPage.aspx?Component=Questionnaire&CycleBeginYear=2011 (accessed February 6, 2017).

Chandler, D. 2015. *Perspective from Department of Veterans Affairs*. Presented at the Committee on Accessible and Affordable Hearing Health Care Meeting, Washington DC, April 27.

Chen, D. S., J. Betz, K. Yaffe, H. N. Ayonayon, S. Kritchevsky, K. R. Martin, T. B. Harris, K. R. Martin, T. B. Harris, E. Purchase-Helzner, S. Satterfield, Q. L. Xue, S. Pratt, E. M. Simonsick, and F. R. Lin for the Health ABC Study. 2015. Association of hearing impairment with declines in physical functioning and the risk of disability in older adults. *The Journals of Gerontology Series A: Biological Sciences and Medical Sciences* 70(5):654-661.

Chien, W., and F. R. Lin. 2012. Prevalence of hearing aid use among older adults in the United States. *Archives of Internal Medicine* 172(3):292-293.

Chisolm, T. H., C. M. Noe, R. McArdle, and H. Abrams. 2007. Evidence for the use of hearing assistive technology by adults: The role of the FM system. *Trends in Amplification* 11(2):73-89.

Ciorba, A., C. Bianchini, S. Pelucchi, and A. Pastore. 2012. The impact of hearing loss on the quality of life of elderly adults. *Clinical Interventions in Aging* 7(6):159-163.

CMS (Centers for Medicare & Medicaid Services). 2016a. *Early and periodic screening, diagnostic, and treatment*. https://www.medicaid.gov/Medicaid-CHIP-Program-Information/By-Topics/Benefits/Early-and-Periodic-Screening-Diagnostic-and-Treatment.html (accessed February 27, 2016).

CMS. 2016b. *Health benefits and coverage: What marketplace health insurance plans cover.* www.healthcare.gov/coverage/what-marketplace-plans-cover (accessed February 27, 2016).

CMS. 2016c. *Your Medicare coverage: Hearing and balance exams and hearing aids.* https://www.medicare.gov/coverage/hearing-and-balance-exam-and-hearing-aids.html (accessed February 28, 2016).

Consumer Reports. 2015. *Hearing aid buying guide.* http://www.consumerreports.org/cro/hearing-aids/buying-guide.htm (accessed December 28, 2016).

Contrera, K. J., J. Betz, D. J. Genther, and F. R. Lin. 2015. Association of hearing impairment and mortality in the National Health and Nutrition Examination Survey. *JAMA Otolaryngology—Head & Neck Surgery* 141(10):944-946.

Cox, R. M., and G. C. Alexander. 1995. The abbreviated profile of hearing aid benefit. *Ear and Hearing* 16(2):176-186.

Cox, R. M., and G. C. Alexander. 1999. Measuring satisfaction with amplification in daily life: The SADL scale. *Ear and Hearing* 20(4):306-320.

Cox, R. M., G. C. Alexander, I. M. Taylor, and G. A. Gray. 1996. Benefit acclimatization in elderly hearing aid users. *Journal of the American Academy of Audiology* 7(6):428-441.

Cox, R. M., G. C. Alexander, and C. M. Beyer. 2003. Norms for the international outcome inventory for hearing aids. *Journal of the American Academy of Audiology* 14(8):403-413.

Cox, R. M., K. S. Schwartz, C. M. Noe, and G. C. Alexander. 2011. Preference for one or two hearing aids among adult patients. *Ear and Hearing* 32(2):181-197.

Cox, R. M., J. A. Johnson, and J. Xu. 2014. Impact of advanced hearing aid technology on speech understanding for older listeners with mild to moderate, adult-onset, sensorineural hearing loss. *Gerontology* 60(6):557-568.

Cruickshanks, K. J., T. L. Wiley, T. S. Tweed, B. E. Klein, R. Klein, J. A. Mares-Perlman, and D. M. Nondahl. 1998. Prevalence of hearing loss in older adults in Beaver Dam, Wisconsin. The Epidemiology of Hearing Loss Study. *American Journal of Epidemiology* 148(9):879-886.

Dawes, P., K. J. Cruickshanks, M. E. Fischer, B. E. Klein, R. Klein, and D. M. Nondahl. 2015. Hearing-aid use and long-term health outcomes: Hearing handicap, mental health, social engagement, cognitive function, physical health, and mortality. *International Journal of Audiology* 54(11):838-844.

Desjardins, J. L., and K. A. Doherty. 2009. Do experienced hearing aid users know how to use their hearing aids correctly? *American Journal of Audiology* 18(1):69-76.

Dillon, H., A. James, and J. Ginis. 1997. Client Oriented Scale of Improvement (COSI) and its relationship to several other measures of benefit and satisfaction provided by hearing aids. *Journal of the American Academy of Audiology* 8(1):27-43.

FCC (Federal Communications Commission). 2016. *Telecommunications relay service.* https://www.fcc.gov/consumers/guides/telecommunications-relay-service-trs (accessed January 9, 2017).

FDA (U.S. Food and Drug Administration). 2013. *Regulatory requirements for hearing aid devices and personal sound amplification products—Draft guidance for industry and Food and Drug Administration staff.* https://www.fda.gov/MedicalDevices/DeviceRegulationandGuidance/GuidanceDocuments/ucm373461.htm (accessed February 22, 2017).

Fischer, M. E., K. J. Cruickshanks, A. Pinto, B. E. Klein, R. Klein, and D. S. Dalton. 2014. Hearing impairment and retirement. *Journal of the American Academy of Audiology* 25(2):164-170.

Gatehouse, S., G. Naylor, and C. Elberling. 2003. Benefits from hearing aids in relation to the interaction between the user and the environment. *International Journal of Audiology* 42(Suppl.1):S77-S85.

Genther, D. J., J. Betz, S. Pratt, S. B. Kritchevsky, K. R. Martin, T. B. Harris, E. Helzner, S. Satterfield, Q. L. Xue, K. Yaffe, E. M. Simonsick, and F. R. Lin. 2015. Association of hearing impairment and mortality in older adults. *The Journals of Gerontology Series A: Biological Sciences and Medical Sciences* 70(1):85-90.

Girard, S. A., T. Leroux, R. Verreault, M. Courteau, M. Picard, F. Turcotte, and J. Baril. 2014. Falls risk and hospitalization among retired workers with occupational noise-induced hearing loss. *Canadian Journal on Aging (La Revue canadienne du vieillissement)* 33(1):84-91.

Gnewikow, D., T. Ricketts, G. W. Bratt, and L. C. Mutchler. 2009. Real-world benefit from directional microphone hearing aids. *Journal of Rehabilitation Research & Development* 46(5):603-618.

Goman, A. M., and F. R. Lin. 2016. Prevalence of hearing loss by severity in the United States. *American Journal of Public Health* 106(10):1820-1822.

Gopinath, B., J. Schneider, C. M. McMahon, G. Burlutsky, S. R. Leeder, P. Mitchell, and L. Chao. 2013. Dual sensory impairment in older adults increases the risk of mortality: A population-based study. *PLOS ONE* 8(3):e55054.

Hawkins, D. B. 2005. Effectiveness of counseling-based adult group aural rehabilitation programs: A systematic review of the evidence. *Journal of the American Academy of Audiology* 16(7):485-493.

Hawkins, D. B., and S. V. Naidoo. 1993. Comparison of sound quality and clarity with asymmetrical peak clipping and output limiting compression. *Journal of the American Academy of Audiology* 4(4):221-228.

Hawkins, D. B., and W. S. Yacullo. 1984. Signal-to-noise ratio advantage of binaural hearing aids and directional microphones under different levels of reverberation. *Journal of Speech and Hearing Disorders* 49(3):278-286.

HLAA (Hearing Loss Association of America). 2008. *Great news on federal employee insurance coverage for hearing aids*. http://www.hearingloss.org/content/great-news-federal-employee-insurance-coverage-hearing-aids (accessed January 13, 2017).

HLAA. 2015. *Medicaid regulations*. http://www.hearingloss.org/content/medicaid-regulations (accessed February 9, 2017).

HLAA. 2016. *Consumer's guide to hearing aids*. www.hearingloss.org/content/consumers-guide-hearing-aids (accessed December 28, 2016).

HLAA. 2017. *Types, causes, and treatment*. http://www.hearingloss.org/content/types-causes-and-treatment (accessed February 7, 2017).

Holmes, A. E., H. S. Kaplan, and J. P. Saxon. 2000. Assistive listening devices and systems: Amplification technology for consumers with hearing loss. *Journal of Rehabilitation* 66(3):56-59.

Horner-Johnson, W., K. Dobbertin, J. C. Lee, and E. M. Andresen. 2014. Disparities in health care access and receipt of preventive services by disability type: Analysis of the Medical Expenditure Panel Survey. *Health Services Research* 49(6):1980-1999.

Humes, L. E., and V. Krull. 2012. Hearing aids for adults. In *Evidence-based practice in audiology: Evaluating interventions for children and adults with hearing impairment*, edited by L. Wong and L. Hickson. San Diego, CA: Plural Publishing. Pp. 61-91.

Humes, L. E., and D. L. Wilson. 2003. An examination of changes in hearing-aid performance and benefit in the elderly over a 3-year period of hearing-aid use. *Journal of Speech, Language, and Hearing Research* 46(1):137-145.

Humes, L. E., D. L. Wilson, N. N. Barlow, and C. Garner. 2002. Changes in hearing-aid benefit following 1 or 2 years of hearing-aid use by older adults. *Journal of Speech, Language, and Hearing Research* 45(4):772-782.

Humes, L., J. H. Lee, and M. P. Coughlin. 2006. Auditory measures of selective and divided attention in young and older adults using single-talker competition. *The Journal of the Acoustical Society of America* 120(5):2926-2937.

Jennings, M. B., and L. Shaw. 2008. Impact of hearing loss in the workplace: Raising questions about partnerships with professionals. *Work (Reading, Massachusetts)* 30(3):289-295.

Johnson, E. E., and H. Dillon. 2011. A comparison of gain for adults from generic hearing aid prescriptive methods: Impacts on predicted loudness, frequency bandwidth, and speech intelligibility. *Journal of the American Academy of Audiology* 22(7):441-459.

Kaiser Family Foundation. 2015. *Medicare advantage.* http://kff.org/medicare/fact-sheet/medicare-advantage (accessed February 27, 2016).

Kamil, R. J., J. Betz, B. B. Powers, S. Pratt, S. Kritchevsky, H. N. Ayonayon, T. B. Harris, E. Helzner, J. A. Deal, K. Martin, M. Peterson, S. Satterfield, E. M. Simonsick, and F. R. Lin. 2016. Association of hearing impairment with incident frailty and falls in older adults. *Journal of Aging and Health* 28(4):644-660.

Keidser, G., H. Dillon, E. Convery, and J. Mejia. 2013. Factors influencing individual variation in perceptual directional microphone benefit. *Journal of the American Academy of Audiology* 24(10):955-968.

Kim, J. S., and C. H. Kim. 2014. A review of assistive listening device and digital wireless technology for hearing instruments. *Korean Journal of Audiology* 18(3):105-111.

Kochkin, S. 2005. *The impact of untreated hearing loss on household income.* Alexandria, VA: Better Hearing Institute. http://www.betterhearing.org/sites/default/files/hearingpedia-resources/M7_Hearing_aids_and_income_2006.pdf (accessed January 22, 2017).

Kochkin, S. 2009. Marketrak VIII: 25-year trends in the hearing health market. *Hearing Review* 16(11):12-31.

Kokx-Ryan, M., J. Cohen, M. T. Cord, T. C. Walden, M. J. Makashay, B. M. Sheffield, and D. S. Brungart. 2015. Benefits of nonlinear frequency compression in adult hearing aid users. *Journal of the American Academy of Audiology* 26(10):838-855.

Kramer, S., T. Kapteyn, and T. Houtgast. 2006. Occupational performance: Comparing normally-hearing and hearing-impaired employees using the Amsterdam checklist for hearing and work. *International Journal of Audiology* 45(9):503-512.

Laplante-Levesque, A., L. Hickson, and L. Worrall. 2011. Predictors of rehabilitation intervention decisions in adults with acquired hearing impairment. *Journal of Speech, Language, and Hearing Research* 54(5):1385-1399.

Larson, V. D., D. W. Williams, W. G. Henderson, L. E. Luethke, L. B. Beck, D. Noffsinger, R. H. Wilson, R. A. Dobie, G. B. Haskell, G. W. Bratt, J. E. Shanks, P. Stelmachowicz, G. A. Studebaker, A. E. Boysen, A. Donahue, R. Canalis, S. A. Fausti, and B. Z. Rappaport. 2000. Efficacy of 3 commonly used hearing aid circuits: A crossover trial. NIDCD/VA Hearing Aid Clinical Trial Group. *Journal of the American Medical Association* 284(14):1806-1813.

Lee, D. J., D. L. Carlson, H. M. Lee, L. A. Ray, and K. S. Markides. 1991. Hearing loss and hearing aid use in Hispanic adults: Results from the Hispanic Health and Nutrition Examination Survey. *American Journal of Public Health* 81(11):1471-1474.

Lin, F. R. 2011. Hearing loss and cognition among older adults in the United States. *The Journals of Gerontology Series A: Biological Sciences and Medical Sciences* 66(10):1131-1136.

Lin, F. R., and L. Ferrucci. 2012. Hearing loss and falls among older adults in the United States. *Archives of Internal Medicine* 172(4):369-371.

Lin, F. R., L. Ferrucci, E. J. Metter, Y. An, A. B. Zonderman, and S. M. Resnick. 2011a. Hearing loss and cognition in the Baltimore Longitudinal Study of Aging. *Neuropsychology* 25(6):763-770.

Lin, F. R., E. J. Metter, R. J. O'Brien, S. M. Resnick, A. B. Zonderman, and L. Ferrucci. 2011b. Hearing loss and incident dementia. *JAMA Neurology* 68(2):214-220.

Lin, F. R., R. Thorpe, S. Gordon-Salant, and L. Ferrucci. 2011c. Hearing loss prevalence and risk factors among older adults in the United States. *The Journals of Gerontology Series A: Biological Sciences and Medical Sciences* 66(5):582-590.

Lin, F. R., J. K. Niparko, and L. Ferrucci. 2011d. Hearing loss prevalence in the United States. *Archives of Internal Medicine* 171(20):1851-1852.

Lin, F. R., K. Yaffe, J. Xia, Q. L. Xue, T. B. Harris, E. Purchase-Helzner, S. Satterfield, H. N. Ayonayon, L. Ferrucci, and E. M. Simonsick. 2013. Hearing loss and cognitive decline in older adults. *JAMA Internal Medicine* 173(4):293-299.

Lorenzi, A., and B. Chaix. 2016. *Hearing aids*. http://www.cochlea.org/en/treatments/hearing-aids (accessed February 8, 2017).

MAA (Military Audiology Association). 2016. *Hearing aids*. http://militaryaudiology.org/aids (accessed February 28, 2016).

Mäki-Torkko, E. M., B. Brorsson, A. Davis, I. W. S. Mair, K. I. Myhre, A. Parving, R. P. Roine, U. Rosenhall, M. J. Sorri, and S. Stilvén. 2001. Hearing impairment among adults—Extent of the problem and scientific evidence on the outcome of hearing aid rehabilitation. *Scandinavian Audiology* 30(3):8-15.

McArdle, R., T. H. Chisolm, H. B. Abrams, R. H. Wilson, and P. J. Doyle. 2005. The WHO-DAS II: Measuring outcomes of hearing aid intervention for adults. *Trends in Amplification* 9(3):127-143.

McCormack, A., and H. Fortnum. 2013. Why do people fitted with hearing aids not wear them? *International Journal of Audiology* 52(5):360-368.

Middleton, A., A. Niruban, G. Girling, and P. K. Myint. 2010. Communicating in a healthcare setting with people who have hearing loss. *British Medical Journal* 341:726-729.

Mitchell, P., B. Gopinath, J. J. Wang, C. M. McMahon, J. Schneider, E. Rochtchina, and S. R. Leeder. 2011. Five-year incidence and progression of hearing impairment in an older population. *Ear and Hearing* 32(2):251-257.

Moore, B. C., M. A. Stone, and J. I. Alcántara. 2001. Comparison of the electroacoustic characteristics of five hearing aids. *British Journal of Audiology* 35(5):307-325.

Morton, C. C., and W. E. Nance. 2006. Newborn hearing screening—A silent revolution. *New England Journal of Medicine* 354(20):2151-2164.

Most, T., L. Adi-Bensaid, T. Shpak, S. Sharkiya, and M. Luntz. 2012. Everyday hearing functioning in unilateral versus bilateral hearing aid users. *American Journal of Otolaryngology* 33(2):205-211.

Mueller, H. G. 2001. Probe microphone measurements: 20 years of progress. *Trends in Amplification* 5(2):35-68.

Mueller, H. G. 2005. Fitting hearing aids to adults using prescriptive methods: An evidence-based review of effectiveness. *Journal of the American Academy of Audiology* 16(7):448-460.

Mueller, H. G., J. Weber, and B. W. Hornsby. 2006. The effects of digital noise reduction on the acceptance of background noise. *Trends in Amplification* 10(2):83-93.

Mulrow, C. D., C. Aguilar, J. E. Endicott, M. R. Tuley, R. Velez, W. S. Charlip, M. C. Rhodes, J. A. Hill, and L. A. DeNino. 1990. Quality-of-life changes and hearing impairment. A randomized trial. *Annals of Internal Medicine* 113(3):188-194.

Nachtegaal, J., J. M. Festen, and S. E. Kramer. 2012. Hearing ability in working life and its relationship with sick leave and self-reported work productivity. *Ear and Hearing* 33(1):94-103.

NASEM (National Academies of Sciences, Engineering, and Medicine). 2016. *Hearing health care for adults: Priorities for improving access and affordability*. Washington, DC: The National Academies Press.

Nash, S. D., K. J. Cruickshanks, G. H. Huang, B. E. Klein, R. Klein, F. J. Nieto, and T. S. Tweed. 2013. Unmet hearing health care needs: The Beaver Dam Offspring Study. *American Journal of Public Health* 103(6):1134-1139.

Neuwahl, S., E. P. Fraher, H. C. Pillsbury, M. C. Weissler, T. C. Ricketts, and K. Gaul. 2012. Trends in the otolaryngology workforce in the U.S. *Bulletin of the American College of Surgeons* 97(3):30-34.

NIDCD (National Institute on Deafness and Other Communication Disorders). 2013. *Hearing aids*. http://www.nidcd.nih.gov/health/hearing/pages/hearingaid.aspx (accessed December 28, 2016).

Nieman, C. L., N. Marrone, S. L. Szanton, R. J. Thorpe, Jr., and F. R. Lin. 2016. Racial/ethnic and socioeconomic disparities in hearing health care among older Americans. *Journal of Aging and Health* 28(1):68-94.

Nilsson, M., D. Gelnett, J. Sullivan, S. D. Soli, and R. L. Goldberg. 1992. Norms for the hearing in noise test: The influence of spatial separation, hearing loss, and English language experience on speech reception thresholds. *The Journal of the Acoustical Society of America* 92(4):2385.

Noble, W., and S. Gatehouse. 2006. Effects of bilateral versus unilateral hearing aid fitting on abilities measured by the Speech, Spatial, and Qualities of Hearing Scale (SSQ). *International Journal of Audiology* 45(3):172-181.

Noffsinger, D., G. B. Haskell, V. D. Larson, D. W. Williams, E. Wilson, S. Plunkett, and D. Kenworthy. 2002. Quality rating test of hearing aid benefit in the NIDCD/VA clinical trial. *Ear and Hearing* 23(4):291-300.

Northern, J., and C. Beyer. 1999. Reducing hearing aid returns through patient education. *Audiology Today* 11(2):10-11.

Oeding, K., and M. Valente. 2013. Sentence recognition in noise and perceived benefit of noise reduction on the receiver and transmitter sides of a BICROS hearing aid. *Journal of the American Academy of Audiology* 24(10):980-991.

Oh, S. H., and J. Lee. 2016. General framework of hearing aid fitting management. *Journal of Audiology & Otology* 20(1):1-7.

Pandhi, N., J. R. Schumacher, S. Barnett, and M. A. Smith. 2011. Hearing loss and older adults perceptions of access to care. *Journal of Community Health* 36(5):748-755.

Preminger, J. E. 2011. Group audiologic rehabilitation for adults and their communication partners. *The ASHA Leader* 16(8):14-17.

Popelka, M. M., K. J. Cruickshanks, T. L. Wiley, T. S. Tweed, B. E. Klein, and R. Klein. 1998. Low prevalence of hearing aid use among older adults with hearing loss: The Epidemiology of Hearing Loss Study. *Journal of the American Geriatrics Society* 46(9):1075-1078.

Roth, T. 2015. Chapter 20: Aging of the auditory system. In *Handbook of clinical neurology*, Vol. 29, edited by G. G. Celesia and G. Hickok. Edinburgh, U.K.: Elsevier. Pp. 357-373.

Rouse, M. 2016. *Signal-to-noise ratio*. http://searchnetworking.techtarget.com/definition/signal-to-noise-ratio (accessed February 8, 2017).

Shanks, J. E., R. H. Wilson, V. Larson, and D. Williams. 2002. Speech recognition performance of patients with sensorineural hearing loss under unaided and aided conditions using linear and compression hearing aids. *Ear and Hearing* 23(4):280-290.

Shi, L. F., K. A. Doherty, T. M. Kordas, and J. T. Pellegrino. 2007. Short-term and long-term hearing aid benefit and user satisfaction: A comparison between two fitting protocols. *Journal of the American Academy of Audiology* 18(6):482-495.

Southall, K., J.-P. Gagné, and M. B. Jennings. 2010. Stigma: A negative and a positive influence on help-seeking for adults with acquired hearing loss. *International Journal of Audiology* 49(11):804-814.

Strom, K. E. 2014. *HR 2013 hearing aid dispenser survey: Dispensing in the age of Internet and big box retailers.* http://www.hearingreview.com/2014/04/hr-2013-hearing-aid-dispenser-survey-dispensing-age-internet-big-box-retailers-comparison-present-past-key-business-indicators-dispensing-offices (accessed February 9, 2017).

Sweetow, R., and C. V. Palmer. 2005. Efficacy of individual auditory training in adults: A systematic review of the evidence. *Journal of the American Academy of Audiology* 16(7):494-504.

Thibodeau, L. 2014. Comparison of speech recognition with adaptive digital and FM remote microphone hearing assistance technology by listeners who use hearing aids. *American Journal of Audiology* 23(2):201-210.

TRICARE. 2015. *Hearing aids.* http://www.tricare.mil/CoveredServices/IsItCovered/HearingAids.aspx (accessed February 28, 2016).

Turner, C. W., L. E. Humes, R. A. Bentler, and R. M. Cox. 1996. A review of past research on changes in hearing aid benefit over time. *Ear and Hearing* 17(Suppl. 3):14S-25S.

Tye-Murray, N., J. L. Spry, and E. Mauzé. 2009. Professionals with hearing loss: Maintaining that competitive edge. *Ear and Hearing* 30(4):475-484.

University of Arkansas Rehabilitation Research and Training Center. 2008. *Model state plan for vocational rehabilitation services to persons who are deaf, deaf-blind, heard of hearing, or late deafened.* Little Rock, AR: University of Arkansas.

U.S. Department of Education. 2016. *Welcome to RSA.* http://www2.ed.gov/about/offices/list/osers/rsa/index.html (accessed February 28, 2016).

VA (U.S. Department of Veterans Affairs) Office of the Inspector General. 2014. *Audit of VA's hearing aid services.* Washington, DC: VA.

Valente, M., H. Abrams, D. Benson, T. Chisolm, D. Citron, D. Hampton, and R. Sweetow. 2006. Guidelines for the audiologic management of adult hearing impairment. *Audiology Today* 18(5):32-37.

van Eyken, E., G. Van Camp, and L. Van Laer. 2007. The complexity of age-related hearing impairment: Contributing environmental and genetic factors. *Audiology and Neurotology* 12(6):345-358.

van Vliet, D. 2005. The current status of hearing care: Can we change the status quo? *Journal of the American Academy of Audiology* 16(7):410-418.

Ventry, I. M., and B. E. Weinstein. 1982. The Hearing Handicap Inventory for the Elderly: A new tool. *Ear and Hearing* 3(3):128-134.

Wahl, H. W., V. Heyl, P. M. Drapaniotis, K. Hörmann, J. B. Jonas, P. K. Plinkert, and K. Rohrschneider. 2013. Severe vision and hearing impairment and successful aging: A multidimensional view. *The Gerontologist* 53(6):950-962.

WHO (World Health Organization). 2001. *International Classification of Functioning, Disability and Health.* Geneva, Switzerland: WHO.

WHO. 2015. *Deafness and hearing loss fact sheet.* http://www.who.int/mediacentre/factsheets/fs300/en (accessed December 20, 2016).

Wu, Y. H., E. Stangl, R. A. Bentler, and R. W. Stanziola. 2013. The effect of hearing aid technologies on listening in an automobile. *Journal of the American Academy of Audiology* 24(6):474-485.

Yamasoba, T., F. R. Lin, S. Someya, A. Kashio, T. Sakamoto, and K. Kondo. 2013. Current concepts in age-related hearing loss: Epidemiology and mechanistic pathways. *Hearing Research* 303(Suppl.):30-38.

Yueh, B., P. E. Souza, J. A. McDowell, M. P. Collins, C. F. Loovis, S. C. Hedrick, S. D. Ramsey, and R. A. Deyo. 2001. Randomized trial of amplification strategies. *Archives of Otolaryngology—Head & Neck Surgery* 127(10):1197-1204.

ANNEX TABLE 5-1
Selected Hearing Technologies Taxonomy

Device	Cost Range	Prevalence of Use (%)[a] (age range)	Intended Use	Requirements for Use	
Hearing Aid(s)	$1,000–$4,000 / ear (Kochkin, 2009)	15–30%[d] of adults with hearing loss (Blackwell et al., 2014)	Situational to all waking hours (Chien and Lin, 2012)	• Mild to profound hearing loss • Ability to insert for use • Ability to manage daily care (cleaning, battery change)	
Remote Microphone Systems (Hearing Assistive Technology)	$1,000–$3,000[e]	2–3% of adults with hearing loss (CDC, 2011)	High in noise (Thibodeau, 2014)	• Mild to profound hearing loss • Ability to manage on/off switch and controls • Ability to keep track of device	
PSAPs Personal Sound Amplification Products	$25–$400 (Breitbart et al., 2014)	10% of adults with hearing loss (Abrams and Kihm, 2015)	Low (Breitbart et al., 2014)	• Mild to moderate hearing loss • Ability to manage controls • Ability to keep track of device	

NOTE: FDA = U.S. Food and Drug Administration.

[a]Prevalence of use data based on number of adults with hearing loss who report using devices.

[b]Most devices require limited training or adaptation to use.

[c]Limitations of device vary based on degree of hearing loss, age, and other factors.

[d]Based on calculations by NIDCD Epidemiology and Statistics Program staff using data collected by (1) the National Health Interview Survey (NHIS) annually for number of persons who have ever used a hearing aid [numerator], and (2) periodic NHANES hearing exams for representative samples of the U.S. adult and older adult population [denominator].

[e]Range of retail prices on June 1, 2016.

	Training and Adaption[b]	Benefits of Device	Limitations of Device[c]	Life Span of Device (years)	Maintenance	Other Considerations
	Immediate to short term (Cox et al., 1996)	• Benefit may be limited by degree of hearing loss • Benefit in noise may be limited	High in noise; Low in quiet (Ciorba et al., 2012; McArdle et al., 2005)	4–6 years	2–4 check-ups annually to maintain small parts	• t-coil should be required to access public loop and hearing aid compatible phones • Routine hearing evaluations to reprogram as needed • Cost also includes professional services to fit, program, verify, and counsel client
	Immediate to short term	• Benefits limited to a single talker with the microphone	Low in noise (Thibodeau, 2014)	4–6 years	1–2 check-ups annually to maintain small parts	• Portability of the device may make it more prone to breakdown
	Immediate to short term	• Benefit may be limited by degree of hearing loss • Benefit in noise may be limited	• Amplification may not be customized to degree of loss • Microphone may still receive noise	1–3 years	Annual check to verify function	• Not FDA approved to mitigate hearing loss (at this time)

ANNEX TABLE 5-2
Selected Hearing Technologies Function

Device	One-on-One Communication in Quiet	Small Group Discussions in Quiet	Large Group Discussions in Quiet	Distance Listening in Quiet	Communication via Telephone with One Person in Quiet	
Hearing Aid(s)[a] Varying levels of technology	1	2	3	2-3	3-4	
Remote Microphone Hearing Assistive Technology						
Connectivity system with hearing aid	1	1	2-3	1	Varies	
FM/DM system with hearing aid	1	1	1-2	1-2	Varies	
Independent microphone system (aka PocketTalker)	1	3-5	5	NA	NA	
Select Personal Sound Amplification Products (non-customized ear-level devices)[b]	1	1-2	3	3-4	3-4	

NOTES: Ranking scale 1–5, 1, most if not all, will benefit to 5, less likely to receive benefit. NA = not accessible.

[a]Assumes hearing devices are programmed and fitting is completed using real ear probe microphone measurements and prescriptive targets to verify maximum audibility of the speech spectrum has been achieved. Maximum benefit also includes proper counseling regarding the care and use of the technology after the fitting. An audiologist is the most qualified professional to provide rehabilitation for the nonmedical/nonsurgical treatment of hearing loss.

[b]Not specifically approved for treatment of hearing loss. PSAP products are highly heterogeneous. While some select products that are properly designed could offer benefit, most others will not.

	Communication via Telephone (conference call) in Quiet	One-on-One Communication in Noise	Small Group Discussions in Noise	Large Group Discussions in Noise	Distance Listening in Noise	Listening Without Visual Cues (videos, phone)	Sound Localization (as required for safety at work/home)
	4-5	3-4	4-5	5	5	3-5	3-4
	Varies	3-5	3-5	4-5	4-5	Varies	Varies
	Varies	2-5	2-5	3-5	3-5	Varies	Varies
	NA	4-5	4-5	NA	NA	NA	NA
	4-5	3-4	4-5	5	5	3-5	3-4

6

Augmentative and Alternative Communication and Voice Products and Technologies

The ease and simplicity of use of typical natural speech mask the complexity of a speech production process that involves precise control and coordination of respiration, voice, articulation, and language comprehension and expression (van der Merwe, 2009). For many, speech is the external expression of language, and the motor skills involved are performed with accuracy and speed, without conscious control (Netsell, 1982). With impairment, alterations in speech subsystems become apparent and the complexity revealed. The primary rationale for individuals' electing to use augmentative and alternative communication (AAC) is the inability of their natural speech to meet all of their daily communication needs. Although the severity of impairment plays a role in determining AAC needs and appropriate interventions, other factors include level of communication complexity, skills of communication partners, communication environments and environmental factors, rate of communication, and proficiency at strategic communication, among others. The delicate balance that yields automaticity of natural speech planning, programming, and execution is not replaced by AAC systems, nor does AAC fully mitigate impairments in natural speech production.

Although the primary focus of this chapter is AAC systems, the discussion also briefly addresses voice restoration technologies that support communication associated with head and neck cancer treatments. AAC refers to all types of communication other than oral speech (e.g., pictures, symbols, writing, hand gestures) (ASHA, 2016a). AAC systems may be *unaided* (e.g., signing, gestures) or *aided* (Beukelman and Mirenda, 2013). Aided AAC systems include nontechnology assistive products (e.g., communication boards, books) and technology-based products (e.g., speech-generating devices [SGDs], mobile technologies). This chapter begins with an overview of the conditions benefiting from the use of AAC technologies, which is followed by a detailed taxonomy of AAC and voice products and technologies. Next is a review of the clinical considerations entailed in comparing natural speech and technology-based voice output systems. Evaluation and monitoring, training and adaptation, and access and availability are then addressed in turn. The chapter next considers voice restoration following head and neck surgery. The final section presents findings and conclusions. Before proceeding, it is important to note that the research in this field often has focused on specific areas and populations, making generalizations across studies problematic and highlighting the need for AAC-specific research across adult populations (Bourgeois, 2013).

OVERVIEW OF CONDITIONS BENEFITING FROM AAC TECHNOLOGIES

Prevalence of AAC Need

An estimated 1.3 percent of Americans (about 4 million people) cannot reliably meet their daily communication needs using natural speech (Beukelman and Mirenda, 2013), and the prevalence and complexity of communication disorders increase with age (Yorkston et al., 2010a). Additionally, many individuals with other disabilities (e.g., developmental, physical) have co-occurring communication disabilities (Lawthers et al., 2003; Perry et al., 2004). Although datasets on the prevalence of AAC use are limited, increases in the number of individuals requiring AAC have been observed (Light and McNaughton, 2012). Factors contributing to this increase include the rising incidence of autism spectrum disorders (CDC, 2011, 2014); advances in medical intervention that have resulted in improved survival, albeit with lifelong disability (Durkin et al., 2016; Hustad and Miles, 2010; Vincer et al., 2006); increased life spans of individuals with communication disability (Balandin and Morgan, 2001); and increased overall life expectancy (Gaskin et al., 2016; Segalman, 2011). Improvements in AAC technology that better account for the unique cognitive and linguistic skills of persons with physical and cognitive disabilities have resulted in new opportunities for the appropriate provision of AAC services (Beukelman and Mirenda, 2013; Light and McNaughton, 2012).

Medical Conditions Benefiting from AAC

Prevalent conditions leading to a need for AAC include Alzheimer's disease, Parkinson's disease, autism spectrum disorder, learning difficulties, stroke, cerebral palsy, head/brain injury, profound and multiple learning disabilities, and motor neuron disease/amyotrophic lateral sclerosis (ALS) (Perry et al., 2004; Wodka et al., 2013). Other conditions include, but are not limited to, head and neck cancers (Sullivan et al., 2007b), aphonia/ voice impairment (Rousseau et al., 2015), progressive illnesses (e.g., multiple sclerosis, Huntington's disease) (Beukelman et al., 2007c), dementia (Bourgeois, 1992; Bourgeois et al., 2001), primary progressive aphasia (King et al., 2007), brainstem impairment/locked-in syndrome (Culp et al., 2007), genetic associations/syndromes (e.g., Prader-Willi, William's, Rett, Angelman, Fragile X, Down, 22q.11 deletion) (Brady et al., 2006; McDuffie et al., 2016), and other neuromuscular diseases (e.g., muscular dystrophy, spinal muscular atrophy) (Ball et al., 2012, 2016a; Fried-Oken et al., 2015). In an Australian sample, the age range of the largest number of people with complex communication needs was 19 to 40 years. Most individuals with such needs as a result of congenital conditions were in the same age range, with cerebral palsy (46 percent), genetic/congenital syndromes (37 percent), and autism spectrum disorder (48 percent) predominating. The same study found that some conditions associated with complex communication needs increase with age (e.g., stroke, dementia, laryngectomy, Parkinson's disease, Huntington's disease) (Perry et al., 2004).

Data on 2014 Medicare services (see Appendix C) indicate that the majority (168/227, or 73 percent) of SGDs funded were in the E2510 category (SGD, synthesized speech output, multiple message formulation methods). Although the reason for the predominance of this category is unknown, funding, professional training, availability of AAC assessment teams, and public awareness likely contribute. Many individuals use this type of AAC device to produce complex language, while others use the sophisticated features of the device to support beginning communication skills (Brock et al., 2017; Ganz et al., 2015).

A potential misalignment exists between clinician perceptions of the need for AAC and actual need (Hustad and Miles, 2010). This misalignment may produce underestimated numbers of individuals who would benefit from AAC based on clinician (e.g., speech-language pathologist [SLP], physician) identification alone. There is no evidence to support the idea that persons with complex communication needs who undergo AAC evaluation receive no recommendation for AAC technology. The greater challenge is that there are few SLPs to provide AAC evaluation and treatment services, as is discussed later in this chapter.

TAXONOMY

AAC systems are used to establish functional communication when natural speech methods are insufficient to achieve daily communication goals and meet communication needs (Beukelman and Mirenda, 2013). Aided AAC systems can be categorized into nontechnology and technology-based products. Nontechnology products are nonelectronic boards or books that contain images that the individual selects to convey messages (e.g., picture symbols, alphabet boards, photograph books). Technology-based systems employ hardware and software to produce visual output, that is, digitally displayed messages (i.e., dynamic or static displays) or voice output (verbal messages [SGDs and mobile AAC technologies]). For the purposes of this report, the term "AAC technology" refers generally to technology-based communication systems with voice output, and it includes both SGDs and mobile AAC technologies. Voice output may be digitized, synthesized, or a combination of the two. Box 6-1 summarizes the definitions relevant to the AAC taxonomy used in this chapter (see also Table 6-1 and Annex Table 6-1 at the end of this chapter).

Technology-based AAC systems include a number of features that need to be considered when these systems are selected for particular individuals (see Table 6-1). Table 6-2 summarizes the ways in which vocabulary and messages are represented and generated for communication using technology-based AAC systems. To optimize a particular individual's communication performance, any number of features may need to be personalized or customized by an SLP or other qualified team member. While careful selection of these features may partially mitigate a communication impairment, training in use of the selected AAC technology alone cannot eliminate environmental and personal barriers that may impact use.

AAC Software

Important features of AAC software include (1) language/message representation methods, (2) vocabulary selection and organization based on communication needs and personal preferences, and (3) language/message generation options (Hill and Corsi, 2012). The features shown in Table 6-2 are not mutually exclusive, and multiple methods are often integrated into communication (e.g., a combination of direct selection for typical use and scanning for selection when fatigued; word-by-word message formulation strategies for novel utterances combined with preformulated messages for rapid access to frequently used utterances). One consideration in the selection of software features is the additional cognitive tasks associated with each option or combination of options; successful communication in the context of the cognitive, visual, and learning demands of complex AAC systems is influenced by an individual's language and cognitive status (Light and McNaughton, 2013; Rowland et al., 2003). While extensive evidence supports the benefits of some software and apps for language and access methods, little evidence exists for others as yet (Caron and Light, 2016) (see also Annex Table 6-2 at the end of this chapter).

BOX 6-1
Augmentative and Alternative Communication (AAC) Systems

Unaided Communication Systems: Systems that enable communication that relies on the user's body (language) to deliver messages. Examples include gestures, eye gaze, vocalizations, sign language, and facial expressions (adapted from ASHA [2016a]).

Aided AAC Systems: Systems that "require the use of tools or equipment in addition to the user's body. Aided communication methods can range from paper and pencil to communication books or boards to devices that produce voice output (speech generating devices or [AAC technologies, mobile technologies]) and/or written output. Electronic communication aids allow the user to use picture symbols, letters, and/or words and phrases to create messages. Some devices can be programmed to produce different spoken languages" (ASHA, 2016a).

- ***Nontechnology Products:*** Communication aids that do not need batteries or an electric power source to meet users' needs. Most are simple aids such as communication boards or books.
- ***Technology-Based Products***
  - **Visual output:** Used primarily to support messages when natural, digitized, or synthesized speech is not understood or available. Examples include aided symbols and text viewed on a display.
  - **AAC technologies:** Technology-based communication systems that may include speech-generating devices and mobile AAC technologies.
  - **SGDs:** Essential durable medical equipment that provides speech output using digitized, synthesized, or combined digitized and synthesized speech (adapted from Drager et al. [2010]).
  - **Mobile AAC technologies:** Mainstream technology (e.g., iOS, Android, Windows) with software or applications that provide speech output using digitized, synthesized, or combined digitized and synthesized speech output.
    - **Digitized voice output:** Generated by communication devices that reproduce messages consisting of a recording of natural speech that is converted to digital format. The voice output on the device is recorded by another person, as opposed to the computer (adapted from Beukelman and Mirenda [2013]).
    - **Synthesized voice output:** Generated by communication devices that convert typed text to digital speech.

Software Message Management Features

To communicate with AAC, individuals employ formulation, storage, and retrieval (words, codes, messages) strategies (Beukelman and Mirenda, 2013). A variety of software options are used to manage and generate messages, including but not limited to spelling letter-by-letter, using symbols

TABLE 6-1
Communication-Related Features of Aided AAC Systems

Feature	No-Technology AAC	Digitized SGD				Synthesized SGD		Mobile AAC Technology
Minutes of recording time		≤8	9–20	21–40	>40	>40	>40	>40
Digitized voice output		X	X	X	X			X
Synthesized voice output						X	X	X
Message banking		X	X	X	X	X	X	X
Voice banking					X	X	X	X
Visual output	X		X	X	X	X	X	X
Preprogrammed messages	X	X	X	X	X	X	X	X
Message formulation	X				X	X	X	X
Battery operated		X	X	X	X	X	X	X
Rechargeable			X	X	X	X	X	X
Fixed display	X	X	X	X	X			
Dynamic display						X	X	X
Physical contact/direct selection	X	X	X	X	X	X	X	X
Scanning	X		X	X	X	X	X	X
Multiple access options	X				X	X	X	X
Eye gaze access	X						X	X
Graphic/symbol representation	X	X	X	X	X	X	X	X
Text representation	X				X	X	X	X
Photo/visual scene representation	X	X	X	X	X	X	X	X

Rate acceleration: encoding	X	X	X	X	X	X	X	X
Rate acceleration: prediction						X	X	X
Visual adjustments (spacing, font, brightness)	X			X	X	X	X	X
Auditory adjustments (volume)		X	X	X	X	X	X	X
Funding (Medicare/Medicaid, insurers, VA)		X	X	X	X	X	X	
Assessment and Training	X	X	X	X	X	X	X	

NOTE: AAC = augmentative and alternative communication; SGD = speech-generating device; VA = U.S. Department of Veterans Affairs.

TABLE 6-2
Components of AAC Technology

LANGUAGE COMPONENTS		
Language Representation	**Vocabulary**	**Method of Utterance Generation**
• Alphabet or text • Single-meaning pictures/ symbols • Multimeaning icons	• Core—high frequency words • Extended—low frequency or topic specific words	• Novel utterance generation • Prestored utterances
HARDWARE AND SOFTWARE COMPONENTS		
Display Features	**Control and Selection Methods**	**Outputs**
• Symbol type • Display type and size • Number of grid locations • Number of pages • Encoding, color	• Direct selection: keyboard, head pointing, eye gaze, Morse code, brain-computer interfaces • Scanning: one or two switches, scanning pattern	• Speech: synthesized, digitized, individually created digital voices • Other: display, electronic/ infrared/radio frequency, Bluetooth, data logging
OTHER COMPONENTS AND SERVICES		
System Options	**Manufacturer Options**	**Other Supports**
• External computer access • Internet, Wi-Fi • Phone access • Switches • Mounting systems • Carrying cases	• Technical support • Repairs • Equipment loans • Warranties • Funding support • Device training	• Equipment loan closets • Funding requests, appeals • System training • Communication programming • Communication participation training (speech-language pathologist)

SOURCES: Adapted from Hill, 2010; Hill and Corsi, 2012.

to represent words and messages, sequencing icons to represent words and messages, selecting individual words from a display to generate word-by-word messages, and selecting partial and full messages that have been programmed and stored for retrieval. Each variation is appropriate for some individuals, and given the complex cognitive demands of these systems, careful consideration is required across a wide range of technologies to match individuals with the most appropriate systems (Higginbotham et al., 2007; Light and McNaughton, 2013; Mizuko et al., 1994; Ratcliff, 1994; Rowland et al., 2003; Thistle and Wilkinson, 2013; Wagner and Jackson, 2006).

Aided symbol representation includes the visual, auditory, or tactile presentation of communicative messages, symbols, and codes from which the individual selects (Beukelman and Mirenda, 2013). Aided symbols include two-dimensional symbols that can represent other items, and may include tangible objects (e.g., miniatures, partial objects), textures (e.g., a piece of spandex to represent swimming/a swimming suit), picture symbols (e.g., photographs, drawings, codes), and orthographic symbols (e.g., alphabet, Braille) (Beukelman and Mirenda, 2013). Most AAC technologies use aided symbols with visual displays of pictures, alphabet, pictorial symbols, or codes. For individuals with visual or other impairments, AAC technologies may present spoken messages or offer tactile representation of items (e.g., objects, textures, shapes). Although a wide array of strategies is used with communication software, methods for representing language or messages can be identified as (1) alphabet- or text-based methods, (2) single-meaning picture symbols, (3) visuals scenes, or (4) multimeaning icons or semantic compaction (Beukelman et al., 2015; Ganz et al., 2015; Gevarter et al., 2014; Light and McNaughton, 2012; Therrien and Light, 2016).

Keystroke and Rate Manipulation

People who rely on AAC often select components of messages one at a time from the display. A number of strategies have been developed to reduce the time and effort this process requires (Beukelman and Mirenda, 2013; Hoag et al., 2009).

Encoding Considered sequential building of sounds in words (Hartsuiker et al., 2005), encoding in the case of AAC technologies involves converting electronic data into a standard format that can be sent within the device and later decoded as communication output (Barrett and King, 2005). Encoding strategies typically found in AAC technologies involve word and message features in the communication software.

Stored words Alphabet- or text-based methods, including alpha, alphanumeric, letter-category, and numeric codes, may be used to represent words. Alpha codes typically employ truncation (e.g., use the first few letters of a word, such as *sched* = *schedule*) or contraction (e.g., use the most salient letters, such as *schdl* = *schedule*). Alphanumeric codes use letter–number combinations (e.g., *sched1* = *work schedule*, *sched2* = *travel schedule*, *sched3* = *home schedule*). Letter-category codes involve indicating a category with the first letter and then the word with the second letter (e.g., *S* = *my schedules*, *SW* = *work schedule*, *ST* = *travel schedule*). Numeric codes have limited use but are helpful when display space is limited (e.g., assignment of an arbitrary number, such as *15* = *work schedule*). Morse code is another encoding system available in some AAC technologies; dot and dash combinations are used to access the alphabet, punctuation, numbers, and computer functions (King, 2000).

Symbols Symbols and icons may be used to represent words. In the case of single-meaning symbols, one symbol represents one word. Symbol representation of words may result in keystroke savings over the course of a conversation. Since an individual's vocabulary typically includes several thousand words, however, this method requires the availability of an equal number of symbols. Sequencing two or three icons to access a word is another keystroke-saving approach that offers rate enhancement value for some individuals with severe physical disabilities, such as cerebral palsy (McNaughton et al., 2002). Use of multimeaning icons or semantic compaction (Baker, 1986; Chang et al., 1992) entails combining teachable icon sequences based on semantic relationships to represent a word. This representation method involves sequencing a small set (single display) of icons to reduce navigation among symbols/text.

Messages Alpha, alphanumeric, letter-category, and numeric codes and single- and multimeaning symbols/icons also may be used to represent phrases and messages. Some individuals use salient letter codes to indicate the relevant message content (e.g., *OD* = *please open the door for me*). Color encoding also may represent contextual (e.g., red = body parts, blue = work supplies) or linguistic (e.g., green = nouns, orange = verbs) categories (Thistle and Wilkinson, 2009). Communication software programs using symbols and icon sequences may contain prestored messages. Thus, one picture symbol or icon sequence may produce a greeting, provide the individual's name/address, or access a prestored presentation for a workplace meeting or conference.

Prediction Letter, word, and message prediction involves active retrieval in which options change according to the portion of the word/message already formulated. As with the now commonplace texting keyboard on many smartphones and tablets, algorithms predict content based on the probability of letter occurrence, letter combinations, and linguistic context to provide a set of options for the target message. Types of prediction include word completion, next-word prediction, linguistic prediction, message prediction, and icon prediction (Dowden, 2016).

Hardware Components

AAC technologies offer myriad hardware options for the message display, selection method, and output and input.

Display

Those AAC system components used to present the language components to the person with communication needs are commonly referred to as the display. AAC displays generally are of one of four types: fixed, dynamic, visual scenes, or hybrid (Beukelman and Mirenda, 2013).

Fixed display In fixed, or static, displays, graphic symbols are displayed in fixed locations, typically in a grid layout with symbols shown in cells that have fixed locations (Drager et al., 2003). The number of symbols or messages that a fixed display can present to the individual is limited (fewer than 150 in the largest displays) because each available item is visible at all times; as a result, some AAC systems utilize multiple, often hierarchical displays to accommodate various communication needs, environments, and listeners (Bruno and Trembath, 2006; Hochstein et al., 2003). Nonelectronic-aided AAC systems and most digitized AAC technologies employ fixed displays.

Dynamic display AAC technologies typically employ computer-based dynamic displays that change to a new set of symbols (pages) automatically when activated. Multiple levels of displays accommodate myriad individual vocabulary and linguistic needs (Drager et al., 2003). As with fixed displays, the majority of dynamic displays are presented in a grid or matrix, with items arranged in rows and columns. In contrast with fixed displays, however, the number of symbols or messages that a dynamic display can present to the individual is not limited by what is visible; such displays offer symbols that are not visible but can be accessed through page linking (Drager et al., 2003). Dynamic displays provide a range of organizational strategies that make complex language constructions possible (Bruno and Trembath, 2006; Drager et al., 2003). Some digitized AAC technologies and most synthesized devices employ dynamic displays (Beukelman and Mirenda, 2013).

Visual scene display In contrast with the grid format of many dynamic displays, visual scene displays provide context for the user by integrating a picture, photograph, or virtual environment within a visual image (e.g., showing people, objects, and events against the background in which they occur) (Beukelman et al., 2015; Dietz et al., 2006; Thistle and Wilkinson, 2015). Visual scene displays may be used across a wide range of AAC technologies (e.g., photographic images placed on a digitized device, digital images placed on devices that support programming "hot spots"). Visual scene displays support interactive communication across a variety of ages and disability groups (Beukelman et al., 2015; Brock et al., 2017; Ganz et al., 2015; Gevarter et al., 2014; Therrien and Light, 2016; Ulmer et al., 2016).

Hybrid display Hybrid displays typically consist of a fixed display with a dynamic component (e.g., indicator lights that highlight items, word prediction on alphabetic displays) (Beukelman and Mirenda, 2013). In other cases, a visual scene display may be embedded with dynamic hotspots that move the display away from the visual scene to a text or grid display (Gevarter et al., 2016). Hybrid displays may be used across the full range of AAC technology types.

Selection Method

AAC systems typically provide two methods for selecting elements on the display and producing messages: direct selection and scanning.

Direct selection Direct selection, available as an option on most AAC systems, allows the user to select a desired item without intervening supports. The most common form of direct selection involves a finger point or pressure (i.e., physical contact); however, direct selection may also involve pointing with another body part or activating an item without physical contact (e.g., head/mouth stick, eye gaze, head mouse, eye-safe laser) (Ball et al., 2010b; Fager et al., 2012; Hanson et al., 2016). Brain–computer interfaces show promise but are still under study; they are currently available only in selected clinics primarily as components of research programs (Akcakaya et al., 2014; Barreto et al., 2000; Fried-Oken et al., 2015; Hill et al., 2014; Wolpaw et al., 2000).

Scanning Scanning is an alternative selection method commonly used by individuals who are unable to choose items directly, most commonly because of impaired motor control (Beukelman and Mirenda, 2013). Scanning involves presenting items on the display by moving progressively through a predetermined pattern (e.g., row-column, circular, linear, group-item). Scanning requires that the user wait while the system sequentially presents undesired items before reaching the item of choice; a switch is used to activate the scanning movement and select the item/message (Beukelman and Mirenda, 2013).

Output Capabilities

Aided AAC systems provide a variety of message output modes, including digitized and synthetized speech, nonelectronic-aided symbols, and print (Beukelman and Mirenda, 2013). Visual output (e.g., aided symbols or text viewed on a display) is used primarily to support messages when natural, digitized, or synthesized speech is not understood or available. Individuals with impaired natural speech may use synthesized or digitized speech to gain listeners' attention, produce utterances at a distance, communicate in group conversations, and talk on the telephone, among many other activities (Alamsaputra et al., 2006; Hanson et al., 2016; Hill, 2010).

AAC technologies provide speech output using digitized, synthesized, or combined digitized and synthesized speech (Drager et al., 2010). Digitized and synthesized speech incorporated into electronic communication devices has resulted in significant advances in AAC (Alamsaputra et al., 2006).

Digitized speech Digitized speech refers to human voice stored as segments of sound waves (Schlosser, 2003). It consists of natural speech that has been recorded with a microphone, converted to a digital signal, and stored and retrieved in word or message form (Beukelman and Mirenda, 2013). Message banking, a strategy that involves storing digitized speech, is used primarily by individuals who, retaining intelligible speech but anticipating its loss (e.g., because of degenerative disease or head/neck cancer), want to record their own voice for use in future communication systems (Costello, 2011, 2014). Message banking strategies are not effective for individuals who are referred late for AAC evaluation, already presenting with moderate to severe speech impairment (Nordness et al., 2010). Although most technology-based AAC systems provide a feature for digitally recording a message, many provide a limited amount of storage space for such recordings (see Table 6-1). Prerecorded stored messages cannot be modified for spontaneous or real-time communication.

Synthesized speech Synthesized speech is computer-generated according to a set of rules in a mathematical algorithm (Drager et al., 2010). Text-to-speech synthesis, a common method for generating synthetic speech for AAC technologies, involves extracting speech sound components from words and then combining them to form natural-sounding synthetic voices (Beukelman and Mirenda, 2013; Drager et al., 2010). In contrast with the stored messages from digitized speech, synthesized speech systems allow the user to generate speech for each utterance and therefore provide greater novel message flexibility.

New options for creating a personalized synthetic voice that combine components of digitized and synthesized output have emerged and appear promising. However, the intelligibility and effectiveness of these options currently remain under study (Bunnell et al., 2015; Jreige et al., 2009; Patel et al., 2015; Yamagishi et al., 2012).

CLINICAL CONSIDERATIONS

Overall, people who rely on AAC for daily interactions value situational flexibility, reliability, learning ease, and intelligibility of output in their communication devices, as reflected in characteristics described by individuals who use AAC and their facilitators as research priorities (O'Keefe et al., 2007). In the study by O'Keefe and colleagues (2007),

AAC consumers with cerebral palsy and spinal cord injury indicated as priority needs (1) preparing people who use AAC to participate and have success in social relationships (e.g., friendships, dating) and employment; (2) improving AAC technologies and optimal, rapid service delivery; and (3) improving literacy among people who use AAC (O'Keefe et al., 2007). SLPs typically measure the function of speech subsystems, including intelligibility, comprehensibility, and efficiency, in conducting evaluations (ASHA, 2004c). One method for evaluating AAC systems and factors impacting their use involves comparing the effectiveness of natural speech with AAC options. Evidence from pediatric populations suggests that the extent of AAC use is directly related to the extent of communication need that is managed effectively with natural speech (Oommen and McCarthy, 2014). Although research is lacking for the full range of populations that may benefit from AAC (Light and Drager, 2007), considerations for comparing natural speech and technology-based voice output are summarized below for message and overall communication intelligibility, comprehensibility and listener comprehension, efficiency, and effectiveness.

Intelligibility

Broadly considered the measured understandability of speech, intelligibility is defined as the degree to which a person's natural speech is understood by a communication partner (Yorkston et al., 1992). Intelligibility is a key criterion for determining the severity of speech-production disorders (Yorkston et al., 2010b), as reduced intelligibility may critically limit vocational, educational, and social participation (Hustad, 2008). It follows that intelligibility is a key criterion for AAC output, as reductions result in increases in communication breakdowns (Ball et al., 2001, 2002). Many AAC speakers retain some functional natural speech with limited degrees of intelligibility; as a result, they may use AAC technology in some speaking situations and natural speech in others.

Standard procedures for intelligibility assessment commonly involve transcription (identification) of individual sounds, words, or sentences from decontextualized utterances (Yorkston et al., 1992). Each intelligibility assessment type yields task-specific information: phoneme intelligibility measures the understandability of discrete sound productions; word intelligibility measures the understandability of single-word utterances; and sentence intelligibility measures speech production in longer utterances characteristic of typical occupational interactions (Kent et al., 1989; Yorkston and Beukelman, 1981; Yorkston et al., 1992). Research has identified factors contributing to the intelligibility of synthesized speech, including quality of synthesis (Greene et al., 1986; McNaughton et al., 1994), message length (Mirenda and Beukelman, 1987, 1997), and rate

(Higginbotham et al., 1994). Continued advances in the quality of synthesized speech are expected to result in output that is increasingly comparable to natural speech.

Comprehensibility and Listener Comprehension

In contrast with intelligibility, in which the speech signal is extracted from context, comprehensibility is the degree to which speech is understood when combined with available relevant information (e.g., linguistic context, physical environment, gestures, and conversational topic) (Duffy, 2013; Yorkston et al., 1996). Assessment of comprehensibility, like that of intelligibility, involves transcribing verbal productions, except for the supplementation of verbal productions with contextual information (Hustad, 2008). When speech impairment is present, the addition of this contextual information usually results in comprehensibility scores superior to those for intelligibility (Hustad, 2008). Research has identified factors contributing to the comprehensibility of synthesized speech, including environment (noise, quiet) (Nelson et al., 2005), native language (Alamsaputra et al., 2006; Reynolds et al., 1996), message predictability and meaningfulness (Hoover et al., 1987; Oshrin and Siders, 1987; Slowiaczek and Nusbaum, 1985), and linguistic context (Beukelman and Mirenda, 2013; Drager and Reichle, 2001; Marics and Williges, 1988). Quantifying the comprehensibility of AAC output involves providing structured opportunities for transcription of messages in specific, functional contexts that are relevant to the individual (e.g., employment environments, topics, messages).

Separately, comprehension measures the ability of listeners to interpret the meaning of messages produced, which is evaluated by examining a listener's ability to answer questions about the message or utterance content (Hustad, 2008). Unlike scores on intelligibility and comprehensibility, comprehension scores do not reflect the severity of speech impairment; indeed, these scores tend to be higher than intelligibility scores, particularly for individuals with moderate to severe speech disability (Hustad, 2008).

Efficiency

Communication efficiency, often quantified by measures of speaking rate (i.e., intelligible words per minute [wpm], comprehensible wpm), refers to the rate at which understandable information is conveyed (Duffy, 2013). Measures of communication efficiency are key indicators of perceived normalcy of communication in social contexts because intelligibility efficiency reflects functional limitations, while comprehensibility efficiency reflects the ability to participate effectively in daily interactions (Duffy, 2013). Little research has addressed efficiency of comprehension for natural, digitized, or synthesized speech, although it likely influences such participation.

Typical speaking rates for people unaffected by speech-language disability (i.e., unimpaired intelligibility and comprehensibility) vary by task: paragraph reading rates range from 160 to 170 wpm (Fairbanks, 1960); sentence reading rates are approximately 190 wpm (Yorkston and Beukelman, 1981); and a much wider range of 150 to 250 wpm is noted for conversational utterances (Goldman-Eisler, 1986) because these utterances are influenced by the cognitive load of the task at hand (Yorkston et al., 2010b). Speakers with dysarthria tend to speak at slower rates, reflected in mean syllable durations of 246-249 milliseconds, relative to unimpaired speakers, with a typical rate of 198 milliseconds (Darley et al., 1975; Yorkston et al., 2010b).

Efficiency of AAC output also is impacted by measures of rate, which are influenced by the same factors associated with spoken messages but also by the interaction with AAC technology and by physical (e.g., motor, sensory, perceptual) ability and access methods (Higginbotham et al., 2007). AAC communication rates reflect such factors as message formulation and message delivery time. Communication rates 15-25 times slower than those of spoken speech are common for AAC (Beukelman and Mirenda, 2013), with a speaking rate of 10 wpm having been reported when alphabet-based rate acceleration strategies are combined (Newell et al., 1998). A significant objective in selecting an individual's optimal AAC system is to heighten message communication rates to those typical of natural speech and permit more efficient communication (Wisenburn and Higginbotham, 2009). The ideal balance of rate and content for AAC selection remains under study (Haidet et al., 2012; Lesher et al., 1998; Trnka et al., 2008; Wisenburn and Higginbotham, 2009).

Effectiveness

Considered a component of participation in daily interactions, self-perceived communication effectiveness also may reflect efficiency (McAuliffe et al., 2010). Ratings of communication effectiveness have demonstrated a positive correlation with intelligibility (Ball et al., 2004). However, efficiency and intelligibility factors are not the sole contributors to effectiveness (Donovan et al., 2008; Dykstra et al., 2015; McAuliffe et al., 2010). In some research, speakers with ALS and their listeners have expressed similar perceptions of communication effectiveness (Ball et al., 2004), whereas speakers with Parkinson's disease and traumatic brain injury have perceived their communication effectiveness as higher relative to listeners and expressed the view that intelligibility is not significantly related to effectiveness (Donovan et al., 2008; McAuliffe et al., 2010). Additionally, speakers with ALS have rated their communication effectiveness as poor even though the intelligibility of their utterances remained above 90 percent, potentially a reflection of the influence of effort and fatigue on perceptions of communication effectiveness (Ball et al., 2004). A research focus on the effectiveness of AAC communication is emerging (Beukelman et al., 2015; Fried-Oken et al., 2012; Higginbotham et al., 2007). Focus group participants in a study by O'Keefe and colleagues (2007, p. 95) highlighted the need for emphasis on aspects of participation, stating, "Don't make the use of technology an end goal; instead show me how to communicate satisfactorily to get and keep a job." and "Don't make the design and use of [AAC] our center of attention; concentrate on how I use communication to find a wife."

EVALUATION AND MONITORING

The ultimate goal of an AAC assessment is to recommend an AAC system and design treatment that will assist the individual in achieving "the most effective interactive communication possible" (ASHA, 2016b). Successfully matching an individual to the appropriate communication technology is a complex process. The following subsections describe required elements of comprehensive evaluation and monitoring of the achievement of functional communication goals.

Team Approach

The dynamic and multidimensional nature of disability results in complexities that are best addressed by interdisciplinary assessment teams (Fried-Oken and Granlund, 2012; Raghavendra et al., 2007; WHO, 2002). The members of the AAC team vary depending on individual user abilities, expectations, and communication needs and the availability of services. At a minimum, AAC team members include the individual with a communication disability; key communication partners (e.g., caregivers, partner, adult children); an SLP; and the individual's physician (Beukelman et al., 2008; Binger et al., 2012; Dietz et al., 2012). The SLP typically is the lead professional in the AAC team evaluation process and is likely to provide the intervention with AAC technology. The roles of the team members in AAC may be filled by many different people and may overlap. Importantly, the team approach makes the individual and family central contributors, interacting with the rest of the team to ensure their full participation and information sharing (Binger et al., 2012; Hill et al., 1998). Table 6-3 illustrates the roles of personnel involved in AAC assessment and treatment beyond the individual with communication needs, who is involved in every aspect listed in the table (Beukelman et al., 2008; Binger et al., 2012).

TABLE 6-3
Personnel Involved in AAC Assessment and Treatment

Personnel	Assessment and Treatment Involvement
AAC Finder	Identify and refer Report case history
General-practice speech-language pathologist	Identify and refer Acquire and evaluate case history Evaluate speech-language capacity and related domains Identify and recommend AAC options Acquire funding Establish and provide treatment
AAC clinical specialist	Evaluate case history Determine diagnostic questions[a] Identify and recommend AAC options Acquire funding Establish and provide treatment Provide AAC technical support
AAC facilitator (communication partner)	Identify and refer Report case history Contribute to diagnostic questions Participate in evaluation and treatment Advocate for individual Provide support across transitions Provide AAC technical support
Collaborating professional (e.g., occupational therapist; physical therapist; vision, hearing, rehabilitation medicine specialists)	Identify and refer Report/evaluate case history Contribute to diagnostic questions Participate in evaluation and treatment Access troubleshooting
AAC manufacturer/vendor	Identify AAC options Assist in evaluation process Provide equipment loans/trials Facilitate funding of selected AAC Provide AAC devices and accessories Provide AAC technical support
AAC technology training agency	Facilitate AAC evaluation and intervention Identify and recommend AAC options Establish and provide treatment Provide equipment loans/trials Provide AAC training Provide AAC technical support

[a]AAC clinical specialists may perform testing associated with a collaborating professional (e.g., vision, hearing, physical skills, cognition) as related specifically to communication and access.

Assessment

An AAC assessment requires integration of a broad scope of information to determine an appropriate recommendation and its implementation (Beukelman and Mirenda, 2005). The complexity of the assessment is influenced by such factors as the user's characteristics (e.g., skills, communication needs, environments), AAC team dynamics, rapidly occurring changes in technology, limited preprofessional training, and limited research on AAC clinical decision making (Dietz et al., 2012).

AAC assessment identifies daily communication needs, details functional communication goals, outlines individual/family supports, and generates treatment recommendations (Beukelman and Mirenda, 2013; Light and McNaughton, 2013; Williams et al., 2008). To enable comprehensive participation, evidence supporting communication needs for educational endeavors, vocational training, transition activities, and employment is integrated into the assessment. In addition, many funding sources require a medical necessity for communication; therefore, interactions needed for medical/health interactions are often identified. A sequential process of AAC assessment includes: (1) identifying communication needs and completing subsequent referral, (2) collecting information relevant to communication status and needs, (3) determining diagnostic questions and communication goals, (4) developing and completing evaluation procedures, (5) ascertaining and recommending AAC interventions, (6) securing funding, and (7) repeating steps 2-6 as additional needs arise (Binger et al., 2012). Assessments typically involve dynamic procedures designed to identify individual skills and strengths that can be used to support functional communication, gauge the impact of modifications on performance, and determine effort required for successful interactions (King et al., 2015). Although various models, frameworks, and guidelines are used in AAC assessments, feature matching (i.e., matching the user to AAC technology) and system trials are standard components (Beukelman and Mirenda, 2013; Cook and Polgar, 2008; Hill, 2004; Scherer and Craddock, 2002; Zabala et al., 2005). A brief description of typical assessment processes used to determine communication abilities, needs, and AAC options follows. Medical and communication diagnosis, prognosis, communicative needs, and functional abilities provide the basis for matching individuals with appropriate AAC systems by creating a customized system that supports communication based on the individual's skills. There are no prerequisite skills (e.g., cognitive, motor, language/literacy) for using AAC technologies (Light and McNaughton, 2012; Snell et al., 2010).

Demographics, Background, and Communication Needs

In addition to demographic and diagnostic information, the individual's educational, vocational, and previous clinical experiences are noted; this history informs assessment procedures and the AAC options presented. For example, an individual with long-standing developmental disabilities (e.g., cerebral palsy, cognitive impairment) may have previous experience with AAC systems that will reveal prior successes/failures with specific devices, while other individuals may have no prior AAC experience. For some individuals (e.g., those with ALS), a delay in referral for an AAC assessment creates an urgency to identify an immediate means for communicating (Nordness et al., 2010). Interviews and questionnaires provide information about the individual's (and his or her primary communication partners') values, beliefs, motivations, and expectations regarding AAC; current communication status and communication necessary to support daily communication activities; and environmental factors that may influence successful AAC implementation (Binger et al., 2012; Romski and Sevcik, 2005).

Speech/Oral Motor Skills

Individuals are candidates for AAC intervention if their natural speech is not sufficiently functional to meet all of their daily communication needs (Beukelman and Mirenda, 2013). A person may find that his or her dysarthric natural speech is functional for interactions with a spouse at home in a quiet or context-rich environment, but that this same speech will not support vocational interactions; therefore, natural speech fails to meet all of the person's communication needs. Unintelligible speech or significantly reduced rate of speech influences functionality, thus supporting a person's need for AAC technology.

Cognitive–Linguistic Considerations

Beyond current language ability, conversational needs, and communication contexts, AAC techniques and symbols and/or strategies are evaluated to identify optimal communication performance (Hill and Corsi, 2012; Hill et al., 2010; Romich et al., 2005). Frequently, linguistic evaluations are conducted prior to the AAC assessment as part of a standard speech-language evaluation. Important considerations include the individual's

- receptive (comprehension), expressive (speaking and writing), and pragmatic (social) language skills, which influence the selection of an optimal language representation and messaging system; and

- cognitive and executive functioning skills (e.g., attention, focus, orientation, organization, and sequencing), which influence the selection of an optimal AAC system and the individual's functional and strategic implementation of that system.

Fine/Gross Motor Skills and Mobility

Assessment of physical skills in the context of an AAC system includes identifying input selection techniques, transporting the device, and ensuring proper seating and positioning (Cooper et al., 2009; Costigan and Light, 2010). The identification of appropriate input selection techniques is influenced by body or extremity (e.g., finger, hand, knee, toe, head) range of motion, accuracy and consistency of movement, degree of force required to activate the device or a switch, the speed at which the individual can activate and release the device or switch, and the length of time and frequency with which the individual can repeat the movement before becoming fatigued. Assessment of input selection may entail evaluating the person's access to the device using available movements (e.g., digit of the hand, foot, eye gaze, stylus, mouse or head mouse, joystick, head stick or mouth stick). Many device features may be modified to improve selection accuracy and efficiency (e.g., accept or release time, display size or orientation, touch guides, key guards). Likewise, assessment includes identifying impacts of such modifications on communication performance, device transport (e.g., weight, size), and effective interactions. When direct selection is ineffective as an access technique, the individual's ability to scan using one or multiple switches is assessed, which entails evaluating access to AAC technologies indirectly by means of switch activation. Options include activation using body part movement or function (e.g., hand or arm, foot or leg, head, blink, motion, voice). Device features may be modified to improve selection accuracy and efficiency (e.g., scan method, scan rate, highlighting, repeat scans), and the assessment includes comparing positive and negative impacts of the various options.

Although many individuals who communicate with AAC ambulate independently, many have complex disability that requires the use of rollators, wheelchairs, or alternative seating and positioning. Many changes in AAC technologies that have occurred in recent years influence how they are both used and transported (McNaughton and Light, 2013). Alternative seating may require a means of mounting the AAC system to enable access as the person is positioned throughout the day and during transport; the AAC team makes such decisions about enhanced access as part of the assessment process (Beukelman et al., 2008; Binger et al., 2012). Mounting systems can be fitted to a wheelchair, and commercial mounting products offer a variety of features (e.g., swing-away, folding, rolling). The assessment includes making comparisons to identify features that will benefit an individual or are needed to maximize use of the AAC.

Vision and Hearing

Assessment of functional vision and hearing influences the selection and use of an AAC system: visual skills inform decisions regarding the size, type, and placement of symbols, while hearing informs decisions regarding voice output system needs (Beukelman and Mirenda, 2013; Hill, 2010; Hill and Corsi, 2012). Assessment includes identifying the appropriate number of locations on a display to accommodate vision abilities and needs and controls for auditory output (e.g., volume, voice output, speech rate, or pitch).

Choice of an Appropriate AAC Technology for the Individual

AAC assessment and prescription entails a systematic approach to matching an individual's abilities, communication needs, and expectations to specific AAC features. The assessment team identifies the user's current communication needs and then attempts to anticipate the future by considering potential changing needs and skills (e.g., transitions, skill development, degeneration). The intent is to optimize functional interactions in all communication situations (ASHA, 2004b; Glennen and DeCoste, 1997; Scherer, 2002, 2005; Scherer and Craddock, 2002).

Previous AAC Experience

Identification of previous AAC interventions is helpful in determining categories and features of AAC devices that may meet the individual's abilities, needs, and expectations. The effectiveness of previously implemented features also can be evaluated. In some cases, updates to AAC technologies may impact performance.

Selection of AAC Device Features

Informing the individual and family of various AAC technology options is a critical step in feature matching, helping to remove bias from the selection process. The taxonomy of AAC devices presented earlier and in Annex Tables 6-1, 6-2, and 6-3 at the end of this chapter reveals the complexity of AAC features and their combinations. The AAC team seeks to identify AAC device features that support identified communication goals, which may involve medical, social, educational, and/or vocational interactions. Device features identified as important to effective AAC implementation by SLPs and individuals who use AAC include ease of use (e.g., efficiency, reliability, suitability, adjustability), design (e.g., comfort, size, portability, durability), performance (e.g., battery life, rapid use, simple maintenance, rechargeable during use), integrated software and layout (e.g., ability to find words and messages easily and produce spontaneous messages), and voice output (e.g., rapid speech production, having an alternative output method) (Judge and Townend, 2013; O'Keefe et al., 2007).

The rise in the use of mobile technologies (e.g., smartphones, tablets) in the United States and the vast array of applications available for download have opened the door to the use of such technologies by individuals with complex communication needs (McNaughton and Light, 2013). Mobile AAC technologies may be a good match for some individuals and can offer certain benefits over traditional AAC systems such as SGDs. Often the mobile technologies are smaller and less expensive than traditional AAC systems, and they offer the myriad features typical of such devices that go well beyond the AAC function (McNaughton and Light, 2013). In addition, because they are mainstream technologies, their use as AAC devices promotes social acceptance. As one AAC user noted, "Using an iPad, Blackberry, or iPhone . . . is not another thing that makes me different. It wasn't using a strange, unfamiliar device to communicate with this group" (Hyatt, 2001, p. 25; McNaughton and Light, 2013). Yet, while ease of access to and social acceptance of AAC mobile technologies are benefits attending such devices, they come with a downside. Focusing on the technologies themselves ignores the most important element of any communication device for someone with complex communication needs—its ability "to facilitate effective communication and fuller participation in society" for that individual (McNaughton and Light, 2013, p. 110). Regardless of the category of devices being considered, whether a variety of SGDs or different mobile AAC technologies, it is important that consumers and providers be aware of all of the available options and engage in a process of evaluation and decision making that will result in matching the individual with the most appropriate device to meet his or her communication needs (McNaughton and Light, 2013).

AAC Technology Trials

Practice with an assortment of AAC technologies that have been matched to the user's needs optimizes assessment outcomes for both the individual and the AAC team and illustrates the strengths and weaknesses of various options or combinations thereof. The format and methods used for practice, known as trials, are at the discretion of the SLP, the individual and family, and the other AAC team members. Upon completion of system trials, team members reach informed consensus on the optimal system.

Trial Decisions

As the lead professional on the AAC team, the SLP typically selects an array of AAC technologies to be used during trials. Individuals may have suggestions about products they have heard about, seen, and hope to try, which are integrated into the evaluation process to the extent possible (e.g., based on availability, individual access options, and/or appropriate representation). Trials may reflect professional experience and preferences with respect to AAC technology; therefore they tend to be idiosyncratic across SLPs (Glennen, 2000). Selecting AAC technologies for trial includes ensuring that the individual is aware of various options and the personal abilities and communication needs they address. Summarizing trial results may serve to highlight evidence of individual communication performance with the different technologies and features, thus adding support for device selection by providing a personalized performance profile.

Rationale for AAC Technology Selection

Integrating information on clinical implementation, personal performance, and external participation (e.g., in the community, home, and workplace) gleaned from AAC technology trials guides decision making and optimizes the selection of an AAC system. Clinical and personal evidence are based on comprehensive assessment of communication ability and the domains influencing communication, daily communication needs, functional communication goals, and personal preferences. The trial process allows the AAC team to identify specific components, features, and tools necessary to meet the individual's communication needs.

Monitoring

AAC clinical services are intended to support the myriad communication needs of the augmented communicator (Higginbotham and Engelke, 2013). To enable the user to accomplish the most effective communication, quantitative and qualitative performance measures are gathered intermittently. Performance measurement typically includes examining clinical evidence and communication performance in a clinical setting. Participation and outcome measures also are used to monitor progress toward achieving optimal use of the recommended AAC system (ASHA, 2004b).

AAC outcome measurement involves evaluating AAC technology-based interactions during specific communication activities, then comparing achieved outcomes with the intended results or desired goals. Measuring the effectiveness of AAC communication requires having appropriate measurement instruments and methodologies available (Anderson et al., 2016;

Smith, 1996). Measures of real-time communication functioning and research investigating the impact of AAC technologies on communicative participation are sparse. Various instruments collect measures of satisfaction and self-reported outcomes for various assistive products and technologies; some include AAC, while others can be modified for evaluating AAC results (Anderson et al., 2016; Demers et al., 2002; Jutai et al., 1996; Scherer and Craddock, 2002). Similarly, some AAC devices have a data logging feature that automatically records the communicator's utterances (Higginbotham et al., 2002; Hill, 2004) and provides a file for analysis and tracking of communication trends (Hill, 2010).

Monitoring also includes tracking acceptance and abandonment of AAC devices. High levels of acceptance of AAC technologies have been documented for a variety of individuals across disability groups. Among individuals with communication impairment resulting from traumatic brain injury using devices based on assessment recommendations, acceptance of synthesized high-tech devices was more than 94 percent, and acceptance of digitized low-tech devices was 100 percent (Fager et al., 2006). Likewise, individuals with ALS have been found to have an acceptance rate of synthesized high-tech devices of approximately 96 percent (Ball et al., 2004, 2007). Other individuals with progressive disease also have demonstrated acceptance of AAC technologies (Beukelman et al., 2007a), including those with primary progressive aphasia (Fried-Oken et al., 2015), spinal muscular atrophy (Ball et al., 2012), and dementia (Bourgeois, 1991; Fried-Oken et al., 2015). Among individuals with aphasia, communication partner strategies have been shown to improve acceptance of AAC technologies (Ball and Lasker, 2013).

Prominent factors in acceptance of AAC include intervention timing (e.g., early referral, regular reevaluations, and continual treatment); involvement of communication partners from the onset (e.g., to establish AAC acceptance and use); and ongoing monitoring and adjustment over time (e.g., integration of new strategies, accommodation of changes in technology or personal ability, integration of multiple modalities to capitalize on strengths) (Fried-Oken et al., 2015). Factors potentially influencing acceptance of AAC mobile technologies include functionality and interconnectivity, consumer empowerment in accessing AAC options, social acceptance of AAC in the mainstream, ease of acquisition, and affordability (McNaughton and Light, 2013).

Data are lacking on abandonment, or the inappropriate discontinuation of AAC technology determined appropriate by the AAC team. Factors influencing abandonment have been reported to include communication partners' belief that they can understand natural speech; insufficient opportunities to engage in conversation; lack of communication partners' motivation; individual preference for other communication methods; and insufficient or inadequate education/preparation for use or maintenance of the device (e.g., programming, generation of timely and appropriate messages, system upkeep) (Johnson et al., 2006). Lack of support from a communication facilitator or partner has been cited as influential in the abandonment of AAC interventions for people with traumatic brain injury (Fager et al., 2006). Factors influencing potential abandonment of AAC mobile technologies include a possible shift in the essential focus on communication to a focus on the technology; the lack of a structured assessment process to identify optimal features for communication and support for a wide variety of communication functions and contexts; and access restricted to mainstream options (Kagohara, et al., 2013; McNaughton and Light, 2013).

TRAINING AND ADAPTATION

Based on the complexity of the AAC system, a wide range of training and adaptation requirements exist, from those in which the individual "turns on and uses" to those requiring multiple learning sessions and ongoing system programming to support interactions with new communicative partners, topics, and/or situations. Little information is available regarding specific training needs and adaptation times across AAC systems.

The need to rely on AAC may result from a wide range of developmental, physical, cognitive, and/or social impairments (Ball et al., 2010a). For many individuals, these impairments are chronic, requiring AAC across the life span and through numerous life transitions (Lilienfeld and Alant, 2009; Mirenda, 2003). During transitions, AAC strategies and system features that have been effective in one communication environment may become less effective in new ones (Hamm and Mirenda, 2006; Lund and Light, 2006). Likewise, depending on the type of disability, individuals who rely on AAC to communicate may find that existing AAC strategies become less effective, generally as a result of the natural course of the medical condition that has resulted in limited spoken communication (either degenerative or gradually improving and eventually stabilizing) (Beukelman et al., 2007b). Degenerative conditions include ALS, primary progressive aphasia, and dementia, among others. For individuals with degenerative conditions, AAC systems are managed so as to maintain effective communication through speech, language, cognitive, or motor control decline. Improving and stabilizing conditions include stroke/aphasia, traumatic brain injury, cerebral palsy, cognitive impairment, and locked-in syndrome, among others. As with degenerative conditions, AAC supports interactions across multiple settings in the context of improving speech, language, cognitive, or motor control (Beukelman et al., 2007b).

AAC system adaptations occur after the original evaluation for four primary reasons: (1) physical changes that result in a need for a new access method, (2) cognitive changes that result in a need for new/updated message representations, (3) changes to other equipment that result in a need for new/updated mounting of the AAC system, and (4) living or vocational setting changes that result in the need to interact in new communication contexts with different partners. Individuals with degenerative, improving, and relapsing-remitting conditions require frequent adjustments to AAC access, commonly to accommodate physical changes. Some adjustments to the AAC software presentation may be necessary based on increasing/decreasing vocabulary and linguistic complexity (e.g., someone with Alzheimer's disease wants to maintain a key skill at work, or someone with cognitive impairment is promoted and wishes to train for new interactions).

AAC Use and Prognosis for Occupational Success

Speech and language disorders encompass a wide range of impairments (e.g., congenital, acquired, degenerative) that affect an individual's ability to communicate functionally using natural speech (ASHA, 2016a; Perry et al., 2004; Wodka et al., 2013). Communication competence with AAC is complicated not simply by the need to have knowledge of and skills in a native language but also by the need to learn the language software of the AAC system (Drager et al., 2003).

Although data on the subject are sparse, successful employment among individuals who require AAC tends to be dependent on the discrete job requirements and flexibility of employers; successful employment outcomes have been reported for professional jobs with text-centered interactions (i.e., written or text-generated speech) (Fried-Oken, 1993; McNaughton et al., 2001). Individuals have reported as benefits of employment personal expectations (e.g., desire for success, serving as a model for others with disability), finances (e.g., gaining independence), and positive workplace experiences (e.g., enjoying work activities and workplace interactions) (McNaughton and Richardson, 2013; McNaughton et al., 2002). Telework has been shown to have benefits for some individuals who communicate with AAC (e.g., work efficiency, flexible schedule, coworker interactions), although some problems exist (e.g., slow home Internet speeds, need to purchase one's own office equipment, easy access to distractions) (McNaughton et al., 2014). A growing number of individuals who communicate with AAC (e.g., those with autism spectrum disorder or complex communication needs) expect to participate fully in community and workplace activities but require supports (e.g., training and experience valued by employers, academic and vocational training, identification of jobs that are a good match) (Bryen et al., 2007; Howlin et al., 2005; Light and McNaughton, 2012; McNaughton and Arnold, 2013; Wehman et al.,

2012). AAC technologies have been shown to increase employability ratings compared with natural dysarthric speech based on perceived credibility, strength and knowledgeability involving highly skilled positions, verbal ability, and interactivity (Stern et al., 2017).

Individuals who communicate with AAC can obtain and maintain employment (Hourcade et al., 2004; Light et al., 1996; McNaughton and Bryen, 2007), but this is the case for only a small percentage of these individuals because of a number of barriers to their employment (Feinstein et al., 2013; Light et al., 1996). Successful employment has been documented primarily with government agencies and advocacy organizations (McNaughton et al., 2002). Because AAC technologies are subject to breakdown, they require technical support and repair that results in loss of access to communication, and a loss of effective communication, however temporary, will impact an individual's ability to fulfill work responsibilities.

Language, literacy, and education are critical factors for the employment of individuals with physical disabilities, and communication competence for basic workplace interactions is essential for employment of individuals with developmental disabilities (Collier et al., 2012; McNaughton et al., 2002). Development of these skills must begin at an early age if academic, social, and communication skills are to be integrated successfully into the workplace (McNaughton et al., 2002).

Interpersonal communication (e.g., responding to others, participating in conversations, putting others at ease) is an important work-related social-relational skill (Light and McNaughton, 2014). One model of communication competence cites linguistic, operational, social, and strategic abilities, as well as motivation, attitude, confidence, and resilience, as influencing success with AAC technology (Light, 2003; Light and McNaughton, 2014; Thistle and Wilkinson, 2013). Training in social-relational interactions can have a positive impact on communication competence (Kent-Walsh and McNaughton, 2009; Light et al., 1999). Skill in such interactions is important for the communication partners of AAC speakers as well, yet most individuals in a community are unlikely to have had a conversation with such an individual. The lack of partner skill may limit communication effectiveness as much as, if not more than, the AAC technology. Indeed, as noted above, issues related to partner training and AAC technology supports are associated with abandonment of the technology (Johnson et al., 2006).

Integration of AAC software into mainstream technologies can enable easy and rapid interactions that are required for employment, particularly telework (AAC-RERC, 2011), while also providing access to a wide variety of other information (e.g., online services, entertainment, education, health care, public services, employment, health and safety, tools) (Shane et al., 2012). Barriers to control of mainstream technologies may be encountered by individuals with physical limitations who are unable to perform certain movements (e.g., swipe, pinch, use a keyboard or touch screen) without integration of the alternative access available through the AAC technology or implementation of the adapted access options that are increasingly available (e.g., accelerometers, eye gaze, pattern recognition) (Shane et al., 2012).

Reduced communication rates associated with AAC likely interfere significantly with communication interactions, particularly in educational and employment contexts with speakers accustomed to exchanging information at a rapid pace (Higginbotham et al., 2007; McNaughton and Bryen, 2007). Even if an individual is matched with an appropriate device, receives extensive training, and becomes competent in using an AAC system, he or she may not engage adequately in a real-time discussion in a board room because of limitations imposed by the interrelationship among the method of communication; the AAC technology features; and the individual's physical disability, cognitive/linguistic skills, and skills in interacting with a communication partner (Higginbotham et al., 2007). Similarly, various service industry positions require certain (as yet unestablished) interaction pacing to sustain engagement. Communication inefficiencies (reduced comprehensibility) and message timing limitations (time required to formulate a message) interfere with effective communication on the part of many individuals who rely on AAC to communicate (Hanson et al., 2016; Rodriguez et al., 2016; Trnka et al., 2008). Communication applications with various features and strategies may not enhance the rate of communication sufficiently to support individual participation by generating rapid utterances (Newell et al., 1998), and little research published to date supports the notion that word prediction enhances rate (Yang et al., 2009). Other human factors, moreover, such as increased visual monitoring and motor control, influence communication rates when rate enhancement strategies are employed (Beukelman and Mirenda, 2013).

With few exceptions, digitized speech in AAC is associated with greater intelligibility relative to synthesized speech (Drager et al., 2006). Research has demonstrated that low-quality synthesized speech is sufficiently inferior to human speech to have significantly compromised value for functional AAC; however, the quality of synthesized speech has shown dramatic improvements in recent years (Drager and Reichle, 2001; Fucci et al., 1995; Venkatagiri, 2003). Still, multiple investigations have demonstrated that digitized and synthesized systems are not sufficiently intelligible for all listeners in all environments (Alamsaputra et al., 2006).

Communication with Natural Speech: Effects on Prognosis

Effective speakers produce appropriate messages and are active and efficient in relaying them to control, influence, and direct the environment (Yorkston et al., 2010b). People use speech in their daily environments and have individually unique speaking demands that vary based on such factors as employment, life situation, recreational and community involvement, and particular communication preferences (Anderson et al., 2016). And evidence suggests that communication impairments often result in loss of independence and reduced quality of life (Müller et al., 2001).

The impact of employment cannot be overstated. Employment plays a key role in socioeconomic status, personal self-image, and quality of life (Blackstone, 1993; McCarthy, 1986; McNaughton et al., 2001). Emerging evidence indicates that perceived hireability may be limited when individuals communicate with even mild dysarthric natural speech instead of using AAC technologies for communication (Stern et al., 2017). Evidence indicates further that individuals who work for pay tend to report higher speech usage than those who are nonworking; indeed, a large percentage (74 percent) of those working for pay rank speech usage as the most important activity for work and describe it as either "extremely" or "very" important to their work (Anderson et al., 2016). It is difficult, however, to identify the need for communication associated with various jobs. Positions labeled as requiring no verbal communication may nonetheless have a speaking requirement that was not identified by the employer (e.g., a surveillance system operator may watch monitors to prevent shoplifting in a business, but in some way he or she must report incidents when observed).

Social Security Administration Disability Evaluation: Natural Speech and AAC

Based on regulations, the U.S. Social Security Administration (SSA) considers both natural speech and speech supported by AAC in disability determinations. SSA disability evaluation considers "the use of speech by any means and includes the use of mechanical or electronic devices" in determining whether an individual's speech disorder is "severe enough to prevent an individual from doing any gainful activity" (SSA, n.d., 2.00 Special Senses and Speech). The category of impairment defined as "loss of speech due to any cause, with inability to produce by any means speech that can be heard, understood, or sustained" relates to persistent ineffective speech or communication (e.g., SSA, n.d., 2.09 loss of speech, 11.04A aphasia), significant interference with communication (e.g., SSA, n.d., 11.07 cerebral palsy), or unintelligible speech (e.g., SSA, n.d., 11.11 post-polio syndrome).[1]

The Program Operations Manual System Policy for Evaluation of Speech Impairments (SSA, 2017) identifies three attributes pertinent to

[1]This sentence has been revised to reflect the updated Listing of Impairments for Neurological Disorders.

evaluation of speech proficiency: (1) audibility, (2) intelligibility, and (3) functional efficiency. Audibility encompasses loudness or intensity of speech in such contexts as quiet, noise, and riding in automobiles, as well as voice that becomes inaudible with use (as might be experienced with some conditions impacted by fatigue or respiratory insufficiency). Intelligibility, or the ability to articulate accurately, encompasses frequency of articulation errors, the extent to which the person is asked to repeat utterances, and how well the person is understood by strangers (the policy refers specifically to esophageal speech understood by people unfamiliar with this type of speech production). Finally, functional efficiency encompasses the ability to sustain consecutive speech, the number of words spoken without interruption/hesitancy, and the time lapse prior to speaking fatigue. Although specific measures are not indicated, the policy notes that if at least one of these attributes is missing, overall speech is not considered effective.

ACCESS AND AVAILABILITY

AAC Clinician Expertise

The *Scope of Practice in Speech-Language Pathology* of the American Speech-Language-Hearing Association (ASHA) (ASHA, 2016e) provides the conceptual framework within which SLPs provide clinical services. Although SLP graduate training programs meet multimodal communication standards, many universities do not offer a dedicated course in AAC, many AAC courses are not required components of the curriculum, few programs offer more than one such course, and students often graduate without having a supervised AAC clinical experience.

ASHA's *Knowledge and Skills* document outlines the responsibilities, knowledge, and general skills for SLPs in the area of AAC (ASHA, 2016c). Proficiencies required of an SLP for providing AAC services include the following:

- Knowledge of the broad array of . . . [current] devices that are designed specifically for AAC purposes and their respective features.
- Knowledge of the performance differences of the broad array of [AAC technologies] (e.g., different forms of computer hardware and software, as well as adaptations such as touch screens and expanded keyboards that are intended for purposes that include but are not limited to communication) and their respective features.
- Knowledge of how language is generated on AAC systems during communication.
- Matching features of AAC systems to capabilities of individuals being considered for those same systems.
- Customizing AAC systems to meet individuals' needs and skills.

- Modifying AAC systems as individuals' communication abilities and needs change and new technologies arise. (ASHA, 2016c)

Individuals who communicate with AAC experience significant barriers to obtaining and learning to use AAC technology. As discussed below, funding is a concern for these individuals, but the greater barrier at present appears to be the lack of trained SLPs to provide assessment and intervention services. Persons who provide daily support to these individuals often do not receive needed training (Beukelman et al., 2009; McNaughton et al., 2001; Ratcliff and Beukelman, 1995), and as noted above, many graduates of SLP programs fail to receive sufficient training in AAC (Collier and Blackstein-Adler, 1998; Costigan and Light, 2007; Crema and Moran, 2012; Koul and Lloyd, 1994; Matthews, 2001; Robinson and Sadao, 2005). ASHA's 2015 end-of-year membership report cites 156,254 certified SLP members (ASHA, 2015a), whereas the AAC Special Interest Group had 3,239 members, reflecting approximately 2 percent of the association's total membership.

Few, if any, structured programs offer AAC training to SLPs beyond entry-level (Certificate of Clinical Competence) education (Koul and Lloyd, 1994). As a result, SLPs must obtain such training by attending numerous AAC-specific conferences and workshops, completing training with a variety of AAC technologies, reading AAC journals and periodicals, and participating in professional organizations with a focus on AAC (e.g., the ASHA AAC Special Interest Group, the International Society for Augmentative and Alternative Communication) (Beukelman et al., 2009).

AAC Funding Factors

Chapter 7 addresses major sources of coverage and funding for assistive products and technologies, including AAC. This section highlights a few funding considerations that are specific to AAC technology. Funding policies and practices can affect the adequacy of AAC evaluation, as well as funding approval for prescribed AAC technologies. Funding obstacles also may impact receipt of AAC training to maximize employment potential.

Current Procedural Terminology (CPT) codes for speech-language services are both time- and procedure-based (ASHA, 2016d). The time-based codes relevant to AAC include the first hour of an AAC evaluation, each additional 30 minutes of the evaluation, standardized cognitive performance testing per hour, and aphasia evaluation per hour. All other codes are procedure-based; the CPT code is reported once for the procedure and is based on a typical session regardless of the appointment length. Codes include evaluation of speech sound production; evaluation of language comprehension and expression; behavioral and qualitative analysis of voice and resonance; therapeutic services for the use of non-speech-generating AAC; therapeutic services for the use of AAC technology, including programming and modification; and repair/modification of AAC devices. Although modification, repair, or replacement of unrepairable systems often is fundable, no provision is made for interim communication support while these processes are taking place. As a result, it is important to highlight the fact that as technologies or computer-based equipment, AAC systems are subject to breakdown, thus requiring technical support and repair; as noted earlier, loss of access to communication, albeit temporary, will likely impact an individual's ability to fulfill work responsibilities.

Funding mechanisms for the purchase of prescribed AAC technology may influence the prescription of a particular system. Typical funding sources for adults who would benefit from AAC technology include private insurance companies, the Veterans Health Administration, and Medicare or Medicaid. Additional funding mechanisms available to some individuals include state telephone equipment distribution programs, vocational rehabilitation programs, private pay, and charitable programs. Medicare Advantage plans are implemented under contract with private insurers through policies that provide Medicare (Parts A and B) benefits (CMS, 2017a), and individual policies may differ regarding coverage of SGDs. Medicare Supplemental Insurance (Medigap) policies are designed to cover some health care costs associated with Medicare (e.g., coinsurance, deductibles, copayments); these policies may be purchased from private insurers (CMS, 2017b). For funding of SGDs, Medigap policies cover supplemental costs associated with obtaining items covered by Medicare (Medicare typically covers 80 percent of approved SGD costs, and a Medigap policy will cover the 20 percent copayment). Medigap policies do not cover items not approved by Medicare (e.g., mobile AAC technologies, hearing aids) (CMS, 2017b).

Not all AAC technology solutions have been assigned a Healthcare Common Procedure Coding System (HCPCS) code. Delays in assigning codes may occur when technology innovations are added quickly to the market, as is common for rapidly changing technology. If uncoded technology is identified as the best match for and preferred by the individual, funding for that technology may or may not be available. Moreover, ongoing costs associated with mobile technologies (e.g., data rates, access to the Internet, cellphone fees) reduce the use of these AAC technologies for some individuals who could benefit from them (AAC-RERC, 2011), while others may opt for an SGD because it is covered by insurance even though it provides fewer features and is a poorer match for their communication needs (McNaughton and Light, 2013). Conversely, some individuals may purchase a mobile AAC technology thinking it will save them money, only to discover that it is not a good match for their AAC needs. Regardless of the funding source, a range of appropriate AAC technology solutions are presented as part of the evaluation, with the ultimate goal of achieving the best communication match and meeting personal preferences. It remains the case, however, that funding options, cost, and affordability often influence which device is prescribed.

One benefit of Centers for Medicare & Medicaid Services (CMS) funding programs is the establishment of an assessment procedure and specific requirements (CMS, 2001). Some alternative funding options (e.g., equipment lending libraries, private purchase of mobile AAC technologies) do not link appropriate evaluations with AAC selection, trained providers, communication specialists, or indeed any criteria (AAC-RERC, 2011). At times, obtaining equipment in such a way results in a substantial cost savings and an appropriate communication solution; however, chance often determines whether the individual makes an inappropriate purchase that may ultimately prove more costly in terms of money, motivation, and effort.

One concern associated with CMS funding programs with respect to multimodal communication and employment is the requirement that the individual abandon all other forms of communication before selecting an SGD. The requirement is that all other forms of treatment be "considered and ruled out" prior to selection of an AAC option (CMS, 2001).

Individuals with disabilities also face challenges with funding for AAC technologies as they go through transitions. Youth transitioning from education-based services may face questions regarding ownership of AAC products and technologies; if a school system made the purchase, the AAC technology currently used by the individual may be retained by the school. In such situations, an AAC reevaluation and funding approval are required for the individual to have access to an AAC system that meets his or her communication goals and supports the person's continued education, vocational training, and employment.

Although many individuals in need of communication systems have funding available for the purchase of AAC technology, most clinical providers do not. Notably, many clinical facilities do not provide AAC evaluations because of the high cost of purchasing and maintaining AAC technologies, software, and access options. Anecdotal evidence from providers nationwide indicates that assessment sites maintaining updated equipment most commonly are those affiliated with university educational/research programs. Few hospitals maintain evaluation centers with current equipment. Many individual clinicians will arrange to borrow equipment from other evaluation centers (e.g., state offices for assistive technology, disability-specific loan closets) and manufacturers to gain access to appropriate equipment. These funding factors impact access to appropriate evaluations and equipment needed to implement trials.

VOICE RESTORATION FOLLOWING HEAD AND NECK SURGERY

Prevalence of Need

The American Cancer Society estimated 59,000 cases of head and neck cancer in the United States in 2015 (American Cancer Society, 2015). Individuals with head and neck cancer acquire communication needs as a result of various cancer treatments, including surgical resection, radiation, and chemotherapy. Surgical treatments may involve resection of head/neck structures and tissue that may result in partial or complete removal of the larynx, vocal cords, and articulatory structures, in turn resulting in loss of voice and/or speech.

Voice Restoration Taxonomy

Some individuals with head and neck cancer may benefit from various categories of AAC technology, including mobile technologies, SGDs (HCPCS: E2500-E2510), and communication software and apps (HCPCS: E2511) (Ball et al., 2016b; Beukelman and Mirenda, 2013; Happ et al., 2004; Sullivan et al., 2007a,b):

- **Mobile technologies**—Communication applications are available for use on both iOS and Android platforms, although the number of options is currently greater on the former (Ball et al., 2016b). Such mobile technologies are now intrinsic to daily life for people from many cultures, languages, and traditions, and as such may provide a readily accessible means of supporting communication without adding to visible disability (McNaughton and Light, 2013). These technologies are summarized in Annex Tables 6-1 and 6-3.
- **Speech-generating devices**—Designed specifically for communication, SGDs may provide the most effective means of meeting communication needs through highly customizable and variable features (Beukelman and Mirenda, 2013; McNaughton and Light, 2013). Other SGD features that may be of particular importance for individuals with communication needs relate to available language options and options for connectivity to other computer technologies (Ball et al., 2016b). These technologies are described in detail in Tables 6-1 and 6-2 and Annex Tables 6-1 and 6-3.
- **Communication software and apps**—Communication software programs and apps provide options for individuals with head and neck cancer to communicate using direct access. They also may be used to design and print low-tech communication displays that can often be practical for communicating basic messages in acute

care or other temporary settings. Software may represent language using symbols other than traditional text (e.g., pictures, drawings) and therefore may be helpful to individuals with literacy and/or cognitive limitations (Ball et al., 2016b). The framework for these technologies is described in Table 6-2, while details are provided in Annex Table 6-2.

Although some individuals benefit from the specified AAC technologies, individuals typically are supported with voice restoration after undergoing head/neck cancer interventions (Tang and Sinclair, 2015). Similarly, those having undergone a tracheostomy, who retain the body structures and functions necessary to produce speech but whose respiratory flow is redirected away from the vocal cords, are supported with speech restoration (Lichtman et al., 1995). For some, speech becomes functional when diminished speech intensity is supported by amplification (Andreetta et al., 2016). The various options are described below and summarized in Table 6-4.[2]

Functional Speech Following Head/Neck Cancer Surgery and Radiation

For individuals postsurgery, "speech outcomes are the strongest predictor of health-related quality of life, inhibiting a person's ability to return to work, establish or maintain relationships, or participate in everyday activities" (Bolt et al., 2016, p. E1). Psychosocial quality of life decreases as a result of loss of voice after head and neck cancer treatments. Individuals may experience feelings of solitude, limitations in social relationships that result in social withdrawal, and reduced sexual enjoyment (Babin et al., 2009; Singer et al., 2008; Tang and Sinclair, 2015). Key factors in participation in communication include severity of speech loss, cognitive function (perhaps associated with cancer-related cognitive impairment), and extent of surgical resection (Bolt et al., 2016).

One study found that at 3 months following head/neck cancer treatment, 63 percent of individuals postsurgery (55 percent postsurgery with radiation) described broadly functional speech (i.e., perceived as possibly distorted but 100 percent intelligible) with natural speech or when accessing a tracheoesophageal voice prosthesis (TEP), an artificial/electrolarynx (AL/EL), and/or esophageal speech (ESS) (Perry and Shaw, 2000). Another 22 percent of individuals postsurgery (26 percent postsurgery with radiation) reported at least moderate speech disabilities (i.e., perceived as intelligible only when communication partners knew the message context) using the same assistive methods of communication (i.e., TEP, AL/EL, ESS), citing

[2]The images in Table 6-4 serve as examples of device categories only and should not be considered an endorsement of specific products or manufacturers.

a frequent need to repeat spoken messages and use writing to supplement speech to convey intended meaning (Perry and Shaw, 2000). Finally, 12 percent of individuals postsurgery (19 percent postsurgery with radiation) reported poor speech (occasional to no functional communication and/or at least 50 percent unintelligible) with the same assistive communication methods (i.e., TEP, AL/EL, ESS) (Perry and Shaw, 2000). These reports thus indicate a range of 34-45 percent of individuals undergoing head and neck cancer treatments who, although receiving benefit from voice restoration strategies, will likely require AAC technology to achieve fully functional communication.

Functional Speech Following Laryngectomy

For individuals who produce functional speech following a laryngectomy, four primary voice restoration methods are used: (1) esophageal speech, (2) tracheoesophageal voice prosthesis, (3) artificial or electrolarynx (Perry and Shaw, 2000), and (4) voice amplification (see p. 252).

Esophageal Speech

In ESS (see Figure 6-1), air from the mouth is transferred into the upper esophagus, where the released air causes the pharyngo-esophageal tissue to vibrate and produce a low-pitched voice (Enderby et al., 2009). This voice restoration strategy does not involve assistive technology; instead, ESS is produced by the individual's injecting (essentially swallowing) air into the esophagus and then releasing it in a controlled manner to cause the soft tissue to vibrate and produce voicing (Tang and Sinclair, 2015).

Tracheoesophageal Voice Prosthesis

At present, the most common voice restoration strategy for individuals with a complete laryngectomy is the placement of a one-way valve in the tracheoesophageal wall that allows respiratory air to flow from the lungs to the esophagus, where soft tissue vibrates and produces substitute voicing. This voice restoration method involves fitting a prosthesis through a surgically created puncture (e.g., stoma) between the trachea and the esophagus (Enderby et al., 2009). Voice is created by closing the stoma using one's fingers or a hands-free valve (see Figure 6-2).

Artificial/Electrolarynx

This voice restoration strategy involves an electrolarynx, an external device that produces vibrations in the oral cavity or pharyngeal mucosa

TABLE 6-4
Voice and Speech Restoration and Amplification Taxonomy

Feature	AL/EL (L8500)	TSV (L8501)	TEP_{pt} (L8507)	TEP_{pr} (L8509)	AMP (L8510)	ESS
	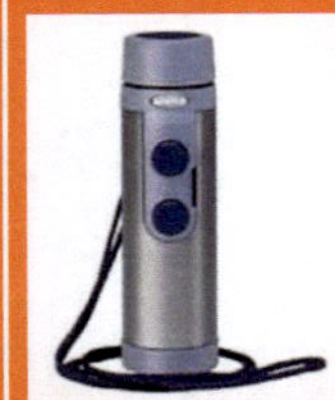 A	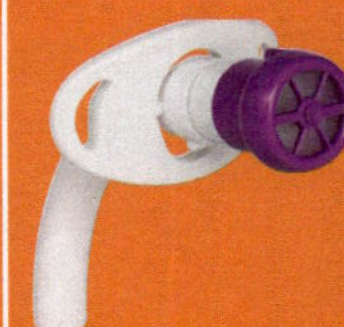 B	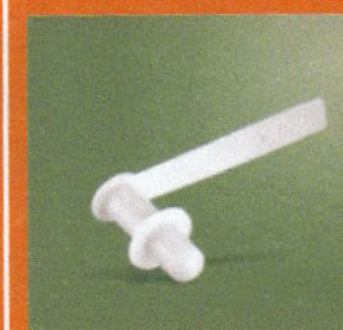 C	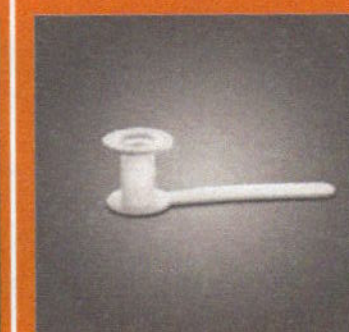 D	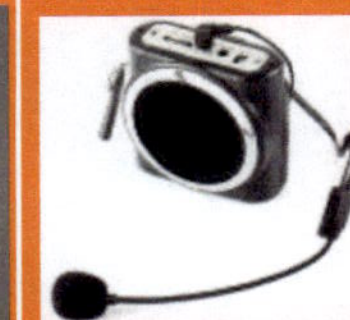 E	
Total laryngectomy	X		X	X	X	X
Partial laryngectomy					X	
Tracheostomy, intact larynx		X				
Professional insertion				X		
Patient insertion			X			
Hands free use		X	X	X	X	X
Hand held use	X				X	
Shunt air into esophagus			X	X		X
Vibrate head/neck tissue	X		X	X		X
Surgical placement			X	X		
Voice amplification					X	
Battery, rechargeable	X				X	

NOTE: AL/EL = artificial/electrolarynx; AMP = voice amplifier; ESS = esophageal speech; TEP = tracheoesophageal voice prosthesis; TEP_{pr} = TEP, provider inserted; TEP_{pt} = TEP, patient inserted; TSV = tracheostomy speaking valve.

SOURCES: A. Servox Digital electrolarynx, Bruce Medical; B. PMV 2001 (purple®), Passy Muir, Inc.; Image courtesy of Passy Muir, Inc. Irvine, CA. C. Blom-Singer® Duckbill–Patient Changeable Voice Prosthesis, InHealth Technologies. Image courtesy of InHealth Technologies, www.inhealth.com; D. Blom-Singer® Classic™ Voice Prosthesis–Clinician Placed (non-sterile), InHealth Technologies. Image courtesy of InHealth Technologies, www.inhealth.com; E. UltraDisk DVA 10W Portable Voice Amplifier, UltraDisk, www.ultradisk.co.uk.

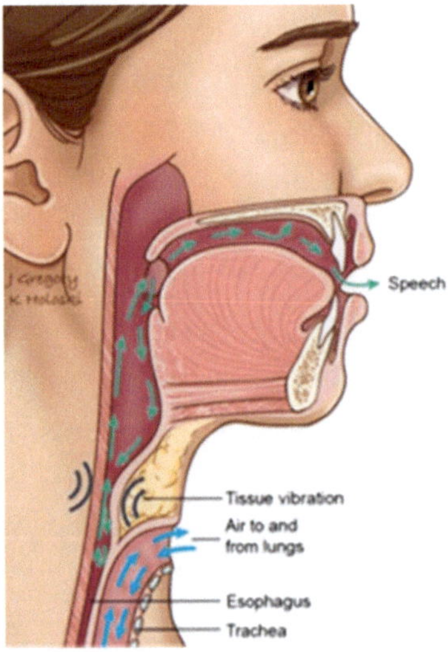

FIGURE 6-1 Illustration of esophageal speech.
SOURCE: THANC Foundation, 2017. Copyright © 2017 Jill Gregory & Kellie Holoski, *Head & Neck Cancer Guide*. All rights reserved. Available at: www.headandneckcancerguide.org.

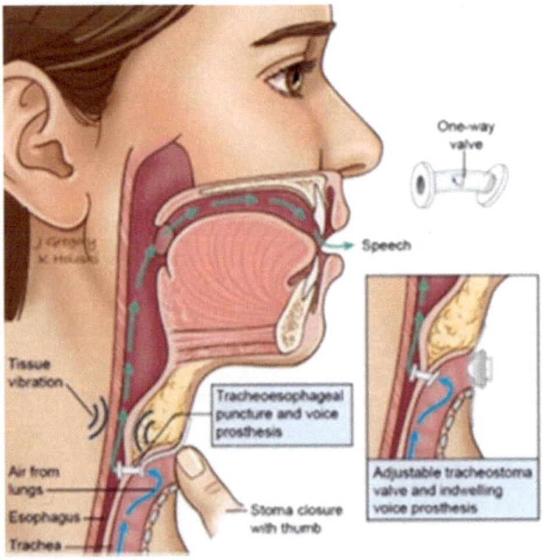

FIGURE 6-2 Tracheoesophageal puncture with prosthesis.
SOURCE: THANC Foundation, 2017. Copyright © 2017 Jill Gregory & Kellie Holoski, *Head & Neck Cancer Guide*. All rights reserved. Available at: www.headandneckcancerguide.org.

(Tang and Sinclair, 2015). An electrolarynx is a small handheld, battery-operated device that, when activated by pressing buttons on the device, vibrates air in the oral cavity to approximate the sound of voicing (Enderby et al., 2009). The device may be positioned on the neck, under the chin (see Figure 6-3), or on the cheek; it also may be used with an oral adapter to vibrate air in the oral cavity.

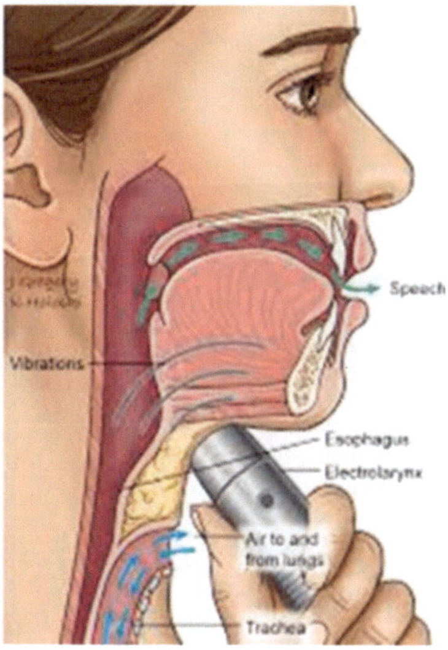

FIGURE 6-3 Chin placement of artificial/electrolarynx.
SOURCE: THANC Foundation, 2017. Copyright © 2017 Jill Gregory & Kellie Holoski, *Head & Neck Cancer Guide*. All rights reserved. Available at: www.headandneckcancerguide.org.

Functional Speech Following Tracheostomy

In tracheostomy, the vocal mechanism typically remains fully functional; however, respiratory air is directed through the tracheostomy tube instead of upward through the vocal cords. As a result, voicing is difficult to impossible without use of a tracheostomy speaking valve (TSV) (Hoffman et al., 2008). A TSV, a small one-way valve prosthesis that is placed on the end of a tracheostomy tube, is designed to redirect exhaled air upward through the vocal cords in the larynx (Hoffman et al., 2008). All TSVs have similar components, but their engineering/design varies. In all TSVs, a diaphragm either (1) remains open and closes on expiration or (2) remains closed and opens when inspiratory effort is applied. All valves close during expiration, and all attach to the hub of a tracheostomy tube (Leder, 1994). Individuals having undergone tracheostomy often benefit from a speaking-valve prosthesis (see Figure 6-4) that uses a one-way valve to redirect exhaled air from the trachea upward through intact vocal cords to produce natural voicing.

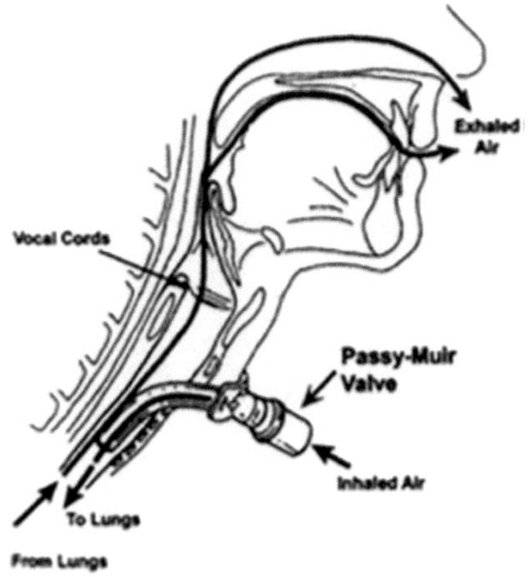

FIGURE 6-4 Tracheostomy speaking valve.
SOURCE: Illustration courtesy of Passy Muir, Inc., Irvine, CA.

Functional Speech with Diminished Vocal Intensity

Voice Amplification

Individuals who retain function of the vocal cords may benefit from voice amplification to address dysphonia or hypophonia (Andreetta et al., 2016). Typically a speaker-type voice amplifier fitted with a head-mounted or lavaliere microphone, this device is designed to amplify the fundamental frequency of voice. It has been shown to increase the intelligibility of speech in noisy situations and when the individual produces insufficiently loud speech (Andreetta et al., 2016). Similarly, those having undergone total laryngectomy who communicate with TEP or ESS often benefit from amplification (Happ et al., 2004; Hilgers et al., 1990).

Functionality of Voice Restoration Technologies

Considered the gold standard, TEPs are deemed effective for many individuals postlaryngectomy and are associated with low occurrence of medical complications (Calkovsky and Hajtman, 2015; Tang and Sinclair, 2015). Still, the resulting voice is sometimes considered monotonous and unpleasant.

Studies have shown that voice restoration with tracheoesophageal puncture is superior to that with an electrolarynx and ESS (Clements et al.,

1999; Eadie et al., 2016; Finzia and Bergman, 2001; Ward et al., 2003). In addition to surgery and radiation, factors associated with head and neck cancer influence speech intelligibility. Decreases in intelligibility are associated with (1) increases in tumor size; (2) increases in the volume of tissue resected; (3) the need for reconstructive surgery; and (4) tumor site, with poorer intelligibility in cases involving the floor of the mouth or lower alveolar crest (Blyth et al., 2014; Borggreven et al., 2007). One recent study found lowest stress and perceived handicap with ESS, followed by an electrolarynx and then tracheoesophageal puncture (Saltürk et al., 2016). One critical consideration is that all voice restoration methods (TEP, ESS, and electrolarynx) rely on the articulatory musculature to produce speech. Thus, loss of articulatory musculature during surgical resection has significant consequences for the production of intelligible speech (Tang and Sinclair, 2015).

Voice Restoration and AAC

Given developments in communication systems for people with unmet communication needs, ESS and electrolarynges are not the sole options available, and in many cases, they may no longer be acceptable to some individuals. The increase in availability and acceptability of these technologies and communication applications for mobile technologies has significantly changed functional communication intervention (e.g., McNaughton and Light, 2013). These factors play an obvious role in determining functional communication interventions using AAC technologies. The situational effectiveness of communication with ESS, an electrolarynx, or both ranges from 80 to 100 percent intelligibility (Sullivan et al., 1993).

Caregivers of adults with complex communication needs have identified as highly important the need for viable modes of communication to (1) regulate the behavior of others for basic wants and needs (e.g., getting needs met, giving instructions/directions, providing clarifications); (2) stay connected with friends and family members (e.g., social closeness); and (3) discuss important issues (e.g., information transfer) (Fried-Oken et al., 2006). AAC supports are necessary given that the overwhelming majority of individuals with severe speech impairments have no access to appropriate communication modalities when hospitalized. They therefore struggle to provide medical information and to have their medical needs met, and they are at increased risk for poor health outcomes (Blackstone et al., 2015; Hemsley and Balandin, 2014).

Factors Affecting Device Use

Speakers have reported using multiple communication methods based on the complexity of communication in various environments, using writing, gestures, and/or interpreters to supplement spoken communication while speaking in situations with background noise or via intercoms (Sullivan et al., 1993). Although written supplementation of spoken communication may be useful in some situations, it does not produce audible output and is limited by literacy skills for some individuals. Indeed, 17.1 percent of individuals with head and neck cancer read at or below the 8th-grade level (Jesse et al., 2015). Because individuals with reduced speech intelligibility tend to experience reduced quality of life, timely identification of such individuals is an important component of their cancer treatment so that they can be provided with appropriate communication options that facilitate their overall recovery (Borggreven et al., 2007).

Voice Restoration Evaluation and Monitoring

Rapid, effective voice and speech restoration is associated with preventing psychosocial and economic consequences of loss of speech (Blom, 2000). Optimal levels of communication support for individuals with head and neck cancer need to be identified throughout the phases of cancer treatment, with consideration of variations/transitions in medical status and personal needs over time. Targeted interventions need to be developed in the context of the cancer site (e.g., tongue, maxilla, larynx), phase of recovery (e.g., presurgical, acute postsurgical, speech restorative), preexisting communication skills and demands, and ongoing communication needs (Sullivan et al., 2007a). Each voice restoration method has specific monitoring and evaluation procedures. To ensure that individuals with head and neck cancer can successfully meet all their communication needs, AAC assessment and intervention procedures are implemented in conjunction with voice restoration strategies (Ball et al., 2016b). AAC service-delivery intervals for these individuals are established to support presurgical care, acute care (immediately postsurgery), initial outpatient care, and ongoing outpatient AAC support (e.g., treatment change or new disease states (Sullivan et al., 2007a).

The goal of *presurgical AAC assessment* is to identify communication needs, determine communication options for implementation immediately postsurgery, and evaluate the potential effectiveness of various AAC options. At this stage, a communication needs assessment is completed, individual patterns of communication are established (e.g., interest in and use of communication), and potential supports and needs following surgery are identified (Ball et al., 2016b). The goal of *acute care AAC assessment* is to evaluate the effectiveness of short-term communication techniques that have been identified and continue to evaluate AAC options for longer-term implementation. The goal of *outpatient AAC assessment* is to identify daily communication needs that are not being met by the selected voice restoration procedures (Ball et al., 2016b). As voice restoration procedures are implemented, communication breakdowns, intelligibility and comprehensibility, and communication efficiency (intelligible words per minute) are monitored (Sullivan et al., 1993). Finally, the goal of *ongoing AAC intervention* is to evaluate new communication needs and any sources of communication breakdown as well as to identify communication options for addressing these issues. Cancer recurrence or new health conditions, for example, may require additional medical treatments that impact communication (Ball et al., 2016b).

AAC assessment for individuals with head and neck cancer often differs from a typical lengthy AAC assessment process that yields a communication system following a series of assessment sessions and trials (Ball et al., 2016b). Instead, the focus is on supporting communication in a rapid, just-in-time manner (i.e., methodically targeting communicative supports as needed). When long-term use of AAC technology is indicated, a comprehensive AAC evaluation may be required.

Individuals with head and neck cancer receiving AAC commonly require (1) lightweight portability (independent, unimpaired ambulation); (2) direct access (full use of hands, sufficiently large keyboard to provide accurate message selection); (3) high-quality display (visibility in multiple environments); (4) traditional orthography (if literacy supports message formulation, native language text); (5) message formulation (few predetermined messages with some repeated/personal messages recorded prior to surgery, formulation of new messages with text-to-speech); (6) rate acceleration (features that speed rate of communication); and (7) ease of use (brief period of time required to learn how to use the device) (Beukelman and Mirenda, 2013). Desired features of mobile communication systems include those mentioned above (e.g., portability, high-quality display). Other desired features include options to obtain extended battery life (e.g., communication during an 8-hour work shift), durability and protection (e.g., a case that increases the durability of the system without compromising access) with screen protection, and voice output amplification. If the user places a high premium on small devices but cannot isolate individual items on the display because of hand/finger size or mobility, it is also important to identify a stylus that will provide access to the keyboard and a means of ensuring its location without loss (i.e., storage slot).

Voice Restoration Training and Adaptation

Individuals report that ESS is more difficult to learn than other communication methods, and success depends on individual motivation and length of time practicing. Other factors include training method, timing of training postsurgery, and type of training (group versus individual) (Kresic et al., 2015; Staffieri et al., 2006).

Individuals with communication problems following head/neck cancer interventions but without other speech/language problems have an undamaged language system (Enderby et al., 2009). These individuals can participate in an AAC assessment to choose a system that best addresses their needs (Fox and Rau, 2001). The goals of AAC for individuals with head and neck cancer are to augment intelligibility, decrease communication breakdowns or miscommunications, enable repair when communication breakdowns occur, and provide alternative means of communication when the voice restoration methods employed result in ongoing unmet communication needs (Ball et al., 2016b).

Often, recommended communication strategies involve simple methods, and clinicians may not see a need for direct instruction; however, not all individuals adapt to their lack of communication and the implementation of new communication methods without instruction (Sullivan et al., 2007b). Moreover, most medical professionals (e.g., nurses, physicians) receive no instruction in interacting with individuals who are unable to communicate effectively via natural speech (Hemsley and Balandin, 2014). Therefore, some form of instruction and therapeutic support for both individuals and providers is likely to yield improved patient–provider communication, which in turn can influence satisfaction with and outcomes of treatment (Downey and Happ, 2013; Hemsley and Balandin, 2014).

Voice Restoration Access and Availability

Caregivers of individuals with head and neck cancer have reported that they primarily taught themselves communication strategies for identifying problems and meeting individual needs, which required intensive effort and creativity on their part. These reports indicate that, postsurgically, these individuals and their caregivers are in critical need of assistance in meeting communication needs (McGrory, 2011). Similarly, nurses have attributed nurse–patient communication breakdowns to the lack of readily manageable and interpretable communication systems (Happ et al., 2004).

The complexity of funding policies impacts access to voice restoration in many cases. Some insurers will not pay for an electrolarynx or voice prosthesis, the latter of which often must be replaced on a routine basis (as often as monthly, although commonly every 2-3 months). As a result, clinicians or treating facilities must provide voice prostheses at their own expense, or the patient must bear the cost. Also, non-indwelling voice prostheses are considered durable medical equipment by CMS, whereas indwelling prostheses are not. The result can be problems with respect to training of SLPs in how to manage non-indwelling prostheses and how to instruct individuals in their insertion and long-term use. Medicare administrative contractors require that a TEP not be distributed directly to an individual but instead directly to a professional, one device at a time, and that a provider visit occur at the time the TEP is distributed and billed (Satterfield, 2015). A separate funding issue is that, at present, Medicare payment for a TEP covers approximately one-half the cost of actually obtaining the device; as a result, many clinical practices no longer provide TEPs (Satterfield, 2015).

Access to voice restoration methods depends on the availability of appropriately trained professionals, which varies by region. ASHA certification (Certificate of Clinical Competence-SLP) is necessary; however, meeting certification requirements is not sufficient to qualify an SLP to perform TEP care as outlined by preferred practice standards (ASHA, 2004a). SLPs require extensive additional training to manage voice restoration options (e.g., anatomy and physiology, instrumentation, TEP and related materials, instruction of individuals in the use of ESS, identification of appropriate TEP candidates, TEP sizing/removal/reinsertion, safety issues) (ASHA, 2004a). Limited numbers of these experts are available, and there have been anecdotal reports of situations in which local surgeons have provided laryngectomy and primary TEP care when no trained SLP was available in the region to provide the necessary pre-/postoperative assessment and interventions, potentially leaving the individual with no voice restoration options. Limited numbers of SLPs specialize in voice assessment and interventions. A survey of providers indicated that 5 percent of SLPs' adult service delivery time was spent in the area of voice (including but not limited to voice restoration), with SLPs in outpatient clinics spending significantly more time, although still negligible (12 percent; $p = .000$), than those in other medical facilities (e.g., skilled nursing facility, U.S. Department of Veterans Affairs facility, hospital, long-term acute care facility) (ASHA, 2015b).

FINDINGS AND CONCLUSIONS

Findings

Need for Augmentative and Alternative Communication

6-1. Severe impairments of natural speech result in complex communication needs that interfere with daily interactions and employment outcomes.

6-2. Research in the field of augmentative and alternative communication (AAC) often focuses on specific areas and populations, making generalizations across studies problematic.

6-3. Individuals with amyotrophic lateral sclerosis (ALS) may be referred for AAC assessment and treatment beyond the time when they could remain at or return to work; this and other factors may increase the urgency of the need for AAC and/or limit AAC acceptance.

6-4. Individuals receiving voice restoration head and neck cancer treatments may also require AAC to achieve fully functional communication.

6-5. The complexity of AAC systems is demonstrated by the multiple features and components that must be identified, evaluated, and manipulated to address the specific abilities, needs, and expectations of each individual.

6-6. Individualized, contextual needs are variable and cannot be generalized within a specific disability group (i.e., individuals have communication skills and needs that are not based on a diagnosis such as cerebral palsy, ALS, or head and neck cancer).

6-7. Individuals who require AAC have complex communication needs, which often change over the course of their impairment (e.g., improving or degenerating communication capabilities) so that individuals require ongoing monitoring and/or intervention to maintain or improve their communication performance.

6-8. Different considerations are entailed in communicating with an electrolarynx or tracheoesophageal voice prosthesis, which requires operational competence, versus AAC, which requires language representation, cognitive and device-based message formulation, and social and operational competencies.

Prognosis for Occupational Success

6-9. Individuals who communicate with AAC can obtain and maintain employment if they are provided early educational preparation; attain high levels of language competence, literacy, and education; and achieve competency in workplace communication interactions.

6-10. Established measures of real-world communicative functioning are sparse, and research investigating the impact of AAC products and technologies on real-world communicative functioning is extremely limited.

6-11. Direct instruction in communication techniques improves clinical outcomes for persons with AAC needs.

6-12. As technologies or computer-based equipment, AAC systems are subject to breakdown, thus requiring technical support and repair; loss of access to communication in the interim will likely impact an individual's ability to fulfill work responsibilities.

6-13. Occupational title listings may indicate no need for speaking, but an occupation often has a speaking requirement nonetheless.

Access and Availability

6-14. Original Medicare benefits are based on medical necessity and cover 80 percent of an approved device's fee schedule, and some individuals may not have the 20 percent copay. The result is that the cost of a speech-generating device (SGD) may remain prohibitive for many people (e.g., a $20,000 AAC system would require a $4,000 out-of-pocket expense). If the SGD is not approved based on the fee schedule, the entire cost falls to the individual.

6-15. Medicaid funding varies by state, with some states having specific criteria for assessments; limiting access to treatment; and/or providing insufficient funding, especially for higher-cost AAC technologies.

6-16. Private health insurance may exclude coverage of AAC systems, even when other types of durable medical equipment are covered.

6-17. Some funding options (e.g., equipment lending libraries, private purchase of mobile technologies) do not link appropriate evaluations with AAC selection, resulting at times in inappropriate recommendations and purchases.

6-18. Some coverage requires that an individual abandon attempts to improve natural speech before qualifying for AAC support.

6-19. School districts that have provided AAC systems for children often retain the devices; as a result, children transitioning from school into postsecondary/vocational settings must navigate the transition while completing the AAC assessment, funding, and new learning processes. Some children may even have to learn entirely new language representation, messaging, and access methods before they can engage in essential communication.

6-20. Required education for preprofessional speech-language pathologists (SLPs) is limited, as a number of university programs still do not have a required AAC course.

6-21. The 2015 American Speech-Language-Hearing Association end-of-year membership report showed that there were 156,254 certified SLP members, although the AAC Special Interest Group comprised only 3,239 members, approximately 2 percent of the total membership. These numbers are indicative of the relatively small number of SLPs with AAC expertise.

6-22. High equipment costs and continual technology developments result in limited availability of AAC systems for use in the assessment, equipment trial, and intervention processes in clinical settings.

Conclusions

Prognosis for Occupational Success

6-1. Data on the prevalence and use of AAC systems by adults are fragmented and limited, resulting in incomplete knowledge of employability, vocational effectiveness, and overall employment outcomes. [Findings 6-2, 6-9]

6-2. Establishing objective measures of real-world communicative functioning will promote improved understanding of the effects of AAC products and technologies on actual practical and interactive communicative function. [Finding 6-10]

6-3. Although great progress has been achieved in AAC systems, use of an SGD does not fully mitigate the impact of a severe communication impairment. In addition, even when provided with optimal assessment, funding resources, AAC systems, interventions, and supports, individuals may not achieve their potential because of any number of environmental and personal factors that influence communication performance in employment contexts. [Findings 6-5, 6-6, 6-11, 6-12]

Access and Availability

6-4. Access to SLPs and other professional members of an AAC team with relevant knowledge, skills, and expertise is necessary and currently limited. [Findings 6-4, 6-5, 6-6, 6-7, 6-10, 6-19, 6-20, 6-21]

6-5. Limited availability of AAC systems in the clinical setting impedes proper assessment, equipment trial, and intervention processes to the detriment of the individual's participation in educational and vocational settings. [Finding 6-22]

6-6. Differences in funding policies among various programs significantly limit access to AAC technology and clinical services. [Findings 6-14, 6-15, 6-16, 6-17, 6-18, 6-20]

REFERENCES

AAC-RERC (Augmentative and Alternative Communication-Rehabilitation Engineering Research Center). 2011. *Mobile devices and communication apps: An AAC-RERC white paper*. http://aac-rerc.psu.edu/index.php/pages/show/id/46 (accessed February 22, 2017).

Akcakaya, M., B. Peters, M. Moghadamfalahi, A. R. Mooney, U. Orhan, B. Oken, D. Erdogmus, and M. Fried-Oken. 2014. Noninvasive brain-computer interfaces for augmentative and alternative communication. *IEEE Reviews in Biomedical Engineering* 7:31-49.

Alamsaputra, D. M., K. J. Kohnert, B. Munson, and J. Reichle. 2006. Synthesized speech intelligibility among native speakers and non-native speakers of English. *Augmentative and Alternative Communication* 22(4):258-268.

American Cancer Society. 2015. *Cancer facts & figures 2015*. Atlanta, GA: American Cancer Society. http://www.cancer.org/content/dam/cancer-org/research/cancer-facts-and-statistics/annual-cancer-facts-and-figures/2015/cancer-facts-and-figures-2015.pdf (accessed January 22, 2017).

Anderson, L., C. R. Baylor, T. L. Eadie, and K. M. Yorkston. 2016. Describing speech usage in daily activities in typical adults. *Journal of Voice* 30(1):42-52.

Andreetta, M. D., S. G. Adams, A. D. Dykstra, and M. Jog. 2016. Evaluation of speech amplification devices in Parkinson's disease. *American Journal of Speech-Language Pathology* 25(1):29-45.

ASHA (American Speech-Language-Hearing Association). 2004a. *Knowledge and skills for speech-language pathologists with respect to evaluation and treatment for tracheoesophageal puncture and prosthesis: Knowledge and skills*. http://www.asha.org/policy (accessed February 13, 2017).

ASHA. 2004b. *Preferred practice patterns for the profession of speech-language pathology [preferred practice patterns]*. http://www.asha.org/policy/PP2004-00191 (accessed November 16, 2016).

ASHA. 2004c. *Roles and responsibilities of speech-language pathologists with respect to augmentative and alternative communication: Technical report*. http://www.asha.org/policy/TR2004-00262 (accessed January 22, 2017).

ASHA. 2015a. *Highlights and trends: Member and affiliate counts, year-end 2015*. http://www.asha.org/uploadedFiles/2015-Member-Counts.pdf (accessed January 18, 2017).

ASHA. 2015b. *SLP Health Care Survey 2015 caseload characteristics*. http://www.asha.org/uploadedFiles/2015-SLP-Health-Care-Survey-Caseload.pdf (accessed February 13, 2017).

ASHA. 2016a. *Augmentative and alternative communication (AAC)*. http://www.asha.org/public/speech/disorders/AAC (accessed October 25, 2016).

ASHA. 2016b. *Augmentative and alternative communication decisions*. http://www.asha.org/public/speech/disorders/CommunicationDecisions (accessed October 25, 2016).

ASHA. 2016c. *Augmentative and alternative communication: Knowledge and skills for service delivery [knowledge and skills]*. http://www.asha.org/policy/KS2002-00067.htm (accessed November 16, 2016).

ASHA. 2016d. *Current procedural terminology (CPT) codes: Speech language pathology*. http://www.asha.org/Practice/reimbursement/coding/SLPCPT (accessed December 31, 2016).

ASHA. 2016e. *Scope of practice in speech-language pathology [scope of practice]*. http://www.asha.org/policy/SP2016-00343 (accessed November 16, 2016).

Babin, E., D. Beynier, D. Le Gall, and M. Hitier. 2009. Psychosocial quality of life in patients after total laryngectomy. *Revue de Laryngologie—Otologie—Rhinologie* 130(1):29-34.

Baker, B. 1986. Using images to generate speech. *Byte* 11(9):160-168.

Balandin, S., and J. Morgan. 2001. Preparing for the future: Aging and alternative and augmentative communication. *Augmentative and Alternative Communication* 17(2):99-108.

Ball, L. J., and J. Lasker. 2013. Teaching partners to support communication for adults with acquired communication impairment. *Perspectives on Augmentative and Alternative Communication* 22(1):4-15.

Ball, L. J., A. Willis, D. R. Beukelman, and G. L. Pattee. 2001. A protocol for identification of early bulbar signs in amytrophic lateral sclerosis. *Journal of the Neurological Sciences* 191(1-2):43-53.

Ball, L. J., D. R. Beukelman, and G. L. Pattee. 2002. Timing of speech degeneration in people with amyotrophic lateral sclerosis. *Journal of Medical Speech-Language Pathology* 10(4):231-235.

Ball, L. J., D. R. Beukelman, and G. L. Pattee. 2004. Communication effectiveness of individuals with amyotrophic lateral sclerosis. *Journal of Communication Disorders* 37(3): 197-215.

Ball, L. J., D. R. Beukelman, and L. Bardach. 2007. Amyotrophic lateral sclerosis. In *Augmentative communication strategies for adults with acute or chronic medical conditions,* edited by D. R. Beukelman, K. L. Garrett, and K.M. Yorkston. Baltimore, MD: Paul H. Brookes Publishing Co. Pp. 287-316.

Ball, L. J., K. Stading, and D. Hazelrigg. 2010a. AAC considerations during the transition to adult life. In *Transition strategies for adolescents & young adults who use AAC*, edited by D. McNaughton and D. R. Beukelman. Baltimore, MD: Paul H. Brookes Publishing Co. Pp. 201-218.

Ball, L., A. Nordness, S. Fager, K. Kersch, B. Mohr, G. L. Pattee, and D. R. Beukelman. 2010b. Eye-gaze access of AAC technology for persons with amyotrophic lateral sclerosis. *Journal of Medical Speech-Language Pathology* 18(3):11-23.

Ball, L. J., S. Fager, and M. Fried-Oken. 2012. AAC in progressive neuromuscular disease. *Physical Medicine and Rehabilitation Clinics of North America* 23(3):689-699.

Ball, L. J., S. Evans, S. Chavez, M. Leach, and K. Smart. 2016a (unpublished). Communication of children diagnosed with spinal muscular atrophy type 1: A parent survey.

Ball, L. J., J. Kent-Walsh, and N. A. Harrington. 2016b. Consideration of communication options in head and neck cancer: Augmentative and alternative. In *Cases in head and neck cancer: A multidisciplinary approach*, edited by B. H. Ruddy, H. Ho, C. Sapienza, and J. J. Lehman. San Diego, CA: Plural Publishing, Inc. Pp. 207-218.

Barreto, A. B., S. D. Scargle, and M. Adjouadi. 2000. A practical EMG-based human-computer interface for users with motor disabilities. *Journal of Rehabilitation Research & Development* 37(1):53-63.

Barrett, D., and T. King. 2005. *Computer networking illuminated.* Sudbury, MA: Jones and Bartlett Publishers.

Beukelman, D. R., and P. Mirenda. 2005. *Augmentative and alternative communication: Supporting children and adults with complex communication needs.* 3rd ed. Baltimore, MD: Paul H. Brookes Publishing Co.

Beukelman, D. R., and P. Mirenda. 2013. *Augmentative and alternative communication: Supporting children and adults with complex communication needs.* 4th ed. Baltimore, MD: Paul H. Brookes Publishing Co.

Beukelman, D. R., S. Fager, L. J. Ball, and A. Dietz. 2007a. AAC for adults with acquired neurological conditions: A review. *Augmentative and Alternative Communication* 23(3): 230-242.

Beukelman, D. R., K. M. Yorkston, and K. L. Garrett. 2007b. An introduction to AAC services for adults with chronic medical conditions: Who, what, when, where, and why. In *Augmentative communication strategies for adults with acute or chronic medical conditions*, edited by D. R. Beukelman, K. L. Garrett, and K. M. Yorkston. Baltimore, MD: Paul H. Brookes Publishing Co. Pp. 1-16.

Beukelman, D. R., K. L. Garrett, and K. M. Yorkston. 2007c. *Augmentative communication strategies for adults with acute or chronic medical conditions*. Baltimore, MD: Paul H. Brookes Publishing Co.

Beukelman, D. R., L. J. Ball, and S. Fager. 2008. An AAC personnel framework: Adults with acquired complex communication needs. *Augmentative and Alternative Communication* 24(3):255-267.

Beukelman, D. R., E. K. Hanson, E. Hiatt, S. Fager, and D. Bilyeu. 2009. AAC technology learning part 3: Regular AAC team members. *Augmentative and Alternative Communication* 21(3):187-194.

Beukelman, D. R., K. Hux, A. Dietz, M. McKelvey, and K. Weissling. 2015. Using visual scene displays as communication support options for people with chronic, severe aphasia: A summary of AAC research and future research directions. *Augmentative and Alternative Communication* 31(3):234-245.

Binger, C., L. J. Ball, A. Dietz, J. Kent-Walsh, J. Lasker, S. Lund, M. McKelvey, and W. Quach. 2012. Personnel roles in the AAC assessment process. *Augmentative and Alternative Communication* 28(4):278-288.

Blackstone, S. W. 1993. Employment in the AAC community: A problem for some . . . but not for everyone. In *Proceedings of the Pittsburgh Employment Conference for Augmented Communicators*, edited by R. V. Conti and C. Jenkins-Odorisio. Pittsburgh, PA: SHOUT Press. Pp. 3-6.

Blackstone, S. W., D. R. Beukelman, and K. M. Yorkston. 2015. *Patient-provider communication: Roles for speech-language pathologists and other health care professionals*. San Diego, CA: Plural Publishing, Inc.

Blom, E. D. 2000. Current status of voice restoration following total laryngectomy. *Oncology* 14(6):915-922.

Blyth, K. M., P. McCabe, R. Heard, J. Clark, C. Madill, and K. J. Ballard. 2014. Cancers of the tongue and floor of mouth: Five-year file audit within the acute phase. *American Journal of Speech-Language Pathology* 23(4):668-678.

Bolt, S., T. Eadie, K. Yorkston, C. Baylor, and D. Amtmann. 2016. Variables associated with communicative participation after head and neck cancer. *JAMA Otolaryngology—Head & Neck Surgery* 142(12):1145-1151.

Borggreven, P. A., I. M. Verdonck-de Leeuw, M. J. Muller, M. L. C. H. Heiligers, R. de Bree, N. K. Aaronson, and C. R. Leemans. 2007. Quality of life and functional status in patients with cancer of the oral cavity and oropharynx: Pretreatment values of a prospective study. *European Archives of Oto-Rhino-Laryngology* 264(6):651-657.

Bourgeois, M. S. 1991. Communication treatment for adults with dementia. *Journal of Speech, Language, and Hearing Research* 34(4):831-844.

Bourgeois, M. S. 1992. Evaluating memory wallets in conversation with persons with dementia. *Journal of Speech, Language, and Hearing Research* 35(6):1344-1357.

Bourgeois, M. S. 2013. Restricted literature base limits interpretation of meta-analysis of the effectiveness of communication-enhancing interventions in dementia. *Evidence-based Communication Assessment and Intervention* 7(1):1-3.

Bourgeois, M. S., K. Dijkstra, L. Burgio, and R. Allen-Burge. 2001. Memory aids as an augmentative and alternative communication strategy for nursing home residents with dementia. *Augmentative and Alternative Communication* 17(3):196-210.

Brady, N., D. Skinner, J. Roberts, and E. Hennon. 2006. Communication in young children with fragile X syndrome: A qualitative study of mothers' perspective. *American Journal of Speech-Language Pathology* 15(4):353-364.

Brock, K., R. Koul, M.Corwin, and R. Schlosser. 2017. A comparison of visual scene and grid displays for people with chronic aphasia: A pilot study to improve communication using AAC. *Aphasiology* 1-25.

Bruno, J., and D. Trembath. 2006. Use of aided language stimulation to improve syntactic performance during a weeklong intervention program. *Augmentative and Alternative Communication* 22(4):300-313.

Bryen, D. N., B. B. Potts, and A. C. Carey. 2007. So you want to work? What employers say about job skills, recruitment and hiring employees who rely on AAC. *Augmentative and Alternative Communication* 23(2):126-139.

Bunnell, H. T., J. Chandlee, J. Lilley, J. Gray, B. Moyers, and B. Warren. 2015. *ModelTalker*. https://www.modeltalker.org (accessed January 24, 2017).

Calkovsky, V., and A. Hajtman. 2015. Primary prosthetic voice rehabilitation in patients after laryngectomy: Applications and pitfalls. *Advances in Experimental Medicine and Biology* 852:11-16.

Caron, J. G., and J. Light. 2016. Social media experiences of adolescents and young adults with cerebral palsy who use augmentative and alternative communication. *International Journal of Speech Language Pathology* 1-13.

CDC (U.S. Centers for Disease Control and Prevention). 2011. *Autism and Developmental Disabilities Monitoring (ADDM) Network*. Atlanta, GA: CDC.

CDC. 2014. Prevalence of autism spectrum disorder among children aged 8 years: Autism and Developmental Disabilities Monitoring Network, 11 sites, United States, 2010. *Morbidity and Mortality Weekly Report* 63(2).

Chang, S. K., G. Costagliola, S. Orefice, G. Polese, and B. R. Baker. 1992. *A methodology for iconic language design with application to augmentative communication*. Proceedings of the 1992 IEEE Workshop on Visual Languages, Seattle, WA, September 15-18.

Clements, K., C. Rassekh, H. Seikaly, J. A. Hokanson, and K. H. Calhoun. 1999. Communication after laryngectomy: An assessment of patient satisfaction. *Archives of Otolaryngology—Head & Neck Surgery* 123(5):493-496.

CMS (Centers for Medicare & Medicaid Services). 2001. *CMS Pub. 100-3, Medicare National Coverage Determinations Manual, Chapter 1, Section 50.1. LCD Title Speech Generating Devices, ID number L108*. Baltimore, MD: CMS.

CMS. 2017a. *Medicare Advantage Plans cover all Medicare services*. https://www.medicare.gov/what-medicare-covers/medicare-health-plans/medicare-advantage-plans-cover-all-medicare-services.html (accessed April 6, 2017).

CMS. 2017b. *What's Medicare supplemental insurance (Medigap)?* https://www.medicare.gov/supplement-other-insurance/medigap/whats-medigap.html (accessed April 6, 2017).

Collier, B., and S. Blackstein-Adler. 1998. Building competencies in augmentative and alternative communication among professionals. *Augmentative and Alternative Communication* 14(4):250-260.

Collier, B., S. W. Blackstone, and A. Taylor. 2012. Communication access to businesses and organizations for people with complex communication needs. *Augmentative and Alternative Communication* 28(4):205-218.

Cook, A. M., and J. M. Polgar. 2008. *Cook & Hussey's assistive technologies: Principles and practice*. St. Louis, MO: Mosby Elsevier.

Cooper, L., S. Balandin, and D. Trembath. 2009. The loneliness experiences of young adults with cerebral palsy who use alternative and augmentative communication. *Augmentative and Alternative Communication* 25(3):154-164.

Costello, J. M. 2011. Last words, last connections how augmentative communication can support children facing end of life. *The ASHA Leader* 1-6.

Costello, J. M. 2014. *Message banking, voice banking and legacy messages.* Boston, MA: Boston Children's Hospital.

Costigan, F. A., and J. Light. 2007. *A research review of preservice training in augmentative and alternative communication for speech-language pathologists, special education teachers, and occupational therapists.* Poster presented at the Annual Convention of the American Speech-Language-Hearing Association, Boston, MA.

Costigan, F. A., and J. Light. 2010. A review of preservice training in augmentative and alternative communication of speech-language pathologists, special education teachers, and occupational therapists. *Assistive Technology* 22(4):200-212.

Crema, C., and N. Moran. 2012. Training speech-language pathologists of adult clients on the implementation of AAC into everyday practice. *Perspectives on Augmentative and Alternative Communication* 21(2):37-42.

Culp, D., D. R. Beukelman, and S. Fager. 2007. Brainstem impairment. In *Augmentative communication strategies for adults with acute or chronic medical conditions,* edited by D. R. Beukelman, K. L. Garrett, and K. M. Yorkston. Baltimore, MD: Paul H. Brookes Publishing Co. Pp. 59-90.

Darley, F., A. Aronson, and J. Brown. 1975. *Motor speech disorders.* Philadelphia, PA: Saunders.

Demers, L., R. Weiss-Lambrou, and B. Ska. 2002. The Quebec User Evaluation of Satisfaction with Assistive Technology (QUEST 2.0): An overview and recent progress. *Technology and Disability* 14(3):101-105.

Dietz, A., M. McKelvey, and D. R. Beukelman. 2006. Visual scene displays (VSD): New AAC interfaces for persons with aphasia. *Perspectives on Augmentative and Alternative Communication* 15(1):13-17.

Dietz, A., W. Quach, S. K. Lund, and M. McKelvey. 2012. AAC assessment and clinical-decision making: The impact of experience. *Augmentative and Alternative Communication* 28(3):148-159.

Donovan, N. J., D. L. Kendall, M. E. Young, and J. C. Rosenbek. 2008. The communicative effectiveness survey: Preliminary evidence of construct validity. *American Journal of Speech-Language Pathology* 17(4):335-347.

Dowden, P. A. 2016. *UW augmentative and alternative communication.* http://depts.washington.edu/augcomm (accessed November 5, 2016).

Downey, D., and M. B. Happ. 2013. The need for nurse training to promote improved patient-provider communication for patients with complex communication needs. *Perspectives on Augmentative and Alternative Communication* 22(2):112.

Drager, K. D., and J. E. Reichle. 2001. Effects of age and divided attention on listeners' comprehension of synthesized speech. *Augmentative and Alternative Communication* 17(2):109-119.

Drager, K. D., J. C. Light, J. C. Speltz, K. A. Fallon, and L. Z. Jeffries. 2003. The performance of typically developing 2 1/2-year-olds on dynamic display AAC technologies with different system layouts and language organizations. *Journal of Speech, Language, and Hearing Research* 46(2):298-312.

Drager, K. D., E. A. Clark-Serpentine, K. E. Johnson, and J. L. Roeser. 2006. Accuracy of repetition of digitized and synthesized speech for young children in background noise. *American Journal of Speech-Language Pathology* 15(2):155-164.

Drager, K. D. R., J. Reichle, and C. Pinkoski. 2010. Synthesized speech output and children: A scoping review. *American Journal of Speech-Language Pathology* 19(3):259-273.

Duffy, J. R. 2013. *Motor speech disorders: Substrates, differential diagnosis, and management.* 3rd ed. St. Louis, MO: Elsevier Mosby.

Durkin, M. S., R. E. Benedict, D. Christensen, L. A. Dubois, R. T. Fitzgerald, R. S. Kirby, M. J. Maenner, K. Van Naardent Braun, M. S. Wingate, and M. Yeargin-Allsopp. 2016. Prevalence of cerebral palsy among 8-year-old children in 2010 and preliminary evidence trends in its relationship to low birthweight. *Paediatric Perinatal Epidemiology* 30(5):496-510.

Dykstra, A. D., S. G. Adams, and M. Jog. 2015. Examining the relationship between speech intensity and self-rated communicative effectiveness in individuals with Parkinson's disease and hypophonia. *Journal of Communication Disorders* 56(2015):103-112.

Eadie, T. L., D. Otero, S. Cox, J. Johnson, C. R. Baylor, K. M. Yorkston, and P. C. Doyle. 2016. The relationship between communicative participation and postlaryngectomy speech outcomes. *Head & Neck* 38(Suppl. 1):E1955-E1961.

Enderby, P., C. Pickstone, A. John, K. Fryer, A. Cantrell, and D. Papaioannou. 2009. *Resource manual for commissioning and planning services for SLCN*. London, UK: Royal College of Speech & Language Therapists. https://www.rcslt.org/speech_and_language_therapy/commissioning/aphasia_plus_intro (accessed January 22, 2017).

Fager, S., K. Hux, D. R. Beukelman, and R. Karantounis. 2006. Augmentative and alternative communication use and acceptance by adults with traumatic brain injury. *Augmentative and Alternative Communication* 22(1):37-47.

Fager, S., L. Bardach, S. Russell, and J. Higginbotham. 2012. Access to augmentative and alternative communication: New technologies and clinical decision-making. *Journal of Pediatric Rehabilitation Medicine* 5(1):53-61.

Fairbanks, G. 1960. *Voice and articulation drillbook*. 2nd ed. New York: Harper & Row.

Feinstein, C. S., J. Lemanowicz, M. Cunningham, R. Whiting, and The Institute on Disabilities. 2013. *Independent monitoring for quality (IM4Q): A statewide summary for the Pennsylvania Office of Developmental Programs Statewide Steering Committee on Independent Monitoring*. Philadelphia, PA: Institute on Disabilities, Temple University.

Finzia, C., and B. Bergman. 2001. Health-related quality of life in patients with laryngeal cancer: A post-treatment comparison of different modes of communication. *The Laryngoscope* 111(5):918-923.

Fox, L. E., and M. T. Rau. 2001. Augmentative and alternative communication for adults following glossectomy and laryngectomy surgery. *Augmentative and Alternative Communication* 17(3):161-166.

Fried-Oken, M. 1993. Do AAC users with degenerative neurological disease remain or return to the work force? In *The First Annual Pittsburgh Employment Conference for Augmented Communicators*, edited by R.V. Conti and C. Jenkins-Odorisio. Pittsburgh, PA: SHOUT Press. Pp. 73-78.

Fried-Oken, M., and M. Granlund. 2012. AAC and ICF: A good fit to emphasize outcomes. *Augmentative and Alternative Communication* 28(1):1-2.

Fried-Oken, M., L. Fox, M. T. Rau, J. Tullman, G. Baker, M. Hindal, N. Wile, and J.-S. Lou. 2006. Purposes of AAC device use for persons with ALS as reported by caregivers. *Augmentative and Alternative Communication* 22(3):209-221.

Fried-Oken, M., D. R. Beukelman, and K. Hux. 2012. Current and future AAC research considerations for adults with acquired cognitive and communication impairments. *Assistive Technology* 24(1):56-66.

Fried-Oken, M., A. Mooney, and B. Peters. 2015. Supporting communication for patients with neurodegenerative disease. *Neurorehabilitation* 37(1):69-87.

Fucci, D., M. Reynolds, R. Bettagere, and M. D. Gonzales. 1995. Synthetic speech intelligibility under several experimental conditions. *Augmentative and Alternative Communication* 11(2):113-117.

Ganz, J. B., E. R. Hong, W. Gilliland, K. Morin, and N. Svenkerud. 2015. Comparison between visual scene displays and exchange-based communication in augmentative and alternative communication for children with ASD. *Research in Autism Spectrum Disorders* 11:27-41.

Gaskin, J., J. Gomes, S. Darshan, and D. Krewski. 2016. Burden of neurological conditions in Canada. *Neurotoxicology* [E-pub ahead of print].

Gevarter, C., M. F. O'Reilly, L. Fojeski, N. Sammarco, J. Sigafoos, G. E. Lancioni, and R. Lang. 2014. Comparing acquisition of AAC-based mands in three young children with autism spectrum disorder using iPad applications with different display and design elements. *Journal of Autism and Developmental Disorders* 44(10):2464-2474.

Gevarter, C., M. F. O'Reilly, M. Kuhn, L. Watkins, R. Ferguson, N. Sammarco, L. Rojeski, and J. Sigafoos. 2016. Assessing the acquisition of requesting a variety of preferred items using different speech generating device formats for children with autism spectrum disorder. *Assistive Technology* 1-8.

Glennen, S. 2000. *AAC assessment myths and realities*. Paper presented at ASHA SID 12 Leadership Conference on Augmentative and Alternative Communication, Sea Island, GA.

Glennen, S., and D. C. DeCoste. 1997. *The handbook of augmentative and alternative communication*. San Diego, CA: Singular Publishing Group, Inc.

Goldman-Eisler, F. 1986. *Cycle linguistics: Experiments in spontaneous speech*. New York: Academic Press.

Greene, B. G., J. S. Logan, and D. B. Pisoni. 1986. Perception of synthetic speech produced automatically by rule: Intelligibility of eight text-to-speech systems. *Behavior Research Methods, Instruments, & Computers* 18(2):100-107.

Haidet, P., R. E. Levine, D. X. Parmelee, S. Crow, F. Kennedy, P. A. Kelly, L. Perkowski, L. Michaelsen, and B. F. Richards. 2012. Perspective: Guidelines for reporting team-based learning activities in the medical and health sciences education literature. *Academic Medicine* 87(3):292-299.

Hamm, B., and P. Mirenda. 2006. Post-school quality of life for individuals with developmental disabilities who use AAC. *Augmentative and Alternative Communication* 22(2):134-147.

Hanson, E. K., E. Goldhammer, and T. Bethard. 2016. Telephone talk: Effects of two access methods on phone call success. *Augmentative and Alternative Communication* 32(3):219-226.

Happ, M. B., T. Roesch, and S. H. Kagan. 2004. Communication needs, methods, and perceived voice quality following head and neck surgery. *Cancer Nursing* 27(1):1-9.

Hartsuiker, R., R. Bastiaanse, A. Postma, and F. Wijnan. 2005. *Phonological encoding and monitoring in normal and pathological speech*. New York: Psychology Press.

Hemsley, B., and S. Balandin. 2014. A metasynthesis of patient-provider communication in hospital for patients with severe communication disabilities: Informing new translational research. *Augmentative and Alternative Communication* 30(4):329-343.

Higginbotham, D. J., and C. Engelke. 2013. A primer for doing talk-in-interaction research in augmentative and alternative communication. *Augmentative and Alternative Communication* 29(1):3-19.

Higginbotham, D. J., A. L. Drazek, K. Kowarsky, C. Scally, and E. Segal. 1994. Discourse comprehension of synthetic speech delivered at normal and slow presentation rates. *Augmentative and Alternative Communication* 10(3):191-202.

Higginbotham, D. J., G. W. Lesher, B. J. Moulton, and G. J. Rinkus. 2002. Automated data logging in augmentative communication. In *Emerging and accessible telecommunications, information and healthcare technologies—engineering challenges in enabling universal access*, edited by J. Winters, C. Robinson, R. Simpson, and G. Vanderheiden. Arlington, VA: Resna Press. Pp. 82-94.

Higginbotham, D. J., H. Shane, S. Russell, and K. Caves. 2007. Access to AAC: Present, past, and future. *Augmentative and Alternative Communication* 23(3):243-257.

Hilgers, F., A. Ackerstaff, N. Aaronson, P. Schouwenburg, and N. Van Zandwijk. 1990. Physical and psychosocial consequences of total laryngectomy. *Clinical Otolaryngology & Allied Sciences* 15(5):421-425.

Hill, K. 2004. Augmentative and alternative communication and language: Evidence-based practice and language activity monitoring. *Topics in Language Disorders* 24(1):18-30.

Hill, K. 2010. Advances in augmentative and alternative communication as quality-of-life technology. *Physical Medicine and Rehabilitation Clinics of North America* 21(1):43-58.

Hill, K., and V. Corsi. 2012. The role speech language pathologists in assistive technology assessments. In *Assistive technology assessment: A handbook for professionals in disability, rehabilitation and health professions*, edited by M. J. Scherer and S. Federici. London, UK: Taylor & Francis Group. Pp. 301-336.

Hill, K., R. Lytton, and S. Glennen. 1998. *The role of manufacturers' consultants in delivering AAC services [poster]*. Paper presented at 1998 International Society for Augmentative and Alternative Communication (ISAAC) Conference, Dublin, Ireland, August 24-27.

Hill, K., B. Romich, and G. Vanderheiden. 2010. Augmentative communication. In *The biomedical engineering handbook*, 4th ed., edited by J. D. Bronzino. Boca Raton, FL: CRC Press.

Hill, K., T. Kovacs, and S. Shin. 2014. Reliability of brain-computer interface language sample transcription procedures. *Journal of Rehabilitation Research & Development* 51(4):579-590.

Hoag, L., J. Bedrosian, and K. McCoy. 2009. Theory-driven AAC practices with adults who use utterance-based systems: The case of conversational rule violations. *Perspectives on Augmentative and Alternative Communication* 18(4):146-153.

Hochstein, D. D., M. A. McDaniel, S. Nettleton, and K. H. Neufeld. 2003. The fruitfulness of a nomothetic approach to investigating AAC: Comparing two speech encoding schemes across cerebral palsied and nondisabled children. *American Journal of Speech-Language Pathology* 12(1):110-120.

Hoffman, L., J. Bolton, and S. Ferry. 2008. Passy-Muir Speaking Valve use in a children's hospital: An interdisciplinary approach. *Perspective on Voice and Voice Disorders* 18:76-86.

Hoover, J., J. Reichle, D. Van Tassel, and D. Cole. 1987. The intelligibility of synthesized speech: Echo II versus votrax. *Journal of Speech, Language, and Hearing Research* 30:s425-s431.

Hourcade, J., T. E. Pilotte, E. West, and P. Parette. 2004. A history of augmentative and alternative communication for individuals with severe and profound disabilities. *Focus on Autism and Other Developmental Disabilities* 19(4):235-244.

Howlin, P., J. Alcock, and C. Burkin. 2005. An 8 year follow-up of a specialist supported employment service for high-ability adults with autism or Asperger syndrome. *Autism* 9(5):533-549.

Hustad, K. C. 2008. Comprehension and intelligibility scores for speakers with dysarthria. *Journal of Speech, Language, and Hearing Research* 51:562-573.

Hustad, K. C., and L. K. Miles. 2010. Alignment between augmentative and alternative communication needs and school-based speech-language services provided to young children with cerebral palsy. *Early Childhood Services (San Diego, California)* 4(3):129-140.

Hyatt, G. W. 2011. The iPad: A cool communicator on the go. *Perspectives on Augmentative and Alternative Communication* 20(1):24-27.

Jesse, M. T., N. Fei, E. Goldstein, I. Rakitin, L. Shama, F. Hall, and T. Ghanem. 2015. Head and neck cancer screenings and human papillomavirus knowledge across diverse suburban and urban populations. *American Journal of Otolaryngology* 36(2):223-229.

Johnson, J. M., E. Inglebret, C. Jones, and J. Ray. 2006. Perspectives of speech language pathologists regarding success versus abandonment of AAC. *Augmentative and Alternative Communication* 22(2):85-99.

Jreige, C., R. Patel, and H. T. Bunnell. 2009. *Vocalid: Personalizing text-to-speech synthesis for individuals with severe speech impairment.* ASSETS '09: Proceedings of the 11th International ACM SIGACCESS Conference on Computers and Accessibility, Pittsburgh, PA, October 25-28.

Judge, S., and G. Townend. 2013. Perceptions of the design of voice output communication aids. *International Journal of Language and Communication Disorders* 48(4):366-381.

Jutai, J., N. Ladak, R. Schuller, S. Naumann, and V. Wright. 1996. Outcomes measurement of assistive technologies: An institutional case study. *Assistive Technology* 8(2):110-120.

Kagohara, D., L. van der Meer, S. Ramdoss, M. F. O'Reilly, G. E. Lancioni, T. N. Davis, M. Rispoli, R. Lang, P. B. Marschik, D. Sutherland, V. A. Green, and J. Sigafoos. 2013. Using iPods® and iPads® in teaching programs for individuals with developmental disabilities: A systematic review. *Research in Developmental Disabilities* 34(1):147-156.

Kent, R. D., G. Weismer, J. F. Kent, and J. C. Rosenbek. 1989. Toward phonetic intelligibility testing in dysarthria. *Journal of Speech and Hearing Disorders* 54(4):482-499.

Kent-Walsh, J., and D. McNaughton. 2009. Communication partner instruction in AAC: Present practices and future directions. *Augmentative and Alternative Communication* 21(3):195-204.

King, T. 2000. *Modern morse code in rehabilitation and education.* Boston, MA: Allyn & Bacon.

King, J. M., N. Alarcon, and M. A. Rogers. 2007. Primary progressive aphasia. In *Augmentative communication strategies for adults with acute or chronic medical conditions*, edited by D. R. Beukelman, K. L. Garrett, and K. M. Yorkston. Baltimore, MD: Paul H. Brookes Publishing Co. Pp. 207-241.

King, M. R., C. Binger, and J. Kent-Walsh. 2015. Using dynamic assessment to evaluate the expressive syntax of children who use augmentative and alternative communication. *Augmentative and Alternative Communication* 31(1):1-14.

Koul, R., and L. Lloyd. 1994. Survey of professional preparation in augmentative and alternative communication (AAC) in speech-language pathology and special education programs. *American Journal of Speech-Language Pathology* 3(3):12-22.

Kresic, S., M. Veselinovic, G. Mumovic, and S. M. Mitrovic. 2015. Possible factors of success in teaching esophageal speech. *Medicinski Pregled Medical Review* 68(1-2):5-9.

Lawthers, A. G., G. S. Pransky, L. E. Peterson, and J. H. Himmelstein. 2003. Rethinking quality in the context of persons with disability. *International Journal for Quality in Health Care* 15(4):287-299.

Leder, S. B. 1994. Perceptual rankings of speech quality produced with one-way tracheostomy speaking valves. *Journal of Speech, Language, and Hearing Research* 37(6):1308-1312.

Lesher, G., B. Moulton, and D. J. Higginbotham. 1998. Techniques for augmenting scanning communication. *Augmentative and Alternative Communication* 14(2):81-101.

Lichtman, S. W., I. L. Birnbaum, M. R. Sanfilippo, J. T. Pellicone, W. J. Damon, and M. L. King. 1995. Effect of a tracheostomy speaking valve on secretions, arterial oxygenation, and olfaction: A quantitative evaluation. *Journal of Speech, Language, and Hearing Research* 38(3):549-555.

Light, J. C. 2003. Shattering the silence: Development of communicative competence by individuals who use AAC. In *Communicative competence for individuals who use AAC: From research to effective practice*, edited by J. C. Light, D. R. Beukelman, and J. Reichle. Baltimore, MD: Paul H. Brookes Publishing Co. Pp. 3-38.

Light, J. C., and K. Drager. 2007. AAC technologies for children with complex communication needs: State of the science and future research directions. *Augmentative and Alternative Communication* 23(3):204-216.

Light, J. C., and D. McNaughton. 2012. The changing face of augmentative and alternative communication: Past, present, and future challenges. *Augmentative and Alternative Communication* 28(4):197-204.

Light, J. C., and D. McNaughton. 2013. Putting people first: Re-thinking the role of technology in augmentative and alternative communication intervention. *Augmentative and Alternative Communication* 29(4):299-309.

Light, J. C., and D. McNaughton. 2014. Communicative competence for individuals who require augmentative and alternative communication: A new definition for a new era of communication? *Augmentative and Alternative Communication* 30(1):1-18.

Light, J. C., B. Stoltz, and D. McNaughton. 1996. Community-based employment: Experiences of adults who use AAC. *Augmentative and Alternative Communication* 12(4):215-229.

Light, J. C., C. Binger, T. L. Agate, and K. N. Ramsay. 1999. Teaching partner-focused questions to individuals who use augmentative and alternative communication to enhance their communicative competence. *Journal of Speech, Language, and Hearing Research* 42(1):241-255.

Lilienfeld, M., and E. Alant. 2009. The social interaction of an adolescent who uses AAC: The evaluation of a peer-training program. *Augmentative and Alternative Communication* 21(4):278-294.

Lund, S. K., and J. Light. 2006. Long-term outcomes for individuals who use augmentative and alternative communication: Part I—What is a "good" outcome? *Augmentative and Alternative Communication* 22(4):284-299.

Marics, M. A., and B. H. Williges. 1988. The intelligibility of synthesized speech in data inquiry systems. *Human Factors* 30(6):719-732.

Matthews, R. 2001. A survey to identify therapists' high-tech AAC knowledge, application, and training. *International Journal of Language and Communication Disorders* 36(Suppl.):64-69.

McAuliffe, M. J., S. Carpenter, and C. Moran. 2010. Speech intelligibility and perceptions of communication effectiveness by speakers with dysarthria following traumatic brain injury and their communication partners. *Brain Injury* 24(12):1408-1415.

McCarthy, H. 1986. Making it in able-bodied America: Career development in young adults with physical disabilities. *Journal of Applied Rehabilitation Counselling* 17(4):30-38.

McDuffie, A., A. Oakes, W. Machalicek, M. Ma, L. Bullard, S. Nelson, and L. Abbeduto. 2016. Early language intervention using distance video-teleconferencing: A pilot study of young boys with Fragile X syndrome and their mothers. *American Journal of Speech-Language Pathology* 25(1):46-66.

McGrory, A. 2011. Communicating with head and neck cancer patients. *ORL—Head and Neck Nursing* 29(3):7-11.

McNaughton, D., and A. Arnold. 2013. Supporting positive employment outcomes for individuals who use AAC. *Perspectives on Augmentative and Alternative Communication* 22(3):164-172.

McNaughton, D., and D. N. Bryen. 2007. AAC technologies to enhance participation and access to meaningful societal roles for adolescents and adults with developmental disabilities who require AAC. *Augmentative and Alternative Communication* 23(3):217-229.

McNaughton, D., and J. Light. 2013. The iPad and mobile technology revolution: Benefits and challenges for individuals who require augmentative and alternative communication. *Augmentative and Alternative Communication* 29(2):107-116.

McNaughton, D., and L. Richardson. 2013. Supporting positive employment outcomes for individuals with autism who use AAC. *Perspectives on Augmentative and Alternative Communication* 22(3):164-172.

McNaughton, D., K. Fallon, J. Tod, F. Weiner, and J. Neisworth. 1994. Effect of repeated listening experiences on the intelligibility of synthesized speech. *Augmentative and Alternative Communication* 10(3):161-168.

McNaughton, D., J. Light, and L. Groszyk. 2001. "Don't give up": Employment experiences of individuals with amyotrophic lateral sclerosis who use augmentative and alternative communication. *Augmentative and Alternative Communication* 17(3):179-195.

McNaughton, D., J. C. Light, and K. Arnold. 2002. "Getting your wheel in the door": Successful full-time employment experiences of individuals with cerebral palsy who use augmentative and alternative communication. *Augmentative and Alternative Communication* 17(2):59-76.

McNaughton, D., T. Rackensperger, D. Dorn, and N. Wilson. 2014. "Home is at work and work is at home": Telework and individuals who use augmentative and alternative communication. *Work* 48(1):117-126.

Mirenda, P. 2003. Toward functional augmentative and alternative communication for students with autism: Manual signs, graphic symbols, and voice output communication aids. *Language, Speech, and Hearing Services in Schools* 34(3):203-216.

Mirenda, P., and D. R. Beukelman. 1987. A comparison of speech synthesis intelligibility with listeners from three age groups. *Augmentative and Alternative Communication* 3(3):120-128.

Mirenda, P., and D. R. Beukelman. 1997. A comparison of intelligibility among natural speech and seven speech synthesizers and listeners from three age groups. *Augmentative and Alternative Communication* 6(1):61-68.

Mizuko, M., J. Reichle, A. Ratcliff, and J. Esser. 1994. Effects of selection techniques and array sizes on short-term visual memory. *Augmentative and Alternative Communication* 10(4):237-244.

Müller, J., G. K. Wenning, M. Verny, A. McKee, K. R. Chaudhuri, K. Jellinger, W. Poewe, and I. Litvan. 2001. Progression of dysarthria and dysphagia in postmortem-confirmed parkinsonian disorders. *Archives of Neurology* 58(2):259-264.

Nelson, P., K. Kohnert, S. Sabur, and D. Shaw. 2005. Classroom noise and children learning a second language: Double jeopardy? *Language, Speech, and Hearing Services in Schools* 36(3):219-229.

Netsell, R.. 1982. Speech motor control and selected neurologic disorders. In *Speech motor control*, edited by S. Grillner, J. Lindblom J. Lubker, and A. Persson. Oxford, UK: Pergamon Press. Pp. 247-261.

Newell, A., S. Langer, and M. Hickey. 1998. The role of natural language processing in alternative and augmentative communication. *Natural Language Engineering* 4(1):1-16.

Nordness, A. S., L. J. Ball, S. Fager, D. R. Beukelman, and G. L. Pattee. 2010. Late AAC assessment for individuals with amyotrophic lateral sclerosis. *Journal of Medical Speech-Language Pathology* 18(1):48-54.

O'Keefe, B. M., N. B. Kozak, , and R. Schuller. 2007. Research priorities in augmentative and alternative communication as identified by people who use AAC and their facilitators. *Augmentative and Alternative Communication* 23(1):89-96.

Oommen, E., and J. McCarthy. 2014. Natural speech and AAC intervention in childhood motor speech disorders: Not an either/or situation. *Perspectives on Augmentative and Alternative Communication* 23(3):117-123.

Oshrin, S. E., and J. A. Siders. 1987. The effect of word predictability on the intelligibility of computer synthesized speech. *Journal of Computer-Based Instruction* 14(3):89-90.

Patel, R., G. Meltzner, M. Suen, A. Nilsson, G. Rahhal, S. Bhandari, and R. Schweiker. 2015. *VocaliD™ human voicebank app*. Belmont, MA: VocaliD™.

Perry, A. R., and M. A. Shaw. 2000. Evaluation of functional outcomes (speech, swallowing and voice) in patients attending speech pathology after head and neck cancer treatment(s): Development of a multi-centre database. *The Journal of Laryngology & Otology* 114(8):605-615.

Perry, A., S. Reilly, S. Cotton, K. Bloomberg, and H. Johnson. 2004. A demographic survey of people who have a disability and complex communication needs in Victoria, Australia. *Asia Pacific Journal of Speech, Language, and Hearing* 9(3):259-271.

Raghavendra, P., J. Bornman, M. Granlund, and E. Björck-Åkesson. 2007. The World Health Organization's International Classification of Functioning, Disability, and Health: Implications for clinical and research practice in the field of augmentative and alternative communication. *Augmentative and Alternative Communication* 23(4):349-361.

Ratcliff, A. 1994. Comparison of relative demands implicated in direct selection and scanning: Considerations from normal children. *Augmentative and Alternative Communication* 10(2):67-74.

Ratcliff, A., and D. R. Beukelman. 1995. Pre-professional preparation in augmentative and alternative communication: State-of-the-art report. *Augmentative and Alternative Communication* 11(2):61-73.

Reynolds, M. E., Z. S. Bond, and D. Fucci. 1996. Synthetic speech intelligibility: Comparison of native and non-native speakers of English. *Augmentative and Alternative Communication* 12(1):32-36.

Robinson, N. B., and K. C. Sadao. 2005. Person-focused learning: A collaborative teaching model to prepare future AAC professionals. *Augmentative and Alternative Communication* 21(2):149-163.

Rodriguez, C. S., M. Rowe, L. Thomas, J. Shuster, B. Koeppel, and P. Cairns. 2016. Enhancing the communication of suddenly speechless critical care patients. *American Journal of Critical Care* 25(3):e40-e47.

Romich, B., G. Vanderheiden, and K. Hill. 2005. Augmentative communication. In *The biomedical engineering handbook*, 3rd ed., edited by J. D. Bronzino. Boca Raton, FL: CRC Press.

Romski, M. A., and R. A. Sevcik. 2005. Augmentative communication and early intervention: Myths and realities. *Infants and Young Children* 18(3):174-185.

Rousseau, B., M. Gutmann, I. F. T. Mau, D. Francis, J. Johnson, C. K. Novaleski, K. N. Vinson, and C. G. Garrett. 2015. Randomized controlled trial of supplemental augmentative and alternative communication versus voice rest alone after phonomicrosurgery. *Otolaryngology—Head and Neck Surgery* 152(3):494-500.

Rowland, C., P. D. Schweigert, J. C. Light, D. R. Beukelman, and J. Reichle. 2003. Cognitive skills and AAC. In *Communicative competence for individuals who use AAC: From research to effective practice*, edited by J. C. Light, D. R. Beukelman, and J. Reichle. Baltimore, MD: Paul H. Brookes Publishing Co. Pp. 241-275.

Saltürk, Z., A. Arslanoglu, E. Özdemir, G. Yildirim, I. Ayodogdu, T. L. Kumral, G. Berkiten, Y. Atar, and Y. Uyar. 2016. How do voice restoration methods affect the psychological status of patients after total laryngectomy? *HNO* 64(3):163-168.

Satterfield, L. 2015. Voice of reimbursement: Medicare coverage for vocal disorders. *Perspectives on Voice and Voice Disorders* 25(3):116-123.

Scherer, M. J. 2002. *Assistive technology: Matching device and consumer for successful rehabilitation*. Washington, DC: American Psychological Association.

Scherer, M. J. 2005. *Living in the state of stuck: How assistive technology impacts the lives of people with disabilities*. 4th ed. Brookline, MA: Brookline Books.

Scherer, M. J., and G. Craddock. 2002. Matching person and technology (MPT) assessment process. *Technology and Disability* 14(3):125-131.

Schlosser, R. W. 2003. Outcome measurement in AAC. In *Communicative competence for individuals who use AAC,* edited by J. Light, D. R. Beukelman, and J. Reichle. Baltimore, MD: Paul H. Brookes Publishing Co. Pp. 479-513.

Segalman, R. 2011. AAC, aging, and telephone relay access technology. *Disability Studies Quarterly* 31(4).

Shane, H., S. Blackstone, G. Vanderheiden, M. Williams, and F. DeRuyter. 2012. Using AAC technology to access the world. *Assistive Technology* 24(1):3-13.

Singer, S., H. Danker, A. Dietz, B. Hornemann, S. Koscielny, J. Oeken, C. Matthaus, H. J. Vogel, and O. Krauss. 2008. Screening for mental disorders in laryngeal cancer patients: A comparison of 6 methods. *Psychooncology* 17(3):280-286.

Slowiaczek, L. M., and H. C. Nusbaum. 1985. Effects of speech rate and pitch contour on the perception of synthetic speech. *Human Factors* 27(6):701-712.

Smith, R. O. 1996. Measuring the outcomes of assistive technology: Challenge and innovation. *Assistive Technology* 8(2):71-81.

Snell, M. E., N. Brady, L. Mclean, B. T. Ogletree, E. Siegel, L. Sylvester, B. Mineo, D. Paul, M. A. Romski, and R. Sevcik. 2010. Twenty years of communication intervention research with individuals who have severe intellectual and developmental disabilities. *American Journal of Intellectual and Developmental Disabilities* 115(5):364-380.

SSA (U.S. Social Security Administration). 2017. DI 24535.015 Evaluation of speech impairments. *Program Operations Manual System (POMS)*. https://secure.ssa.gov/poms.nsf/lnx/0424535015 (accessed January 18, 2017).

SSA. n.d. *Disability evaluation under Social Security—listing of impairments—adult listings (Part A)*. https://www.ssa.gov/disability/professionals/bluebook/AdultListings.htm (accessed January 18, 2017).

Staffieri, A., B. E. Mostafea, B. T. Varghese, E. D. Kitcher, M. Jalisi, J. J. Fagan, C. Staffieri, and G. Marioni. 2006. Cost of tracheoesophageal prostheses in developing countries. Facing the problem from an internal perspective. *Acta Oto-Laryngologica* 126(1):4-9.

Stern, S. E., C. M. Chobany, A. A. Beam, B. N. Hoover, T. T. Hull, M. Linsenbigler, C. Makdad-Light, and C. N. Rubright. 2017. Use of speech generating devices can improve perception of qualifications for skilled, verbal, and interactive jobs. *Work* [E-pub ahead of print].

Sullivan, M., D. Beukelman, and P. Mathy-Laikko. 1993. Situational communicative effectiveness of rehabilitated individuals with total laryngectomies. *Journal of Medical Speech-Language Pathology* 1(1):73-80.

Sullivan, M., C. Gaebler, and L. J. Ball. 2007a. AAC for people with head and neck cancer. In *Augmentative communication strategies for adults with acute or chronic medical conditions*, edited by D. R. Beukelman, K. L. Garrett, and K. M. Yorkston. Baltimore, MD: Paul H. Brookes Publishing Co. Pp. 347-367.

Sullivan, M., C. Gaebler, and L. J. Ball. 2007b. *Supporting persons with chronic communication limitations: Head & neck cancer*. Paper presented at American Speech-Language-Hearing Association Convention, Boston, MA.

Tang, C. G., and C. F. Sinclair. 2015. Voice restoration after total laryngectomy. *Otolaryngologic Clinics of North America* 48(4):687-702.

THANC (Thyroid Head & Neck Cancer) Foundation. 2017. *Head & neck cancer guide—Speech and swallowing rehabilitation*. http://www.headandneckcancerguide.org/adults/cancer-diagnosis-treatments/surgery-and-rehabilitation/surgeries-to-aid-breathing-and-eating/speech-and-swallowing-rehabilitation/ (accessed April 6, 2017).

Therrien, M. C., and J. C. Light. 2016. Using the iPad to facilitate interaction between preschool children who use AAC and their peers. *Augmentative and Alternative Communication* 32(3):163-174.

Thistle, J. J., and K. M. Wilkinson. 2009. The effects of color cues on typically developing preschoolers' speed of locating a target line drawing: Implications for augmentative and alternative communication display design. *American Journal of Speech-Language Pathology* 18(3):231-240.

Thistle, J. J., and K. M. Wilkinson. 2013. Working memory demands of aided augmentative and alternative communication for individuals with developmental disabilities. *Augmentative and Alternative Communication* 29(3):235-245.

Thistle, J. J., and K. M. Wilkinson. 2015. Building evidence-based practice in AAC display design for young children: Current practices and future directions. *Augmentative and Alternative Communication* 31(2):124-136.

Trnka, K., J. McCaw, C. Pennington, and K. McCoy. 2008. *Word prediction and communication rate in AAC*. Proceedings of the IASTED International Conference on Telehealth/Assistive Technologies, Baltimore, MD, April 16-18.

Ulmer, E., K. Hux, J. Brown, T. Nelms, and C. Reeder. 2016. Using self-captured photographs to support the expressive communication of people with aphasia. *Aphasiology* 1-22.

van der Merwe, A. 2009. A theoretical framework for the characterization of pathological speech sensorimotor control. In *Clinical management of sensorimotor speech disorders*, 2nd ed., edited by M. R. McNeil. New York: Thieme. Pp. 3-18.

Venkatagiri, H. S. 2003. Segmental intelligibility of four currently used text-to-speech synthesis methods. *Journal of the Acoustical Society of America* 113(4 Pt. 1):2095-2104.

Vincer, M. J., A. C. Allen, K. S. Joseph, D. A. Stinson, H. Scott, and E. Wood. 2006. Increasing prevalence of cerebral palsy among very preterm infants: A population-based study. *Pediatrics* 118(6):e1621-e1626.

Wagner, B., and H. M. Jackson. 2006. Developmental memory capacity resources of typical children retrieving picture communication symbols using direct selection and visual linear scanning with fixed communication displays. *Journal of Speech, Language, and Hearing Research* 49(1):113-126.

Ward, E. C., S. K. Koh, J. Frisby, and R. Hodge. 2003. Differential modes of alaryngeal communication and long-term voice outcomes following pharyngolaryngectomy and laryngectomy. *Folia Phoniatrica et Logopaedica* 55(1):39-49.

Wehman, P., S. Lau, A. Molinelli, V. Brooke, K. Thompson, C. Moore, and M. West. 2012. Supported employment for young adults with autism spectrum disorder: Preliminary data. *Research and Practice for Persons with Severe Disabilities* 37(3):160-169.

WHO (World Health Organization). 2002. *Towards a common language for functioning, disability and health: ICF*. http://www.who.int/classifications/icf/training/icfbeginnersguide.pdf (accessed November 16, 2016).

Williams, M. B., C. Krezman, and D. McNaughton. 2008. "Reach for the stars": Five principles for the next 25 years of AAC. *Augmentative and Alternative Communication* 24(3):194-206.

Wisenburn, B., and D. J. Higginbotham. 2009. Participant evaluations of rate and communication efficacy of an AAC application using natural language processing. *Augmentative and Alternative Communication* 25(2):78-89.

Wodka, E. L., P. Mathy, and L. Kalb. 2013. Predictors of phrase and fluent speech in children with autism and severe language delay. *Pediatrics* 131(4):e1128-e1134.

Wolpaw, J. R., N. Birbaumer, W. J. Heetderks, D. J. McFarland, P. H. Peckham, G. Schalk, E. Donchin, L. A. Quatrano, C. J. Robinson, and T. M. Vaughan. 2000. Brain-computer interface technology: A review of the first international meeting. *IEEE Transactions on Neural Systems and Rehabilitation Engineering* 8(2):164-173.

Yamagishi, J., C. Veaux, S. King, and S. Renals. 2012. Speech synthesis technologies for individuals with vocal disabilities: Voice banking and reconstruction. *Acoustical Science and Technology* 33(1):15.

Yang, C. S., C. H. Yang, L. Y. Chuang, and C. H. Yang. 2009. A wireless Internet interface for person with physical disability. *Mathematical and Computer Modelling* 50(1-2):72-80.

Yorkston, K. M., and D. R. Beukelman. 1981. Communication efficiency of dysarthric speakers as measured by sentence intelligibility and speaking rate. *Journal of Speech and Hearing Disorders* 46(3):296-301.

Yorkston, K. M., P. A. Dowden, and D. R. Beukelman. 1992. Intelligibility measurement as a tool in the clinical management of dysarthric speakers. In *Intelligibility in speech disorders: Theory, measurement and management*, edited by R. D. Kent. Philadelphia, PA: John Benjamin Publishing Company. Pp. 265-285.

Yorkston, K. M., E. A. Strand, and M. R. T. Kennedy. 1996. Comprehensibility of dysarthric speech. *American Journal of Speech-Language Pathology* 5(1):55.

Yorkston, K. M., M. S. Bourgeois, and C. R. Baylor. 2010a. Communication and Aging. *Physical Medicine and Rehabilitation Clinics of North America* 21(2):309-319.

Yorkston, K. M., D. R. Beukelman, E. A. Strand, and M. Hakel. 2010b. *Management of motor speech disorders in children and adults*. 3rd ed. Austin, TX: ProEd.

Zabala, J., G. Bowser, and J. Korsten. 2005. SETT and ReSETT: Concepts for AT implementation. *Closing the Gap* 23(5):1, 10-11.

ANNEX TABLE 6-1*
Summary of Aided Augmentative and Alternative Communication (AAC) Products and Technologies[a]

	Cost Range	
NO TECHNOLOGY *Healthcare Common Procedure Coding System (HCPCS) not applicable (NA)* Examples: Alphabet board Symbol sets Transparent gaze board/eye transfer (ETRAN) Topic boards	$1–$100	

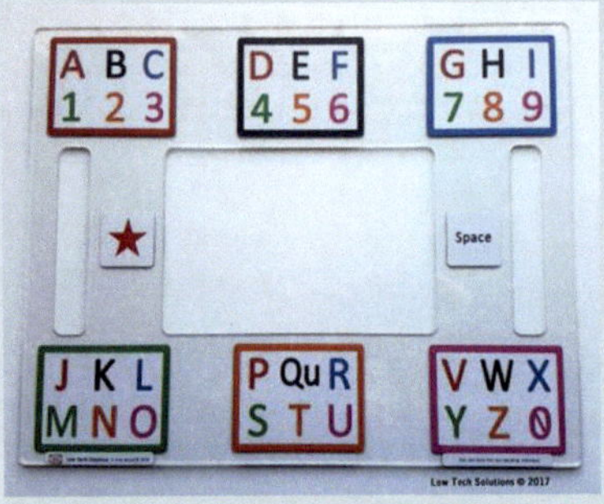

A. E-TRAN Topic Board

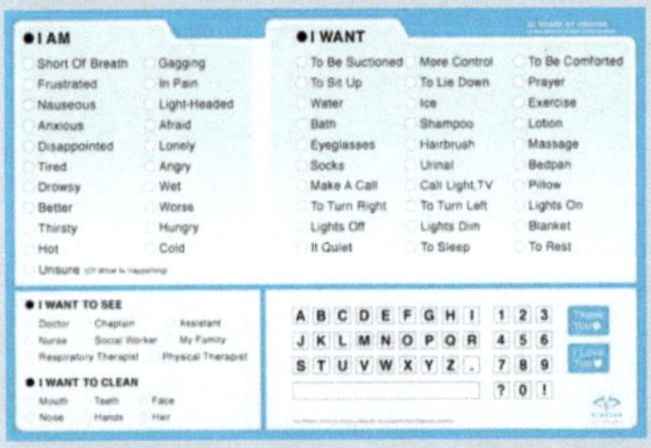

B. EZ Board™

*The images in Annex Table 6-1 serve as examples of device categories only and should not be considered an endorsement of specific products or manufacturers.

	Indications for Use	Relative Contraindications	Benefits	Limitations
	Basic messaging Visual output Establish topic Spell messages Partner-supported communication	Visual impairment Requires verbal output Complex or detailed messaging needs	Lightweight Simple to create, use Replace when damaged Create for multiple contexts Digitized speech is highly intelligible Plexiglass board has increased durability	No voice output No telephone interaction Limited independence Difficult with limited literacy Fixed display Printer required; may require symbol software Limited clinical support available Limited funding available

continued

ANNEX TABLE 6-1
Continued

	Cost Range	
LOW TECHNOLOGY *HCPCS NA* Examples: Megabee Eyegaze Communication Device 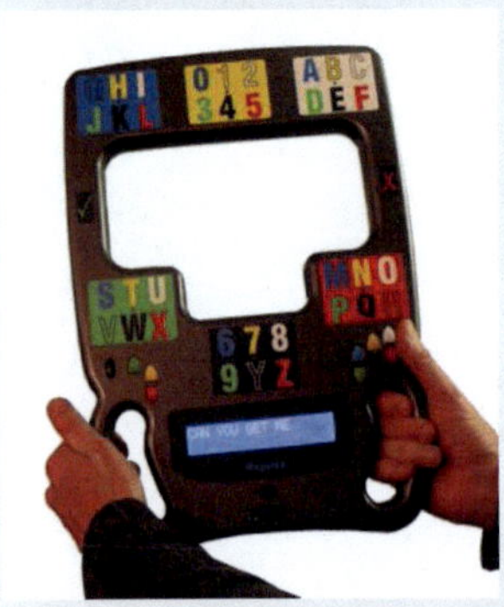 C. MegaBee Eye Gaze Communication Device	$1,260	
AAC/AAC TECHNOLOGY Type *Centers for Medicare & Medicaid Services (CMS) code*	**Cost Range**	
DIGITIZED VOICE OUTPUT		

	Indications for Use	Relative Contraindications	Benefits	Limitations
	Eye gaze selection Text output	Low literacy	Lightweight Portable Battery-operated Dual LCD screen for both communicators to see message Reduces effort of communication partner writing message by displaying on LCD screen	Partner-dependent communication Limited funding available

	Indications for Use	Relative Contraindications	Benefits	Limitations
	Basic, brief messages Prerecorded messages Supports greeting, name/labeling, simple requesting, protesting	Need to formulate novel messages Unimpaired adult cognitive function Literate Complex communication	Lightweight Portable Relatively inexpensive Battery-operated Durable design Multilingual Simple message recording Assessment and treatment codes established for speech-language pathologist (SLP)	Require age/gender-matched communication partner to record messages (partner-dependent) Limited conversations No spontaneous messages

continued

ANNEX TABLE 6-1
Continued

AAC/AAC TECHNOLOGY Type *CMS code*	**Cost Range**	
≤8 minutes recording time *HCPCS E2500* Examples: BIGmack LITTLE Step-by-Step Talking Brix Sequencer 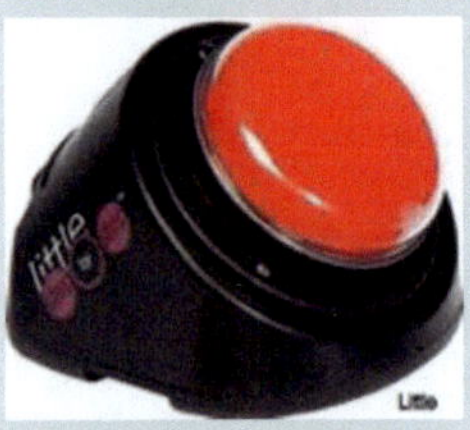 D. LITTLE Step-by Step	\$130–\$3,000	
9–20 minutes recording time *HCPCS E2502* Examples: SuperTalker QuickTalker23 VoicePal Levels 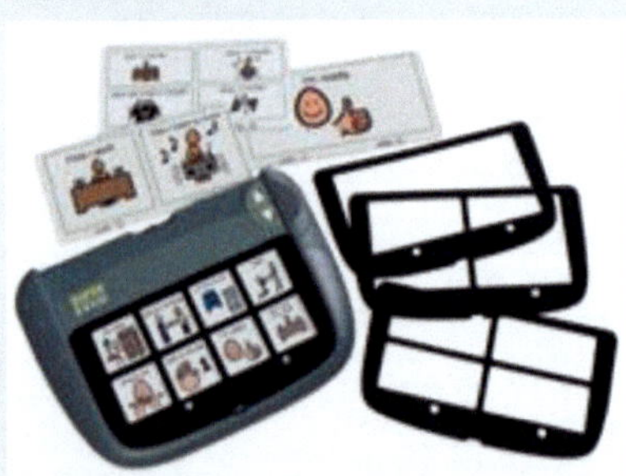 E. SuperTalker	\$300–\$500	

	Indications for Use	Relative Contraindications	Benefits	Limitations
	Single messages Limited communication needs		Initiate interactions Social comments Call attention Familiar communication partners	Long messages Multiple messages Message formulation Multiple environments
	Limited need for multiple messages Supports choice making from array		Combine thoughts into utterances Direct others	Multiple conversation partners

continued

ANNEX TABLE 6-1
Continued

AAC/AAC TECHNOLOGY Type *CMS code*	Cost Range	
21–40 minutes recording time *HCPCS E2504* Examples: GoTalk Express32 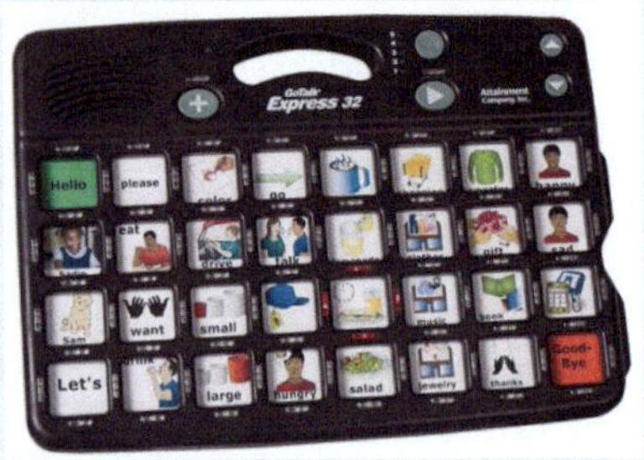 F. Express32	$600–$1,500	
>40 minutes recording time *HCPCS E2506* Examples: Talara32 Logan ProxTalker Smart/128VSD 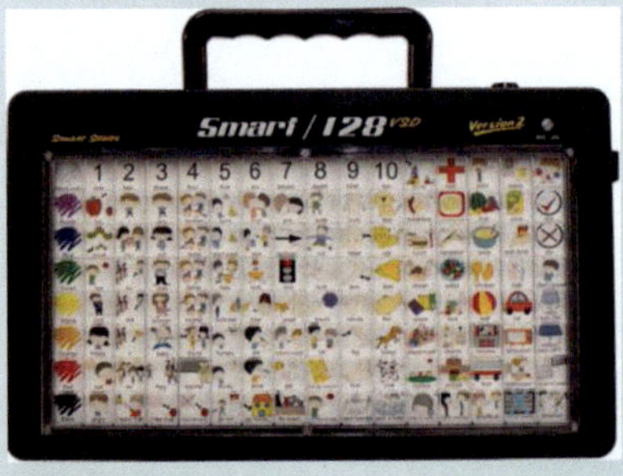 G. Smart/128VSD	$400–$4,100	

	Indications for Use	Relative Contraindications	Benefits	Limitations
	Multiple basic messages Narrative storage and retell		Use messages to describe known places/activities	
	Multiple basic and detailed messages Supports introductions		Lengthier message content	Unknown contexts, activities

continued

ANNEX TABLE 6-1
Continued

AAC/AAC TECHNOLOGY Type *CMS code*	**Cost Range**	
SYNTHESIZED VOICE OUTPUT		
Physical Contact and Spelling *HCPCS E2508* Examples: LightWriter SL40 Allora2 TextSpeak TS04 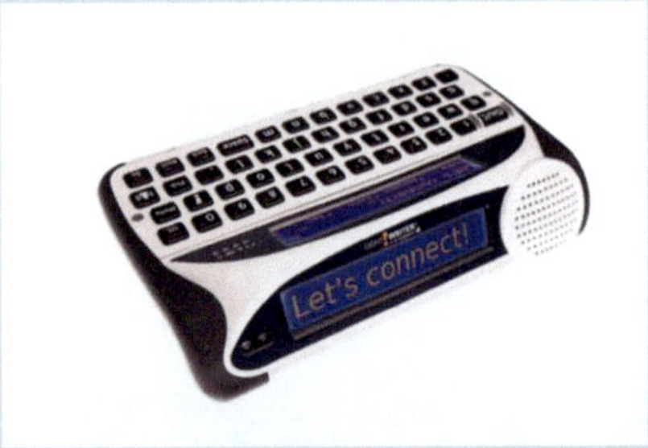 H. LightWriter SL40 Connect	$400–$7,000	

	Indications for Use	Relative Contraindications	Benefits	Limitations
	Provides formulation for individually unique messages Supports telephone interaction, conversation, complex message formulation, personal narratives, past event messaging, clarification, self-talk Benefit from full formulation for individually unique messages	Inability to formulate or comprehend complex interactions Distractibility with dynamic displays	High-quality synthesized voice output Text-to-speech Some multilingual Unlimited messages, contexts, communication partners Independent message formulation Formulate and interact with complex language Personal choice of synthesized voice Rechargeable battery and/or AC connection	Slow communication rate in time-sensitive interactions Some reduction in intelligibility of synthesized speech Wet, dusty conditions problematic
	Keyboard skills (most QWERTY) Typed message formulation Message formulation by (a) spelling every word, (b) device speaking word by word, or (c) person selecting "Enter" to deliver full message	Upper-extremity movement limitations Limited literacy	Familiar format Small, lightweight Portable Minimal training necessary Text representation Rate acceleration Assessment and treatment codes established for SLP (92607, 92608, 92609)	Direct keyboard access Limited accommodation to access in progressive disease Communication rate limited by typing rate Hands occupied for talking, unavailable for other activities

continued

ANNEX TABLE 6-1
Continued

<table>
<tr><th>AAC/AAC TECHNOLOGY Type
CMS code</th><th>Cost Range</th><th></th></tr>
<tr><td>Multiple Formulation and Access
HCPCS E2510

Examples:
Wego
NovaChat
T7-15
Accent
ComLink
ProSlate
Enable Eyes
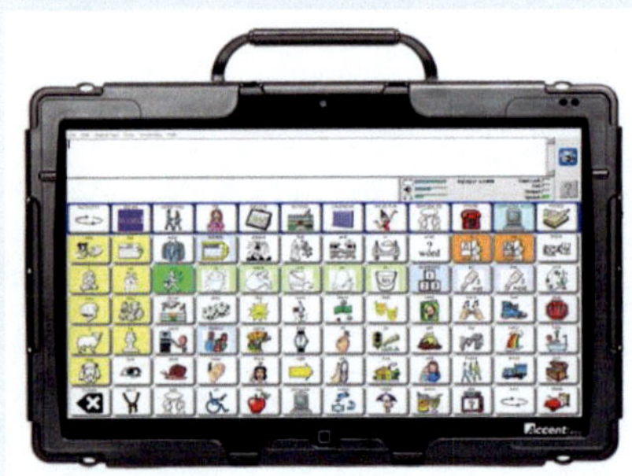
I. Accent 1400</td><td>$2,000-$16,000</td><td></td></tr>
<tr><td>Multiple Formulation and Access
HCPCS NA

Examples:
Apple iPad
Android Tablet
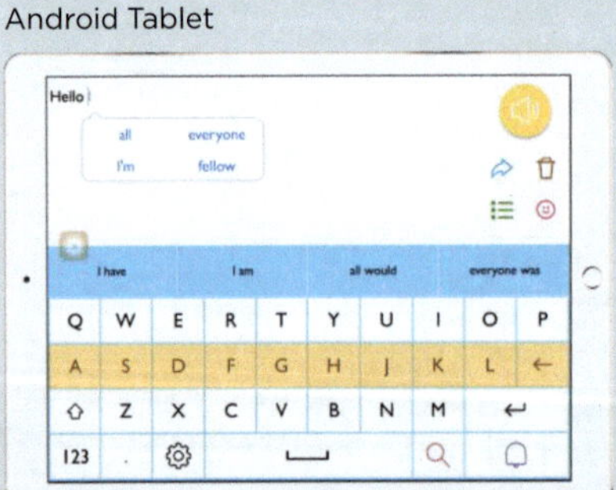

J. iPad running Predictable™</td><td>$50-$1,300</td><td></td></tr>
</table>

	Indications for Use	Relative Contraindications	Benefits	Limitations
	Touchscreen, keyboard, alternative access Display options for visual/cognitive needs Message formulation by spelling, using word prediction, selecting from a message array, device speaking word by word or upon selection to deliver full message	Limited language needs Difficulty navigating dynamic display	Unlimited content Symbol, photo, visual scene, text representation Rate acceleration strategies Dynamic display Direct and scanning access Assessment and treatment codes established for SLP	Many are large with limited portability without mounting to structure (table, wheelchair) and transport Synthesized output can be supplemented with digitized messages Communication software is integrated in speech-generating device (SGD)
	Touchscreen, some alternative access options Mainstream disability access options		Unlimited content Symbol, photo, text representation Rate acceleration strategies Dynamic display Relatively inexpensive	Limited funding options Limited assessment and treatment, professional support Synthesized output can be supplemented with digitized messages Physical disability access options are limited Limited device-app integration support

continued

ANNEX TABLE 6-1
Continued

AAC/AAC TECHNOLOGY Type *CMS code*	Cost Range	
SOFTWARE		

	Indications for Use	Relative Contraindications	Benefits	Limitations
	Provides language supports for communication based on language skills and needs	NA	Provides communication platform for devices Includes interface for alternative access, symbol and message management, and rate acceleration Some multilingual	Some compatibility issues, manufacturer or OS proprietary use Voice synthesizers offered as software Requires device for voice output activation Professional knowledge of communication needs essential to selecting most appropriate software/app

continued

ANNEX TABLE 6-1
Continued

AAC/AAC TECHNOLOGY Type *CMS code*	**Cost Range**	
AAC TECNOLOGY software *HCPCS E2511* Examples: Unity WordPower84 Communicator Speaking Dynamically Pro GoTalk Boardmaker Plus 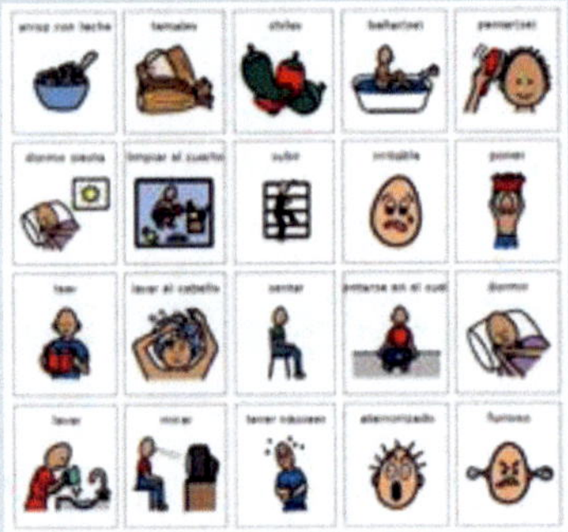 K. Boardmaker Plus 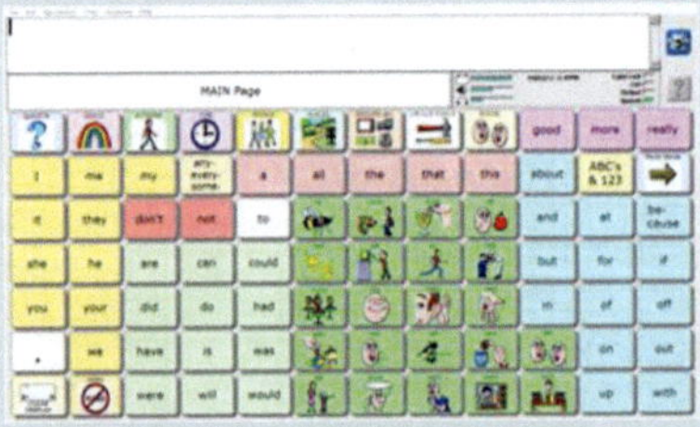 L. WordPower84	$100–$750	

	Indications for Use	Relative Contraindications	Benefits	Limitations
	Require message overlays for digitized devices Communication format on synthesized devices		Provide symbol sets, framework for communication Support digitized and synthesized communication methods Often packaged with SGD	Varied levels of training necessary for use on device Some individuals will require training to understand a new representational system (i.e., using pictures to communicate)

continued

ANNEX TABLE 6-1
Continued

AAC/AAC TECHNOLOGY Type *CMS code*	Cost Range	
Apps *HCPCS NA* Examples: Proloquo2Go Proloquo4Text Verbally Compass Predictable 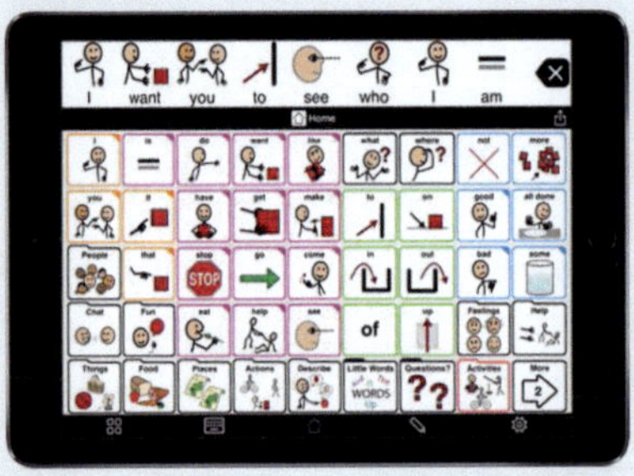 M. Proloquo2Go® 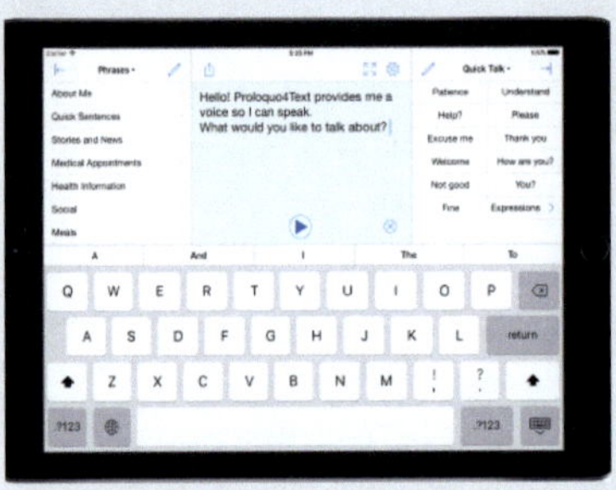 N. Proloquo4Text®	$0–$500	

	Indications for Use	Relative Contraindications	Benefits	Limitations
	Require message overlays for tablet systems	Because of frequent changes to apps, individuals with limited acceptance of new formats or updates may have difficulty	Readily available in online marketplace Relatively low cost	Some apps developed for single individual; varied quality exists in market Limited access to support for use, training, and troubleshooting Large number of apps available; many professionals have difficulty remaining updated on options

continued

ANNEX TABLE 6-1
Continued

AAC/AAC TECHNOLOGY Type *CMS code*	**Cost Range**	
ACCESSORIES *HCPCS E2599*		
Access Switches 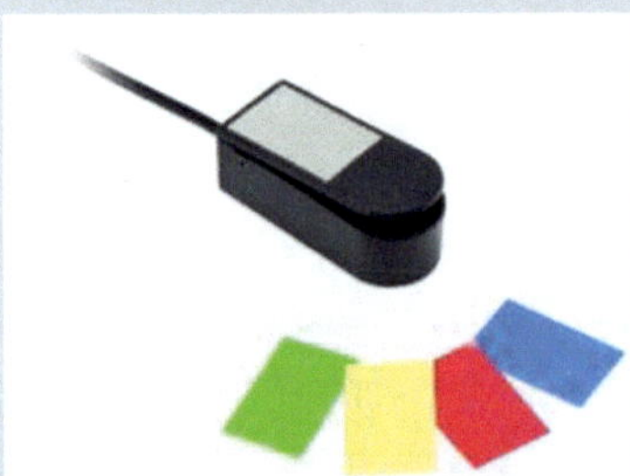 O. Micro Light switch 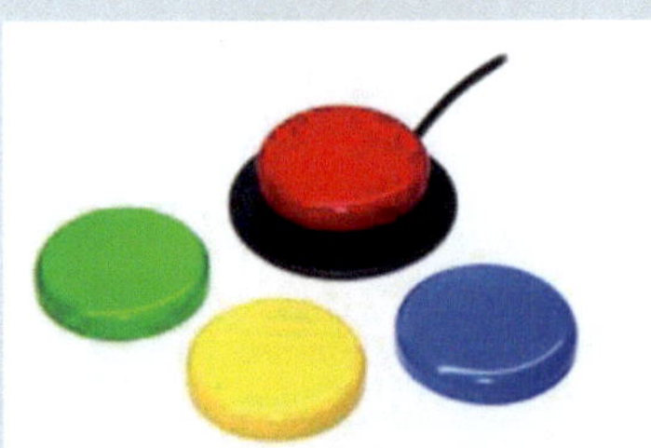 P. Jelly Bean Twist switch	$20–$2,000	

	Indications for Use	Relative Contraindications	Benefits	Limitations
	Provide access to messaging Support for evaluating multiple access method needs (e.g., fatigue, disease progression, context) (Fager et al., 2012)		Accommodate multiple physical disabilities to gain access to communication	Limited professional support available (e.g., SLP with AAC specialization, occupational/physical therapist [OT/PT] with switch experience)
	Indirect access through scanning by activating a switch when desired message is reached Direct access through Morse code by activating one or two switches to formulate message Direct access through head movement and dwell on desired message	May be cognitively taxing (scanning)	Relatively inexpensive	Slow message formulation, particularly with scanning May need supports during transfers to remove accessories or mounts Minimal repairs and maintenance available; most must be replaced when damaged

continued

ANNEX TABLE 6-1
Continued

AAC/AAC TECHNOLOGY Type *CMS code*	**Cost Range**	
Eye Gaze Access Examples: Eyespeak 12HD I-series (12+/15+) NuEye™ Tracking System 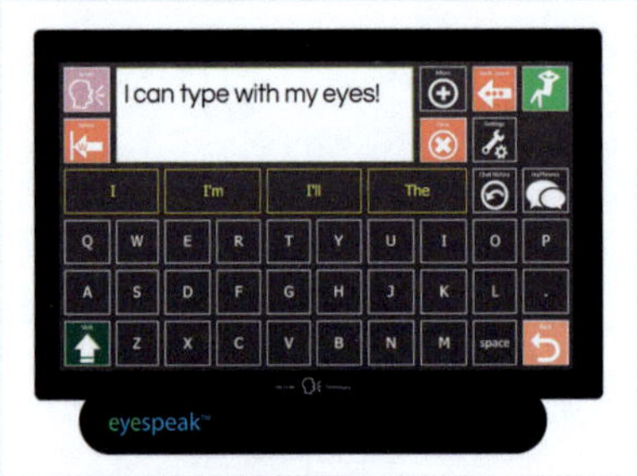 Q. Eyespeak 12HD	$2,000-$8,000	

AAC/AAC TECHNOLOGY Type *CMS code*	**Cost Range**	
MOUNTING SYSTEMS *HCPCS E2512*		

	Indications for Use	Relative Contraindications	Benefits	Limitations
	Direct access through eye gaze selection	Blindness Eye movement impairment (e.g., apraxia) Consistent inability to calibrate the gaze system	Enables individuals to control an AAC device using eye gaze interaction	Extraneous movements (e.g., not under personal control, such as chorea/ hyperkinetic movement) may interfere with calibration and accuracy
	Indications for Use	**Relative Contraindications**	**Benefits**	**Limitations**
	Provide access to device in various environments (e.g., wheelchair, desk, workstation) Secure AAC technology and accessories to mobility devices, seating systems in home/workplace	Direct access to touchscreen with body Portable device	Transport communication device Limit fatigue associated with device transport Provide optimal position for access to device	Limited professional support available (e.g., SLP with AAC specialization, OT/PT with AAC technology mounting experience) Minimal repairs and maintenance available, most must be replaced when damaged May require support to remove/ reposition for safe transfers

continued

ANNEX TABLE 6-1
Continued

AAC/AAC TECHNOLOGY Type *CMS code*	Cost Range	
Device Mounts Examples: Wheelchair mount Desk mount Rolling floor mount 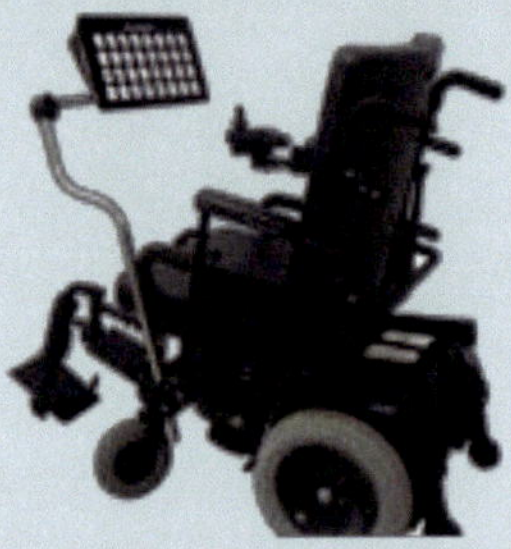 R. DaeSSy Rigid Mount Tech/Talk, Speak & Scan Devices	$400–$1,500	
Switch/Accessory Mounts 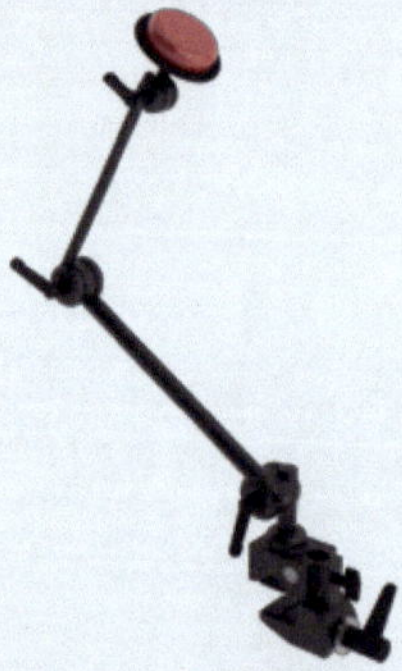 S. LIGHT-3D Table mount with two tubes and three joints with lever (14.4052)[b]	$50–$400	

NOTE: NA = not applicable.

[a]Technologies depicted in these images were current at the time of this writing.

[b]REHAdapt Engineering does not manufacture and has no claim to the switch shown on the mount.

SOURCES: A. Low Tech Solutions 2017; B. Vidatak, LLC; C. E2L Limited; D. AbleNet, Inc. Photo courtesy of AbleNet, Inc.; E. AbleNet, Inc. Photo courtesy of AbleNet, Inc.; F. Attainment Company, Inc.; G. Advanced Multimedia Devices, Inc.; H. Tobbi Dynavox. I. Prentke Romich

	Indications for Use	Relative Contraindications	Benefits	Limitations
	Secure SGD to mobility devices, seating systems in home and community	Handheld portable device in use	Provide effective transport of heavy AAC devices	May require partner set-up for daily access and repositioning as body shifts location
	Secure switches/ eye gaze to AAC technology, mobility devices, seating systems in home and community	Flexible switch placement needed (e.g., on clothing, bedding)	Provide stable, consistent base of support for switch access	Limited switch placement flexibility when in use May require partner set-up for daily access and with movement that removes person from switch proximity

ANNEX TABLE 6-2
Augmentative and Alternative Communication Software and Hardware

	AAC Language Representation				
	Text, Alphabetic Symbols				
	Letter-by-Letter Spelling	Word Prediction	Whole Word Display	Letter Coding	Morse Code
Communication Proficiency	YES	YES	YES	YES	YES
Literacy Proficiency	YES	YES	YES	YES	YES
Prerecorded Utterances	NO	NO	NO	NO	NO
Novel Utterances	YES	YES	YES	YES	YES
Vocabulary Selection	Individual Recall memory	Individual recall and recognition memory supported by software-embedded dictionaries	Individual recognition memory supported by display of high-frequency words	Individual recall memory Typically personalized for individual	Individual recall memory Often supported with visual display of the code
Software and Hardware Features					
Symbol Set/ System	Language-specific alphabet or characters, numbers, and punctuation	Alphabetic whole-word options presented dynamically based on the letter(s) entered	Whole words integrated with alphabet, numbers, and punctuation	Letters and numbers are used to create codes representing messages (e.g., asap = as soon as possible)	Dot and dash sequences represent alphabet, numbers, punctuation, and computer functions

	Single-Meaning Picture Symbols				Multiple-Meaning Icons	
	One Display	Levels with Changeable Displays	Multiple Displays	Multiple Methods	Icon Sequencing	Multiple Methods
	NO	YES	YES	YES	YES	YES
	NO	NO	NO	NO	NO	NO
	YES	YES	YES	YES	YES	YES
	NO	NO	NO	NO	YES	YES
	Professional/ communication partner Selection based on high-frequency vocabulary and/or customized based on personal choice, context, activity	Professional/ communication partner Selection based on high-frequency vocabulary and/or customized based on personal choice, context, activity	Professional/ communication partner Selection based on high-frequency vocabulary and/or customized based on personal choice, context, activity	Professional/ communication partner Selection based on high-frequency vocabulary and/or customized based on personal choice, context, activity	Individual recall and recognition memory supported by high-frequency words Extended vocabulary selected based on personal choice, context, activity	Individual recall and recognition memory supported by high-frequency words Extended vocabulary selected based on personal choice, context, activity
	Photos, line drawings, or color graphic drawings represent words, messages	Photos, line drawings, or color graphic drawings represent words, messages	Photos, line drawings or color graphic drawings represent words, messages	Photos, line drawings, or color graphic drawings represent words, messages, paired with alphabet	Color graphic drawings that represent words and messages with more than one meaning	Color graphic drawings that represent words and messages with more than one meaning with alphabet configurations

continued

ANNEX TABLE 6-2
Continued

	AAC Language Representation				
	Text, Alphabetic Symbols				
	Letter-by-Letter Spelling	Word Prediction	Whole Word Display	Letter Coding	Morse Code
Number of Symbols	Language-specific letters or characters, numbers, punctuation, and other keyboard symbols	Not applicable (NA)	NA	NA	Based on language-specific symbol set
Organization	Language-specific organization: QWERTY, ABCDEF, AEIOU, DVORAK, etc.	Selection options may be positioned at different display locations	Typically organized based on frequency, with the alphabet on the same or a different page	Customized letter codes, most on a separate page or section of a page	Language-specific organization
Number of Display Locations	Based on individual letters or groupings Typically, 26 or more as numbers, punctuation, and control options are available	Typically in addition to the main display Groups of 6, 8, 12, or more words may be presented	Displays with 20 to 144 locations are common	Some are memorized and not displayed	Often a sheet of codes is used to support recall during learning

	Single-Meaning Picture Symbols				Multiple-Meaning Icons	
	One Display	Levels with Changeable Displays	Multiple Displays	Multiple Methods	Icon Sequencing	Multiple Methods
	Based on the number of display locations and individual's vocabulary needs Typically, several thousand symbols are available in communi-cation software, and more may be added	Based on the number of display locations and individual's vocabulary needs Typically, several thousand symbols are available in communi-cation software, and more may be added	Based on the number of display locations and individual's vocabulary needs Typically, several thousand symbols are available in communi-cation software, and more may be added	Based on the number of display locations and individual's vocabulary needs Typically, several thousand symbols are available in communi-cation software, and more may be added	A limited icon set is combined in sequences to represent core vocabulary Several thousand single-meaning symbols represent words	A limited icon set is combined in sequences to represent core vocabulary Several thousand single-meaning symbols represent words, including letters and numbers
	Based on individual communi-cation needs: frequency, grammar, activity, topics of conversation	Based on individual communi-cation needs: frequency, grammar, activity, topics of conversation	Based on individual communi-cation needs: frequency, grammar, activity, topics of conversation	Based on individual communi-cation needs: frequency, grammar, activity, topics of conversation	Does not change with selections. Icon sequences represent core vocabulary and parts of speech	Does not change with selections Icon sequences represent core vocabulary and parts of speech paired with other functions
	Number of locations ranges from 1 to 144 per display or page	Number of locations ranges from 2 to 144 per display or page	Number of locations ranges from 2 to 144 per display or page	Number of locations ranges from 2 to 144 per display or page	Number of locations ranges from 26 to 144 per display or page	Number of locations ranges from 26 to 144 per display or page

continued

ANNEX TABLE 6-2
Continued

	AAC Language Representation				
	Text, Alphabetic Symbols				
	Letter-by-Letter Spelling	Word Prediction	Whole Word Display	Letter Coding	Morse Code
Visual Scene	NA	NA	NA	NA	NA
Color Coding	Not typically; individual-ized color coding is possible	NA	May custom color code (parts of speech, importance, visual needs, etc.)	NA	NA
Navigation; Number of Pages/ Displays	Limited; typically a small number—1-6 pages/ displays	None; predictions appear on the current page/ display	Range; depending on organization of words, multiple pages may be required based on activities or topics	None; NA	None; NA
Rate Enhance-ment	NA	Likely; reduced keystrokes	Likely; reduced keystrokes	Yes	Yes

	Single-Meaning Picture Symbols				Multiple-Meaning Icons	
	One Display	Levels with Changeable Displays	Multiple Displays	Multiple Methods	Icon Sequencing	Multiple Methods
	Visual scenes may support single messages	Visual scenes may support single or multiple messages with embedded hotspots	Visual scenes may support single or multiple messages with embedded hotspots	Visual scenes may support single or multiple messages with embedded hotspots and may be paired with text or symbols	NA	Visual scenes may support single or multiple messages with embedded hotspots and may be paired with multi-meaning icons
	May custom color code (importance, visual needs, etc.)	May custom color code (parts of speech, importance, visual needs, etc.)	May custom color code (parts of speech, importance, visual needs, etc.)	May custom color code (parts of speech, importance, visual needs, etc.)	May custom color code (parts of speech, importance, etc.)	May custom color code (parts of speech, importance, visual needs, etc.)
	None; NA	Range; depending on organization of symbols, multiple pages may be required based on activities or topics	Range; depending on organization of symbols, multiple pages may be required based on activities or topics	Range; depending on organization of symbols, multiple pages may be required based on activities or topics	Range; icon sequencing minimizes navigation, but multiple pages may be required based on activities or topics	Range; icon sequencing minimizes navigation, but multiple pages may be required based on activities or topics
	Possible; performance data are not available	Possible; performance data are not available	Possible; performance data are not available	Word prediction evidence indicates keystroke savings, but not rate enhance-ment	Yes	Yes

continued

ANNEX TABLE 6-2
Continued

	AAC Language Representation					
	Text, Alphabetic Symbols					
	Letter-by-Letter Spelling	Word Prediction	Whole Word Display	Letter Coding	Morse Code	
The following features depend on additional needs of the individual.						
Computer, Environmental Controls	Yes	Yes	Yes	Yes	No	
Training and Support	Varies depending on manufacturer and/or distributor, clinical professional access					
Peripherals	Touch guides, key guards, switches, mounting systems, external speakers, protective c					

	Single-Meaning Picture Symbols				Multiple-Meaning Icons	
	One Display	Levels with Changeable Displays	Multiple Displays	Multiple Methods	Icon Sequencing	Multiple Methods
	Yes	Yes	Yes	Yes	Yes	Yes

ANNEX TABLE 6-3
Augmentative and Alternative Communication Technology Function

AAC Technology Category Descriptors	Common Message Characteristics	Common Message/ Language Functions
Digitized Device ≤8 minutes recording Single display	• Single basic messages • Brief message content • Partner-dependent message formulation • Partner-dependent message recording • Multilingual	• Greet, depart • Name/label • Request (attention, help, food, break, objects, activities) • Existence/nonexistence • Cessation • Protest/reject
Digitized Device 9–20 minutes recording Display modified manually by changing communication overlays	• Multiple basic, few detailed messages • Brief message content • Partner-dependent message formulation • Partner-dependent message recording • Multilingual	• Greet, depart • Name/label • Request (attention, help, food, break, objects, activities) • Comment • Protest/reject • Choices (from array)
Digitized Device 21–40 minutes recording Display modified manually by changing communication overlays	• Multiple basic, detailed messages • Brief or lengthy message content • Partner-dependent message formulation • Partner-dependent message recording • Multilingual	• Greet, depart • Request (attention, help, food, break, objects, activities) • Comment • Protest/reject • Retell narratives • Choices (from array)
Digitized Device >40 minutes recording Display modified manually by changing communication overlays	• Multiple basic, detailed messages • Brief or lengthy message content • Partner-dependent message formulation • Partner-dependent message recording • Multilingual • Minimal message combinations for novel interactions	• Greet, introduce • Request (attention, help, food, break, objects, activities) • Comment • Protest/reject • Retell narratives • Choices (from array)

	Common Communication Contexts	Primary Communication Purposes	Communication Control	Communication Barriers Limitations
	Home Workplace Car/public transport Community	Express wants and needs Engage in social etiquette Information transfer Social closeness/ relationships	Initiate communication Direct action of another Social comments Call attention to self-achievement	No long interactions or conversational dialogue Prerecorded messages Poor fit for spontaneous utterances
	Home Workplace Car/public transport Community	Express wants and needs Engage in social etiquette Information transfer Social closeness/ relationships	Initiate communication Direct action of another Social comments Call attention to self-achievement Combine thoughts into longer utterances	No long interactions or conversational dialogue Prerecorded messages Poor fit for spontaneous utterances
	Home Workplace University Car/public transport Community	Express wants and needs Engage in social etiquette Gain and share information Build and sustain relationships Information transfer	Initiate communication Direct action of another Social comments Call attention to self-achievement Use words to describe location Ask simple questions	Few long interactions, limited conversational dialogue Prerecorded messages Poor fit for spontaneous utterances
	Home Workplace Car/public transport Community	Express wants and needs Engage in social etiquette Gain and share information Build and sustain relationships Information transfer	Initiate communication Direct action of another Social comments Call attention to self-achievement Use words to describe location Ask simple questions	Limited long interactions and conversational dialogue Prerecorded messages Poor fit for spontaneous utterances

continued

ANNEX TABLE 6-3
Continued

AAC Technology Category Descriptors	Common Message Characteristics	Common Message/ Language Functions	
Synthesized Device Physical contact, spelling Display changes dynamically when activated, based on programming	• Unlimited messages • Unlimited content • Independent message formulation • Unlimited combinations for novel interactions • Some multilingual • Most QWERTY keyboards	• Greet, introduce • Formulate jokes • Request (attention, help, food, break, objects, activities, clarification) • Comment and describe • Protest/reject • Hypothesize, speculate, self-talk • Tell narratives, past events • Manage dialogue	
Synthesized Device Multiple formulation and access Display changes dynamically when activated, based on programming	• Unlimited messages • Unlimited content • Independent message formulation • Unlimited combinations for novel interactions • Some multilingual • Multiple display options for visual needs	• Greet, introduce • Formulate jokes • Request (attention, help, food, break, objects, activities, clarification) • Comment and describe • Protest/reject • Tell narratives, past events • Hypothesize, speculate, self-talk • Manage dialogue	
Synthesized Device Multiple formulation and access Tablet (Android/Win/iOS) Display changes dynamically when activated, based on programming	• Unlimited messages • Unlimited content • Independent message formulation • Unlimited combinations for novel interactions • Some multilingual • Multiple display options for visual needs	• Greet, introduce • Formulate jokes • Request (attention, help, food, break, objects, activities, clarification) • Comment and describe • Protest/reject • Tell narratives, past events • Hypothesize, speculate, self-talk • Manage dialogue	
Software Communication interface	• Provides language format • Provides message formulation, access options • Programmed for display accommodations • Varies by software/app • Some multilingual • Multiple options	*Described based on AAC technology categories above*	

	Common Communication Contexts	Primary Communication Purposes	Communication Control	Communication Barriers Limitations
	Home Workplace University Car/public transport Community	Express wants and needs Engage in social etiquette Gain and share information Build and sustain relationships	Initiate and maintain communication dialogue Social comments Call attention for assistance, interactions Formulate and interact with complex language	Slow message formulation, particularly for time-sensitive interactions (e.g., telephone, business meetings) Requires literacy Requires hand-contact keyboarding Some reduced intelligibility of synthesized speech
	Home Workplace University Car/public transport Community	Express wants and needs Engage in social etiquette Gain and share information Build and sustain relationships Information transfer	Initiate and maintain communication dialogue Social comments Call attention for assistance, interactions Formulate and interact with complex language	Slow message formulation, particularly for time-sensitive interactions (e.g., telephone, business meetings) Some reduced intelligibility of synthesized speech Many are large and heavy, require mount for transport
	Home Workplace University Car/public transport Community	Express wants and needs Engage in social etiquette Gain and share information Build and sustain relationships	Initiate and maintain communication dialogue Social comments Call attention for assistance, interactions Formulate and interact with complex language	Slow message formulation, particularly for time-sensitive interactions (e.g., telephone, business meetings) Some reduced intelligibility of synthesized speech Requires selection of access methods from mainstream options Not considered DME
	Home Workplace University Car/public transport Community	Express wants and needs Engage in social etiquette Gain and share information Build and sustain relationships Information transfer	Initiate and maintain communication dialogue Social comments Call attention for assistance, interactions Formulate and interact with complex language	Slow message formulation, particularly for time-sensitive interactions (e.g., telephone, business meetings) Some reduced intelligibility of synthesized speech Require programming of communication display and messaging Require device for voice output Varying levels of communication based on developer

7

Coverage for Relevant Products and Technologies[1]

This chapter reviews the pathways by which individuals may gain coverage of the costs of the relevant products and technologies in each of the four areas of assistive technology (AT) addressed in this report (wheeled and seated mobility devices, upper-extremity prostheses, products and technologies that pertain to hearing, and products and technologies that pertain to communication and speech). The chapter includes discussion of both public and private funding sources, as well as workplace reasonable accommodations (see Annex Table 7-1 at the end of this chapter). In keeping with the committee's statement of task, the chapter focuses primarily on AT funding for adults, although it includes discussion of youth and young adults who are transitioning from a public school environment to higher education, vocational training, or the workplace since AT may have a profound impact on that transition. As noted elsewhere in this report, however, students often lose access to their AT when they age out of or transition from public school education. Also, as discussed elsewhere in this report, coverage for the *costs* of devices does not guarantee the *availability* in all parts of the country of either the devices themselves or the qualified providers and teams with the knowledge, skill, and expertise necessary to properly evaluate, fit, train, and monitor people in the use of the devices.

The first section of the chapter reviews public funding sources, including Medicaid, Medicare, the Veterans Health Administration (VHA), special education programs (for transition-aged youth), state vocational

[1]Much of this chapter is excerpted or slightly modified from a paper commissioned by the committee for this study (Sheldon and O'Connell, 2016).

rehabilitation (VR) agencies, and state workers' compensation programs. Private funding sources are then addressed, including self-pay, Supplemental Security Income's (SSI's) Plan to Achieve Self-Support (PASS), state alternative financing insurance programs, Achieving a Better Life Experience (ABLE) accounts, charitable programs, and private health insurance and private disability insurance providers. The discussion for each funding source encompasses eligibility for the program, general criteria for funding AT, any specific criteria for each of the above four categories of AT addressed, and the availability of an appeals process if relevant. In addition, workplace reasonable accommodations are addressed with discussion on the Americans with Disabilities Act (ADA) and employer accommodations. The chapter ends with findings and conclusions.

Given the breadth of the discussion in this chapter, only one or two specific devices within each of the four categories of AT are addressed under each funding source. However, the overall discussion within each funding source generally applies to each category. The specific products discussed within each category include the following:

- *Wheeled and seated mobility devices*—power wheelchairs with specialty features (tilt-in-space, a seat elevator, and/or an integrated standing feature) and, to a more limited extent, lightweight and ultra-lightweight wheelchairs
- *Upper-extremity prostheses*—myoelectric prostheses (arm or hand)
- *Products and technologies that pertain to hearing*—hearing aids
- *Products and technologies that pertain to communication and speech*—both speech-generating devices (SGDs) that are dedicated and dual-purpose devices (i.e., laptops or tablets that can be used as SGDs and for personal computing)

The above AT devices, if properly matched to the user and with adequate training, may help reduce or eliminate the effects of impairments and enhance an individual's ability to succeed in some work environments. They also tend to be more expensive than the more basic devices within the four categories, making funding more of a challenge in many cases. The Centers for Medicare & Medicaid Services (CMS) and private insurers have implemented competitive bidding for assistive products and technologies as a means of controlling costs (CMS, n.d.-a). Such competitive bidding may result in insurers covering the lowest-cost products and devices and in clinicians being less able to match the needs of their clients because of limited device options. "Medical necessity" is a typical consideration for insurers in their coverage of assistive devices, but devices that are deemed medically necessary may not include features that are most relevant or needed to pursue and support employment.

PUBLIC FUNDING SOURCES

Medicaid

Medicaid is a joint federal–state program authorized by Title XIX of the Social Security Act.[2] While state participation in Medicaid is optional, state compliance with the Medicaid Act is required.[3] CMS is the agency within the U.S. Department of Health and Human Services that provides federal oversight of state Medicaid programs. CMS promulgates regulations and issues policy guidance concerning federal Medicaid requirements to ensure compliance by the states.[4]

Currently, all 50 states, the District of Columbia, and five U.S. territories (American Samoa, Guam, the Northern Mariana Islands, Puerto Rico, and the U.S. Virgin Islands) participate in Medicaid, making it "the nation's main public health insurance program for people with low income and the single largest source of public health coverage in the U.S." (Paradise, 2015). People with disabilities make up nearly 16 percent of the nearly 70 million individuals eligible for Medicaid nationally (Paradise, 2015). At the state level, a single state Medicaid agency and its designees implement the Medicaid state plan.[5] Each state plan and any state plan amendments must be submitted to CMS for approval. States receive federal Medicaid funding, known as federal financial participation (FFP), for both the provision of health care services and certain administrative functions.[6]

Medicaid Eligibility Groups and Benefit Categories

Medicaid programs vary from state to state with respect to both the individuals who are eligible to enroll and the health care services covered. This variation stems from the Medicaid Act's identifying some eligibility groups and service categories as mandatory and others as optional.

Eligibility groups for individuals with disabilities The Medicaid eligibility groups are of particular relevance to individuals with disabilities.

The first group is *SSI beneficiaries*. In 41 states, the District of Columbia, and the Northern Mariana Islands, SSI beneficiaries who receive a cash payment are automatically eligible for Medicaid. The remaining 9 states, called

---

[2]Social Security Amendments of 1965, Public Law 89-97.

[3]See *Schweiker v. Gray Panthers*, 453 U.S. 34 (1981).

[4]42 USC §§ 1396-1396w-5; 42 CFR § 430 *et seq.*

[5]42 CFR § 431.10(b).

[6]42 CFR § 433.10(b). The amount of federal funding a state may claim is based on a formula that compares the state's per capita income with the national average, and it typically ranges from 50 to 83 percent for health care services.

209(b) states, establish their own Medicaid eligibility criteria, of which at least one criterion is more restrictive than the SSI criteria (SSA, 2014a, 2016a).

The second group is *medically needy beneficiaries*. In many states, this optional eligibility group allows individuals with income exceeding the state's Medicaid limit to qualify for Medicaid through a spend-down or cost-share provision. For example, an individual whose countable monthly income exceeded the state's Medicaid eligibility amount by $200 would face a $200 spend-down/cost-share. Once the spend-down or cost-share amount has been paid or incurred, full Medicaid eligibility is established.[7]

Finally, the *Section 1619(b)* and *Medicaid Buy-In* work incentives allow for Medicaid eligibility at significant levels of earned income and are important for working individuals with disabilities who lack private insurance or Medicare or who have insurance that does not cover needed services, such as home health services or durable medical equipment (DME).

The Section 1619(b) eligibility group, which exists in every state and the District of Columbia, allows Medicaid eligibility to continue when an individual loses SSI cash payments as a result of earned income above the threshold established by the state (SSA, 2015a). The 2016 threshold ranged from a low of $27,075 in Alabama to a high of $66,520 in Connecticut (SSA, 2016b). A higher eligibility threshold can be established if an individual's Medicaid-allowed expenses and/or disability-related work expenses are high enough (SSA, 2014b).

The optional Medicaid Buy-In Program was created by Section 4733 of the Balanced Budget Act Amendments of 1997,[8] with significant changes to the program being enacted as part of the Ticket to Work and Work Incentives Improvement Act of 1999.[9] As of April 2014, 46 states offered a Medicaid Buy-In Program for individuals with disabilities (Center for Workers with Disabilities/American Public Human Services Administration, n.d.). States commonly establish an eligibility threshold for the program of 250 percent of the federal poverty level, with some states having higher or lower thresholds (Kehn, 2013). States may charge a premium for participation in the program, set their own unique countable asset limits, and determine which assets are counted and which are exempt. States are required to determine countable income using the SSI earned income exclusions, meaning that the first $65 and half of remaining earned income each month is excluded. For states such as New York that allow income up to 250 percent of the poverty level (monthly countable income limit of $2,475),

[7]42 USC § 1396a(a)(10)(C).

[8]Public Law 105-33 (August 5, 1997).

[9]42 USC §§ 1396a(a)(10)(A)(ii) and 1396o.

gross earned income in 2016 could have been as high as $5,035 per month ($60,420 per year) (New York State Department of Health, 2016).

Mandatory and optional benefit categories The Medicaid Act lists 15 mandatory benefit categories every state is required to include in its state plan, as well as 28 optional categories (CMS, n.d.-c). Although states may choose which optional categories they include for adult beneficiaries aged 21 and older, all optional services must be available to children and youth under age 21 pursuant to the Early and Periodic Screening, Diagnostic, and Treatment (EPSDT) requirements of the Medicaid Act (see CMS, 2014a).[10] This broader array of services available through EPSDT is critical for all eligible children and youth, but is particularly important for those with disabilities who are preparing to transition from school to adult life. As discussed in greater detail later in this chapter, it is vital that transition planning for these youth take into account the fact that their eligibility for some optional Medicaid benefit categories may end when they turn 21.

Of the mandatory services available to beneficiaries of any age, the home health benefit, which includes medical supplies, equipment, and appliances, is often the primary source of AT for eligible individuals with disabilities.[11] In 2016, CMS defined these services as follows:

> Supplies are health care related items that are consumable or disposable, or cannot withstand repeated use by more than one individual, that are required to address an individual medical disability, illness or injury.[12]
>
> Equipment and appliances are items that are primarily and customarily used to serve a medical purpose, generally are not useful to an individual in the absence of a disability, illness or injury, can withstand repeated use, and can be reusable or removable.[13]

Also defined in federal law are several optional benefits that may be a source of AT devices and services.[14] For example, *prosthetic devices* are defined as

---

[10]42 USC § 1396d(r); 42 USC § 1396a(a)(43);42 USC § 1396d(a)(4)(B).

[11]Medicaid programs typically do not use the term "assistive technology" when describing available benefits. Instead, AT devices are often referred to as DME, medical equipment, or prosthetic and orthotic devices.

[12]42 CFR § 440.70(b)(3)(i).

[13]42 CFR § 440.70(b)(3)(ii). The word "disability" was added to the term "illness or injury" in the final home health regulation to avoid the denial of medical equipment and supplies for individuals with "congenital conditions or developmental disabilities." 81 Fed. Reg. 5540.

[14]The optional nature of a benefit does not lessen the state's legal obligation to provide this benefit to eligible beneficiaries. Once an optional service is included in the state plan, it must be provided in compliance with all federal requirements. See *Lankford v. Sherman,* 451 F.3d 496,

> Replacement, corrective, or supportive devices prescribed by a physician or other licensed practitioner of the healing arts . . . [which will] (1) artificially replace a missing portion of the body; (2) prevent or correct physical deformity or malfunction; or (3) support a weak or deformed part of the body.[15]

States that include this category of service in their state plan may cover a variety of AT devices through this benefit, including prosthetic limbs, orthotic braces, SGDs, and compression therapy products.[16]

Other optional benefits relevant to AT include physical, occupational, and speech therapy; preventive services; and rehabilitative services. Importantly, *physical therapy, occupational therapy,* and *speech therapy* are each defined to include the services of a licensed therapist and "any necessary supplies and equipment."[17] *Preventive services* are those that "prevent disease, disability, and other health conditions or their progression; prolong life; and promote physical and mental health and efficiency."[18] *Rehabilitative services* include services that allow for the "maximum reduction of physical or mental disability and restoration of a recipient to his best functional level."[19] Given these broad definitions, each of these benefits may provide access to AT for eligible beneficiaries.

Finally, optional *home- and community-based services* (HCBS) *waivers* may provide items not otherwise available through state plan benefits, including environmental accessibility adaptations, adaptive aids, specialized medical equipment and supplies, and personal emergency response systems.[20] While 1915(c) HCBS waivers and 1915(i) HCBS state plan option programs can be a good source of AT, CMS has clearly advised states that access to certain medical equipment cannot be limited by offering these items only through waiver programs if they also meet the definition of home health medical equipment.[21] For example, Texas Medicaid previously

504 (8th Cir. 2006); *Tallahassee Memorial Regional Medical Center v. Cook*, 109 F.3d. 693, 698 (11th Cir. 1997); *Weaver v. Reagen*, 886 F.2d 194, 197 (8th Cir. 1989); *Ellis v. Patterson*, 859 F.2d 52, 54 (8th Cir. 1988); *Meyers ex rel. Walden v. Reagan*, 776 F.2d 241, 243-44 (8th Cir. 1985); *Eder v. Beal*, 609 F.2d 695, 702 (3d Cir. 1979).

[15]42 CFR § 440.120(c).

[16]Some overlap exists between prosthetic devices and medical equipment, as certain items meet the definition of both service categories. See *Fred C. v. Texas Health and Human Services Commission,* 924 F. Supp. 788 (W.D. Tex. 1996) and 988 F. Supp. 1032 (W.D. Tex. 1997), affirmed per curium, 167 F. 3d 537 (5th Cir. 1998) (finding that SGDs meet the definition of DME and prosthetic device).

[17]42 CFR § 440.110.

[18]42 CFR § 440.130(c).

[19]42 CFR § 440.130(d).

[20]42 CFR § 440.180. In developing an HCBS waiver program, states can choose from an array of services, several of which may encompass AT devices and services.

[21]81 Fed. Reg. 5538.

limited access to ceiling lifts to HCBS waiver participants, claiming that FFP was not available for this equipment if provided through home health. In 2013, CMS wrote to the Texas Medicaid director to advise that the state's position concerning this equipment was incorrect (CMS, 2013). According to CMS, "medically necessary ceiling lifts will be reimbursed by CMS as part of the Texas home health benefit if these lifts meet the state's definition of DME."[22] CMS subsequently advised all states that such restrictions are unacceptable: "States may not restrict access to equipment that meets the criteria for coverage under the home health benefit by carving certain equipment out of home health and offering it only to individuals who qualify under a state's [HCBS waiver programs]."[23]

The broad definitions of these Medicaid benefits are particularly important to individuals seeking AT, as all service categories within the state plan must be "sufficient in amount, duration, and scope to reasonably achieve [their] purpose."[24] According to CMS, "because of the unique nature of medical supplies, equipment, and appliances, scope limitations within the applicable federal and state definitions are not consistent with the sufficiency of the benefit."[25] This means that states cannot simply exclude items of medical equipment from the home health benefit, claiming that such items are not within the scope of the benefit.

Federal Medicaid requirements also prohibit states from "arbitrarily [reducing] the amount, duration, or scope of a required service solely because of the diagnosis, type of illness, or condition."[26] As explained by one federal appeals court, "a state's failure to provide Medicaid coverage for non-experimental, medically-necessary services within a covered Medicaid category is both per se unreasonable and inconsistent with the stated goals of Medicaid."[27] In fact, the primary goal of this program—"to help families and individuals attain or retain their capability for independence or self-care"[28]—is met when eligible beneficiaries with disabilities are able to access AT devices and services through Medicaid.

The Prior Authorization Process

Like other features of state Medicaid programs, the process for requesting services differs from state to state. Many states, however, utilize some

[22]Equipment that does not meet the new federal definition under home health may be covered under a section 1915(c) waiver or the 1915(i) benefit. 81 Fed. Reg. 5538.

[23]81 Fed. Reg. 5538.

[24]42 CFR § 440.230(b).

[25]81 Fed. Reg. 5539.

[26]42 CFR § 440.230(c).

[27]*Lankford v. Sherman*, 451 F.3d 496, 511 (8th Cir. 2006).

[28]42 USC § 1396-1.

system of prior authorization to consider requests for medical equipment and other AT.[29] To obtain Medicaid prior authorization, eligible beneficiaries, in conjunction with their health care providers and Medicaid-enrolled DME suppliers, may be required to demonstrate that a requested device is (1) covered by Medicaid and (2) medically necessary.

Coverage of medical equipment The central principle governing coverage of medical supplies and equipment is long-standing: an item is covered by Medicaid when it fits within the definition of a category of service included in the state plan.[30] In September 1998, the Health Care Financing Administration (now CMS) clarified this basic principle in policy guidance to the states addressing the scope of medical equipment available through the mandatory home health benefit (Richardson, 1998).[31] Known as the DeSario Letter (Richardson, 1998), this guidance explained that a state's exclusion of items meeting the definition of medical equipment conflicts with several important Medicaid provisions, including the reasonable standards requirement[32]; the amount, duration and scope rule[33]; and in some instances, the prohibition on diagnosis-based decision making.[34] While CMS advised that states may develop a list of preapproved DME items as an "administrative convenience," they must also establish a "reasonable and meaningful procedure" for Medicaid beneficiaries to seek "modifications of or exceptions to [the] State's pre-approved list."[35] This process for determining coverage of medical equipment not on a state's list must permit

[29]In some states, individuals who are dually eligible for Medicare and Medicaid are unable to access the state's Medicaid prior authorization process, making it impossible to obtain certain items of medical equipment. In 2016, CMS sought input from the public concerning the extent of this barrier in the states and possible solutions. 81 Fed. Reg. 42,802, 42,864 (June 30, 2016); see Justice in Aging (2016).

[30]Most Medicaid services relevant to AT are defined in federal law. In the absence of a federal definition, states must define benefit categories consistent with Medicaid's amount duration and scope rule (42 CFR § 440.230(b)) and the prohibition on diagnosis-based decision making (42 CFR § 440.230(c)).

[31]This policy letter was issued in response to the decision in *DeSario v. Thomas,* which erroneously upheld Connecticut Medicaid's lists of covered and excluded items. The Supreme Court relied on this guidance in subsequently vacating the Second Circuit decision. 139 F.3d 80 (2nd Cir. 1998), *cert. granted, vacated and remanded sub. nom., Slekis v. Thomas,* 525 U.S. 1098 (1999).

[32]42 USC § 1396a(a)(17).

[33]42 CFR § 440.230(b).

[34]42 CFR § 440.230(c).

[35]To remain current, a state's preapproved list must be updated periodically to reflect changes in available technology.

timely individualized decisions based on the definition of DME and must be available to Medicaid beneficiaries of any age.[36]

In 2016, CMS revised the home health regulation to codify the principles of the *DeSario* guidance, once again clarifying the prohibition on exclusive coverage lists and lists of DME items that are specifically excluded.[37] Importantly, CMS also advised that states cannot characterize an item of medical equipment under an optional category of service that is not included in the state plan for adults in order to limit the availability of that item to beneficiaries under 21[38]: "To ensure full coverage for medical equipment and appliances, we will require that, to the extent there is overlap in coverage with another benefit, states must nevertheless provide for coverage of these items under the mandatory home health benefit."[39]

For the first time, CMS established a federal definition of medical supplies and equipment, in part to address the many inconsistencies across the states regarding coverage of this benefit.[40] According to CMS, "in the absence of a generally applicable definition of [medical equipment], there has been confusion as to the proper scope of the benefit."[41] Consequently, CMS acknowledged that in some states, "this rule may expand coverage of medical supplies, equipment and appliances under the home health benefit."[42]

Notably absent from this federal definition is the requirement that an item be "suitable for use in the home," a Medicare criterion that some states have historically included as part of their Medicaid DME definition.[43] Because the revised regulation now clarifies that beneficiaries can receive home health services "in any setting in which normal life activities take place," states can no longer apply an "in the home" limitation to restrict the DME items covered by Medicaid.[44] As explained by CMS, "the purpose

---

[36]The addition of a federal definition of medical equipment and supplies provides a regulatory framework for states to follow concerning the DME benefit. 42 CFR § 440.70(b)(3)(i-ii); 81 Fed. Reg. 5538.

[37]42 CFR § 440.70(b)(3)(v).

[38]An example of this prohibited practice is when a state claims to provide SGDs through the speech-language pathology benefit, knowing this optional benefit is not included in the state plan for adults and is available only to children and youth through Medicaid's EPSDT requirement.

[39]81 Fed. Reg. 5535.

[40]42 CFR § 440.70(b)(3)(i-ii).

[41]81 Fed. Reg. 5532.

[42]81 Fed. Reg. 5530.

[43]42 CFR § 440.70(c)(1). This provision codifies the principle established in *Detsel v. Sullivan*, 895 F.2d 58 (2d Cir. 1990), and *Skubel v. Fuoroli*, 113 F.3d 330 (2d. Cir. 1997), that private-duty nursing and home health services cannot be restricted to services furnished in the home.

[44]The only exceptions are hospitals, nursing facilities, intermediate care facilities for individuals with intellectual disabilities, and any setting in which payment is or could be made under Medicaid for inpatient services that include room and board. 42 CFR § 440.70(c)(1); 81 Fed. Reg. 5530, 5532.

of this provision is to ensure the delivery of home health services not only in the home, but also in the community when the beneficiary is participating in normal life activities."[45] This clarification is a critical change for Medicaid beneficiaries seeking certain medical equipment, in particular, certain custom powered wheelchairs, as states can no longer deny these wheelchairs on the basis that they are needed for use outside of the home.

The revised regulation also addresses other barriers to coverage of medical equipment. For example, the rule makes clear that eligibility for medical equipment and supplies is not contingent upon a beneficiary's requiring other home health services, such as nursing services or therapy.[46] Moreover, the new rule reiterates that states cannot restrict medical equipment and supplies to individuals who are "homebound," as the application of this requirement for home health services has long been prohibited.[47] Importantly, CMS also advised that states' coverage of medical equipment must be "updated periodically to reflect changes in available technology" (Richardson, 1998).

Medical necessity The requirement that Medicaid services be "medically necessary" is long-standing, dating back to the inception of the Medicaid program. The beneficiary's physician is the "key figure in determining utilization of health services," and it is this physician who "certifies the medical necessity of the services furnished."[48] In 2016, CMS reaffirmed this fundamental principle in the preamble to the revised home health rule, explaining that approval of medical equipment and supplies must be based on the physician's judgment of medical need, consistent with accepted standards of medical practice.[49]

The Medicaid Act does not define "medical necessity" for beneficiaries aged 21 or older. Typically, state Medicaid programs define this term in

---

[45] 81 Fed. Reg. 5530, 5532.

[46] 42 CFR § 440.70(b).

[47] 42 CFR § 440.70(c)(1). According to policy guidance issued by CMS on July 25, 2000, the provision of Medicaid services must comply with the ADA so that individuals with disabilities can live in the most integrated setting possible. As explained by CMS, conditioning Medicaid home health benefits on a homebound requirement violates Medicaid regulations related to "amount, duration, and scope of services" at 42 CFR § 440.230 and "comparability of services" at 42 CFR § 440.240. See Olmstead Letter No. 3, Attachment 3-g (HHS, 2000a).

[48] See S. Rep. No. 404, 89th Cong., 1st Sess., reprinted in 1965 U.S.C.C.A.N. 1943. See also *Weaver v. Reagan*, 886 F.2d 194, 200 (8th Cir. 1989) ("The Medicaid statute and regulatory scheme create a presumption in favor of the medical judgment of the attending physician in determining the medical necessity of treatment."); *Pinneke v. Preisser*, 623 F.2d 546, 550 (8th Cir. 1980) ("The decision whether or not certain treatment or a particular type of surgery is 'medically necessary' rests with the individual recipient's physician and not with clerical personnel or governmental officials.")

[49] 81 Fed. Reg. 5541; 81 Fed. Reg. 5533.

statute, rule, or policy, often requiring that the requested Medicaid service be appropriate for the beneficiary's medical condition or disability and be provided in conformity with accepted standards of medical practice. For example, Colorado Medicaid describes medical necessity in the context of a good or service that

a. Will, or is reasonably expected to prevent, diagnose, cure, correct, reduce, or ameliorate the pain and suffering, or the physical, mental, cognitive, or developmental effects of an illness, condition, injury, or disability. This may include a course of treatment that includes mere observation or no treatment at all;
b. Is provided in accordance with generally accepted professional standards for health care in the United States;
c. Is clinically appropriate in terms of type, frequency, extent, site, and duration;
d. Is not primarily for the economic benefit of the provider or primarily for the convenience of the client, caretaker, or provider;
e. Is delivered in the most appropriate setting(s) required by the client's condition;
f. Is not experimental or investigational; and
g. Is not more costly than other equally effective treatment options.[50]

For children and youth under age 21, medical necessity is defined in federal law and refers to the requirement that requested health care, diagnostic services, treatment, or other measures be necessary "to correct or ameliorate defects and physical and mental illnesses and conditions."[51] Thus, for children and youth under 21, Medicaid services must be provided if they are needed to correct, compensate for, or improve a condition or prevent it from worsening.[52]

Generally, an item of medical equipment is medically necessary when it addresses an individual's medical or functional needs and there is no less costly, equally effective alternative device. States sometimes go beyond their own general medical necessity standard, however, and establish equipment-specific criteria that dictate the circumstances under which a particular item will be considered medically necessary. When requesting prior authorization, the health care provider and equipment supplier must fully address

[50]10 CCR 2505-10 Sec. 8076.1.8.

[51]42 USC § 1396d(r)(5).

[52]See *Ekloff v. Rodgers*, 443 F.Supp. 2d 1173, 1181 (D. Ariz. 2006) (holding that "the phrase 'to correct or ameliorate' within the EPSDT provision is meant to include incontinence briefs for preventive purposes for Plaintiff children"). See also *A.M.T. v. Gargano*, 781 F. Supp. 2d 798, 806-07 (S.D. Ind. 2011) (adopting the definition of "ameliorate" used by the district court in *Ekloff*—"to make better or more tolerable" in light of "Congress' intent to be inclusive rather than exclusive with EPSDT").

these equipment-specific criteria in the evaluation report or letter of medical justification (see NLS, 2011a). To the extent that these criteria are either overly restrictive or otherwise do not comport with current standards of medical practice, Medicaid beneficiaries may have to seek administrative or judicial remedies. This is particularly true given that, nationally, more than half of all Medicaid beneficiaries are now enrolled with Medicaid managed care organizations (Kaiser Family Foundation, n.d.). Given that many of these managed care entities are insurers that typically establish their own medical necessity criteria in their private insurance contracts, Medicaid beneficiaries and their advocates must ensure that those criteria are consistent with the purpose of the Medicaid program and the federal Medicaid requirements governing home health and other relevant benefits.

Medicaid Coverage of Selected AT Devices

As state Medicaid programs begin to amend their home health benefit to comply with the recently revised federal regulation, access to funding for AT devices should become more uniform across the states.[53] Compliance with the new rule should lessen disagreements about Medicaid coverage of a particular item of equipment, turning the focus to the beneficiary's medical need for the requested device.

Powered wheelchair with tilt, seat elevation, and integrated standing feature A custom powered wheelchair configured in this manner meets the four elements of the home health medical equipment definition as it (1) is primarily and customarily used to serve a medical purpose; (2) generally is not useful to an individual in the absence of disability, illness, or injury; (3) can withstand repeated use; and (4) is reusable or removable. It should not matter that the standing feature may have some ancillary use that is not primarily medical in nature, such as enhancing social interaction or supporting psychosocial development, as this feature is an integral part of a therapeutic program of supported standing and is primarily and customarily used to serve numerous medical purposes. Therefore, a custom powered wheelchair with these specific components theoretically should be covered by every state Medicaid program through the home health benefit. However, at least one state continues to expressly exclude wheelchair standing features from coverage through the home health benefit.[54]

As to the medical necessity of this custom powered wheelchair, evidence

---

[53]Recognizing the "operational and budgetary implications" of this rule, CMS delayed states' compliance with the new provisions to July 1, 2017, or July 1, 2018, depending on when the state legislature meets. 81 Fed. Reg. 5530; 81 Fed. Reg. 5535.

[54]Texas Medicaid policy states that power standing systems on a wheeled mobility device are not a benefit of home health (TMHP, 2016, p. 97).

varies with respect to the medical benefits of supported standing. The Rehabilitation Engineering and Assistive Technology Society of North America (RESNA) supports the position that "wheelchair standing devices are often medically necessary," citing research indicating that frequent standing by wheelchair users can assist in maintaining vital organ capacity and bone mineral density; improving passive range of motion; lessening abnormal muscle tone and spasticity; and reducing the occurrence of pressure sores, contractures, and skeletal deformities (Arva et al., 2009; Dicianno et al., 2016, p. 3). However, a systematic review of literature published between 1980 and September 2015 examined the effectiveness of home-based standing programs in adults with chronic neurological conditions (Paleg and Livingstone, 2015). The review indicated that these programs have an impact on range of motion and activity outcomes, while the evidence was less certain for other outcomes. The review identified 36 studies on the impact of a standing intervention on adults with subacute or chronic neurological conditions, including stroke and spinal cord injury, that met the inclusion criteria. The authors found stronger evidence supporting the positive effects of "home-based supported standing programs on range of motion and activity, primarily for individuals with stroke or spinal cord injury" (Paleg and Livingstone, 2015, p. 1). Evidence supporting the effect of standing programs on bone mineral density was mixed, and the evidence for other outcomes (e.g., strength and spasticity; skin, cardiorespiratory, bowel, and bladder function) and populations was determined to be weak or very weak (Paleg and Livingstone, 2015).

Whether a state Medicaid program will agree that a wheelchair with these custom components is medically necessary for a particular individual likely depends on several factors, including the expertise of the medical professionals conducting the wheelchair evaluation, the quality and thoroughness of the evaluation, the specific medical conditions and functional needs to be addressed by the recommended wheelchair, and an explanation as to why a separate standing device or other alternative equipment is not equally effective in meeting the individual's medical need to stand. Litigation to resolve these types of issues has been necessary in several states.[55]

Myoelectric upper-extremity prostheses Myoelectric limbs also meet the four elements of the federal medical equipment definition and thus, theoretically, should be covered through the mandatory home health benefit,[56] although states vary in this regard. Additionally, these devices meet the federal

[55]See footnote 69.

[56]Myoelectric limbs are controlled by electrical signals generated by the user's own muscles, and in many instances they are considered to be more functional than other replacement limbs. For some individuals with very high-level amputations, myoelectric limb replacement is the only possible alternative.

definition of prosthetic devices and can be covered through this optional category of service if it is included in the state plan for adults.[57] The medical necessity of limb replacement appears straightforward, as such devices are neither experimental nor a matter of convenience. More problematic with respect to coverage is the type of prosthesis for which Medicaid will pay. For example, will Medicaid pay for a myoelectric prosthesis or only a less costly body-powered device? Thus, thorough documentation of the individual's medical and functional need for this specific item by qualified medical professionals is critical to obtaining Medicaid approval and funding. Yet, given that CMS does not have a Local Coverage Determinations (LCDs) document related to upper-limb prosthetics, there exist no clear and agreed-upon "reasonable and necessary conditions of coverage," making recommendation and justification of myoelectric devices difficult.

Hearing aids Under the EPSDT program, states must provide hearing screening and appropriate diagnostic and treatment services, including hearing aids, hearing aid accessories, and related services, to Medicaid beneficiaries under 21 years of age. In addition, such services "must be provided periodically at intervals that meet reasonable standards of medical practice" (HLAA, 2015). For adults aged 21 and older, Medicaid coverage for hearing aids varies from state to state (HLAA, 2015). As of January 2015, only 28 states covered the purchase of hearing aids for adult beneficiaries, and these states varied in their requirements for coverage (e.g., level of hearing loss, type of hearing aid), prescription, repairs, and replacements (HLAA, 2015; NASEM, 2016).

Dual-purpose SGD and personal computing device A dedicated SGD is one that performs the sole function of speech generation. Such devices clearly meet the four elements of the home health medical equipment definition and theoretically should be covered through the mandatory home health benefit in every state.[58] For individuals who may not qualify for home health services, such as those residing in nursing facilities, these devices also meet the definition of prosthetic devices and speech-language pathology services and can be covered through these other benefit categories when included in the state plan.

By contrast, a dual-purpose device is one that both generates speech and performs the functions of a personal computer. State Medicaid programs

[57]As previously explained, CMS has cautioned states that to "ensure full coverage for medical equipment and appliances, we will require that, to the extent there is overlap in coverage with another benefit, states must nevertheless provide for coverage of these items under the mandatory home health benefit." 81 Fed. Reg. 5535.

[58]In fact, access to SGDs through state Medicaid programs has been the subject of extensive litigation in numerous states. See footnote 68.

may attempt to avoid coverage of these dual-purpose devices on the basis that they are useful in the absence of disability, illness, or injury and thus do not meet the definition of medical equipment. In some instances, state Medicaid programs have required the personal computing function of dual-purpose SGDs to be locked when the item is delivered to the beneficiary, thereby limiting its function to speech generation. The personal computing function then can be unlocked after delivery for a nominal cost. As with all high-tech devices, a thorough evaluation of the individual's medical need for the recommended device is required. Importantly, the participation of an occupational or a physical therapist, along with the speech-language pathologist, may be required to conduct the SGD evaluation.

Medicaid Appeal Rights

Medicaid beneficiaries are entitled to timely and adequate notice and the opportunity for a fair hearing when a service request "is denied or is not acted upon with reasonable promptness."[59] Medicaid regulations require that denial notices explain, among other things, why the requested DME was denied, the specific regulations supporting the denial, the right to a fair hearing, how to request this hearing, and the time limit within which one must request the hearing.[60] This notice is also required when a requested service is approved with modification, as the state's changes to the recommended service may not fully meet the individual's medical needs.[61] For example, an individual may seek a custom wheelchair with several seating and positioning components. If the Medicaid agency approves the wheelchair but denies some of the requested components, the beneficiary is entitled to a fair hearing to challenge this partial denial.

States' Medicaid fair hearing systems must be authorized to determine whether an adverse coverage decision is contrary to federal requirements and whether a requested item is medically necessary. In most cases, hearing decisions must be issued within 90 days of the request for a hearing.[62] Typically, Medicaid beneficiaries who receive an adverse hearing decision can seek judicial review of the agency's final decision in state court.[63] Litigation in federal court is also an option for challenging state Medicaid requirements that deprive beneficiaries of the AT devices and services they require.

---

[59] 42 USC § 1396a(a)(3); 42 CFR § 431.200 *et seq.*

[60] 42 CFR § 431.210. The required content of notices sent to beneficiaries enrolled in Medicaid managed care organizations is set forth in 42 CFR § 438.404(b).

[61] See *Ladd v. Thomas*, 962 F. Supp. 284 (D. Conn. 1997) (holding that notice and an opportunity for a fair hearing are required when a request for DME is approved with modification).

[62] 42 CFR § 431.244.

[63] 42 CFR § 431.245.

Access to AT Through Advocacy and Litigation

In 1994, Congress authorized the creation of a Protection and Advocacy for Assistive Technology (PAAT) program in each state. The purpose of these programs is to provide legal representation and other advocacy to individuals with disabilities seeking AT devices and services.[64] During fiscal years (FYs) 2009 and 2010, PAAT programs reported serving a combined 2,255 and 2,317 individuals with disabilities, respectively. Thirty-seven percent of the 2009 cases and 34 percent of the 2010 cases entailed health care issues, typically involving Medicaid, Medicare, or private insurance (U.S. Department of Education, 2014).

In fact, legal representation has been necessary to secure Medicaid coverage and approval of various medical supplies, equipment, and AT over the past three decades. For example, Medicaid beneficiaries in Arizona, Florida, Louisiana, Missouri, and Rhode Island have litigated their right to access incontinence briefs through the home health medical supply benefit.[65] In Indiana and New York, Medicaid beneficiaries have litigated the issue of access to compression stockings and orthopedic shoes.[66] Lawsuits have also been brought in Louisiana, Pennsylvania, Rhode Island, and Vermont to obtain hearing aids and eyeglasses.[67]

For individuals requiring more advanced technology, beneficiaries in Connecticut, Florida, Georgia, Mississippi, Texas, and Utah have had to challenge various barriers to coverage for SGDs in court.[68] The same is true for complex custom wheelchairs, which have been the subject of

---

[64] 29 USC § 3001 *et seq.*

[65] *Alvarez v. Betlach*, 572 F. App'x 519 (9th Cir.) *cert. denied*, 135 S. Ct. 870 (2014); *S.D. ex rel. Dickson v. Hood*, 391 F.3d 581 (5th Cir. 2004); *Hiltibran v. Levy*, 793 F. Supp. 2d 1108 (W.D. Mo. 2011); *Smith v. Benson*, 703 F. Supp. 2d 1262 (S.D. Fla. 2010); *Ekloff v. Rodgers*, 443 F. Supp. 2d 1173, 1181 (D. Ariz. 2006); *Bristol v. R.I. Dept. of Hum. Serv.*, 1997 WL 839884 (R.I. Super. January 30, 1997).

[66] *Davis v. Shah*, No. 14-543-cv (2d Cir. 2016); *Davis v. Shrader*, 687 N.E.2d 370 (Ind. App. 1997).

[67] *Jasset v. R.I. Dept. of Hum. Serv.*, 2006 WL 2169891 (R.I. Super. July 31, 2006); *Ledet v. Fischer*, 638 F. Supp. 1288 (M.D. La. 1986); *Simpson v. Wilson*, 480 F. Supp. 97 (D. Vt. 1979); *White v. Beal*, 555 F. 2d 1146 (3d Cir. 1977).

[68] *Conley v. Dept. of Health*, 287 P.3d 452 (Utah. Ct. App. 2012); *William T. ex rel. Gigi T. v. Taylor*, 465 F. Supp. 2d 1267 (N.D. Ga. 2000); *DeSario v. Thomas*, 139 F. 3d 80 (2nd Cir. 1998), *cert. granted, vacated and remanded sub. nom., Slekis v. Thomas*, 525 U.S. 1098 (1999); *Fred C. v. Texas Health and Human Services Commission*, 924 F. Supp. 788 (W.D. Tex. 1996) and 988 F. Supp. 1032 (W.D. Tex. 1997), affirmed per curium, 167 F. 3d 537 (5th Cir. 1998); *Hunter v. Chiles*, 944 F. Supp. 914 (S.D. Fla. 1996); *Myers v. State of Mississippi*, 3:95 CV 185 LN (Slip Op. S.D. Miss. 1995); *Meyers ex rel. Walden v. Reagan*, 776 F. 2d 241 (8th Cir. 1985).

litigation in at least six states (Florida, Minnesota, New York, North Carolina, Pennsylvania, and Texas).[69]

While challenges remain, CMS's recent revisions to the Medicaid home health regulation are a critical step in addressing the barriers to obtaining medical equipment and AT devices that Medicaid beneficiaries with disabilities often face. Timely implementation and enforcement of the new federal home health regulation may reduce or eliminate many of these barriers. These new requirements, in conjunction with medical necessity determinations that reflect current standards of practice, should increase access to the AT devices individuals with disabilities may require to sustain their health, support their independence, and strengthen their quality of life.

Medicare

Medicare Eligibility

Medicare is a federal health insurance program administered by CMS. More than 55 million people participate in Medicare, including

- individuals aged 65 and older;
- individuals receiving Social Security Disability Insurance (SSDI) payments (including many adults with developmental disabilities who receive SSDI on the earnings record of a parent, and many who receive SSDI as widows or widowers) or railroad retirement benefits based on disability[70];
- persons with end-stage renal disease[71]; and
- certain Medicare-qualified federal employees (CMS, 2015b).[72]

---

[69]*Koenning v. Suehs,* 897 F. Supp. 2d 528, 552-53 (S.D. Tex. 2012) *vacated sub nom. Koenning v. Janek*, 539 F. App'x 353 (5th Cir. 2013); *Correa v. North Carolina Department of Health and Human Services*, 09-CVS-18112 (Gen. Ct. of Justice, Sup. Ct. Div. 2010); *Matter of Sorrentino v. Novello*, 295 A.D.2d 945 (NY AD 4th Dept. 2002); *Esteban v. Cook*, 77 F. Supp. 2d 1256 (S.D. Fla. 1999); *HHSC v. Lukefahr*, 2016 WL 5874871 (October 6, 2016); *Johnson v. Minn. Dept. of Human Serv*., 565 N.W.2d 453, 456 (Minn. App. 1997); *Starkweather v. Wing*, 242 A.D.2d 961, 962 (NY AD 4th Dept. 1997); *Matter of Johnson v. Wing*, 237 A.D.2d 960 (NY AD 4th Dept. 1997); *Matter of Ray v. Wing*, 238 A.D.2d 958 (NY AD 4th Dept. 1997); *Gartz v. Wing*, 236 A.D.2d 890 (N.Y.A.D. 4th Dept. 1997); *Dobson v. Perales*, 175 A.D.2d 628 (N.Y.A.D. 4th Dept. 1991); *Baker v. Commonwealth of Pa. Dept. of Pub. Welfare*, 502 A.2d 318 (Pa. Commw. 1985).

[70]SSDI beneficiaries are eligible for Medicare 24 months after SSDI eligibility. This 24-month waiting period is waived for individuals diagnosed with amyotrophic lateral sclerosis (ALS). SSA Program Operations Manual System (POMS) DI 45605.001.

[71]42 USC § 1395c.

[72]POMS HI 00801.400 *et seq*. During this extended coverage period, an individual can receive cost-free Part A coverage and optional Part B and Part D coverage, with premiums and

As with Medicaid, there are extended Medicare work incentive programs for certain beneficiaries. For example, working SSDI recipients who have completed their 9-month trial work period may continue to receive Medicare for an additional 93 months or more in some cases, even when their SSDI cash benefits have ended (SSA, 2015b,c). This extension is particularly important when Medicare is the only source of health care, including AT, for working beneficiaries.

Medicare Benefits

The Medicare program consists of four parts. As explained below, Parts A, B, and D provide a distinct group of benefits for eligible beneficiaries, while Part C allows Medicare beneficiaries to receive their health care through private managed care organizations.[73]

Medicare Part A, often called hospital insurance, generally covers inpatient hospital care, skilled nursing facility care, home health services following hospitalization, and hospice care (SSA, 2015d). Most beneficiaries pay no premium for Part A coverage but may pay a deductible and copayments for these services.

Medicare Part B, or supplemental medical insurance, covers outpatient services, including physician services, therapy services, DME, prosthetic and orthotic devices, and home health services (SSA, 2014c). To enroll in Part B, beneficiaries must pay a monthly premium ($134.00 if newly enrolled in 2017, but less if receiving Medicare prior to 2017). Part B beneficiaries are also responsible for certain deductibles and copayments. State Medicaid programs may pay the Part B premiums and other costs for some beneficiaries with limited incomes through Medicare Savings Programs, including the Qualified Medicare Beneficiaries, Specified Low-Income Medicare Beneficiaries, and Qualified Individual programs (Center for Medicare Advocacy, n.d.-b; SSA, 2011). Eligibility for these three programs is set at 100, 125, and 135 percent of the federal poverty level, respectively, with corresponding countable income limits of $990, $1,188, and $1,337 for a one-person household in 2016. The state Medicaid agency must use an SSI budgeting methodology in determining countable income, meaning, for example, that the first $65 plus 50 percent of remaining earned income exclusion applies.

---

other out-of-pocket expenses. Following this extended eligibility period, coverage through the Premium Medicare for the Working Disabled program can be purchased.

[73]Note that Medicare Supplemental Insurance (Medigap) policies are designed to cover some health care costs associated with original Medicare (e.g., coinsurance, deductibles, copayments); these policies may be purchased from a private insurer (CMS, 2017). However, Medigap policies do not cover items that are not covered by original Medicare (e.g., mobile augmentative and alternative communication technologies, hearing aids) (CMS, 2017).

Medicare Part C, also called Medicare Advantage plans, is an optional benefit. It allows beneficiaries to choose to purchase a managed care option from Medicare-approved private insurers instead of receiving traditional fee-for-service benefits provided by Medicare Parts A and B (SSA, 2015e). Although most beneficiaries participate in the original Medicare program under Parts A and B, about 30 percent chose the Part C option in 2015 (CMS, 2015b). Individuals may prefer the Part C option if they are able to pay an extra monthly premium to receive a broader range of outpatient services than those available through original Medicare. Hearing aids, for example, an item that is otherwise excluded from Medicare coverage, may be available through a Medicare Advantage plan, depending on the plan selected.

Medicare Part D, the prescription drug benefit, has been a part of the program since 2006. Part D is not administered by the federal government, but by various private health insurance plans. Part D generally is not relevant to the acquisition of AT.

Medicare Coverage of Assistive Technology: DME and Prosthetic Devices

DME Medicare covers DME, including AT devices such as powered wheelchairs and SGDs, through the Part B benefit.[74] Medicare defines DME as equipment that

- can withstand repeated use;
- effective after January 1, 2012, has an expected life of at least 3 years;
- is primarily and customarily used to serve a medical purpose;
- generally is not useful to a person in the absence of an illness or injury; and
- is appropriate for use in the home.[75]

Prosthetic devices Medicare also covers certain AT as prosthetic devices, defined as

> prosthetic devices (other than dental) which replace all or part of an internal body organ (including colostomy bags and supplies directly related to colostomy care), including replacement of such devices, and including one pair of conventional eyeglasses or contact lenses furnished subsequent to each cataract surgery with insertion of an intraocular lens; leg, arm, back,

---

[74] 42 USC §§ 1395x(n), 1395x(s)(6).

[75] 42 CFR § 414.202.

and neck braces, and artificial legs, arms, and eyes, including replacements if required because of a change in the patient's physical condition.[76]

Medicare Claims Processing

Unlike Medicaid, original Medicare typically does not provide prior approval of DME.[77] One exception is the Prior Authorization of Power Mobility Devices Demonstration Project, which CMS implemented in September 2012 and which continues through August 2018. Limited to beneficiaries in 19 states, this demonstration project provides a prior authorization process for those seeking scooters or certain powered mobility devices.[78]

In original Medicare, one of four Durable Medical Equipment-Medicare Administrative Contractors (DME-MACs) processes Durable Medical Equipment Prosthetics, Orthotics, and Supplies claims for a defined geographic area or "jurisdiction" (see CMS, 2016g). This claims process begins when the individual takes delivery of an item from the DME supplier. Once the item has been delivered, the supplier submits a claim to the applicable DME-MAC for payment.[79] For the beneficiary, a critical issue is whether the supplier "accepts assignment." Accepting assignment means the supplier agrees to accept the Medicare-approved payment for the item. Medicare pays 80 percent of this approved amount, with the beneficiary paying the remaining 20 percent. For example, if Medicare pays for a powered wheelchair with an approved rate of $10,000, Part B will pay $8,000, and the beneficiary will be responsible for a $2,000 copayment. For individuals who qualify for the Qualified Medicare Beneficiaries program, state Medicaid agencies pay this copayment (SSA, 2011). This is particularly beneficial for low-income Medicare beneficiaries who otherwise could not afford the copayment for certain AT devices.

In some instances, the Medicare-approved amount is less than what the supplier typically charges for an item of DME. If the supplier refuses to accept this rate, the beneficiary may owe far more than 20 percent of the purchase price.[80] Moreover, if the supplier is not confident that the

---

[76]42 USC § 1395x(s)(8-9).

[77]DME items provided to enrollees in a Medicare Advantage plan typically receive prior authorization from the private company administering the plan.

[78]For a listing of states participating in this demonstration project and other information, see CMS (2015c).

[79]Even though there is generally no prior authorization process for DME in original Medicare, a beneficiary can seek an Advance Determination of Medical Coverage (ADMC) (see CMS, 2016f, Section 5.16). Although a positive ADMC does not guarantee approval of funding by the DME-MAC, it does make that a likely result—something to discuss with the equipment supplier.

[80]For an excellent summary of these and other claims issues, see Center for Medicare Advocacy (n.d.-a).

DME-MAC will ultimately agree that the item is available for payment, the supplier may refuse assignment, meaning that the individual must agree to pay for the item if Medicare does not pay the claim. In Medicare Advantage plans, claims are submitted to the managed care organization in which the individual is enrolled. In most instances, the DME item has received prior authorization from the plan, so there is less risk of nonpayment by Medicare.

National and Local Coverage Determinations

CMS maintains a *National Coverage Determinations (NCD) Manual*, which includes a "Durable Medical Equipment Reference List" (CMS, 2005b). This list identifies more than 100 DME items and indicates whether each (1) is "covered," and under what circumstances it can be approved; (2) must be "denied"; or (3) is subject to coverage criteria listed elsewhere within the NCD Manual. For example, coverage criteria for SGDs are in section 50.1, while those for mobility assistive equipment (MAE) are in section 280.1. In addition to NCDs, the DME-MACs may adopt LCDs that apply to specific DME items. A summary of coverage policy for the four categories of selected equipment follows.

Powered wheelchairs, including those with a seat elevator, tilt-in-space, or integrated standing system Medicare coverage of powered wheelchairs is governed by NCD 280.3 (CMS, 2005c). At the regional level, powered wheelchairs are covered as "power mobility devices" pursuant to LCD 33789, an LCD that has been adopted by all four DME-MACs (see CMS, n.d.-b). NCD 280.3, effective May 5, 2005, states, in part:

> CMS finds that the evidence is adequate to determine that MAE is reasonable and necessary for beneficiaries who have a personal mobility deficit sufficient to impair their participation in mobility-related activities of daily living (MRADLs) such as toileting, feeding, dressing, grooming, and bathing in customary locations within the home. Determination of the presence of a mobility deficit will be made by an algorithmic process, Clinical Criteria for MAE Coverage, to provide the appropriate MAE to correct the mobility deficit.

This national policy sets forth the referenced clinical criteria for MAE coverage, including a series of nine questions geared to connecting the beneficiary's mobility limitation to an inability to complete MRADLs in the home; the ability to use other MAE, a cane or walker, or a caregiver to adequately address any limitations; the suitability of the home environment for use of the MAE; the ability to use a power operated vehicle/scooter rather than a powered wheelchair to complete MRADLs; and the need for any additional features a powered wheelchair offers to accomplish one or more MRADLs.

The goal of this policy is not to ensure that individuals will attain functional mobility in or outside the home. Under NCD 280.3, Medicare will not pay for a powered wheelchair needed for reasons other than to accomplish MRADLs or for one to be used outside the home. This outright exclusion of MAE, including powered wheelchairs, when needed only outside the home greatly limits the ability of many Medicare beneficiaries to participate in the workforce. Notably, once a powered wheelchair has been approved, neither the NCD nor the LCD precludes its use outside the home to go to and from work or to accomplish work-related tasks.[81]

LCD L33789 governs the day-to-day decision making of the four DME-MACs and includes more-detailed policies than NCD 280.3. Specifically, this LCD sets forth criteria for approving Group 1, 2, and 3 wheelchairs for funding. Group 3 powered wheelchairs involve complex rehab technology and are often more expensive than Group 1 or 2 wheelchairs. Noridian, the DME-MAC for Jurisdiction D, explains the basic criteria governing Group 3 wheelchair coverage (Noridian Healthcare Solutions, 2016):

- The beneficiary's mobility limitation must be due to a neurological condition, myopathy or congenital skeletal deformity.
- There must be a specialty evaluation performed by a licensed/certified medical professional, such as a physical therapist, occupational therapist, or physician who has specific training and experience in rehabilitation wheelchair evaluations that documents the medical necessity for the wheelchair and its special features.
- The wheelchair must be provided by a supplier that employs a RESNA-certified assistive technology professional (ATP) who specializes in wheelchairs and who has direct, in-person involvement in the wheelchair selection for the beneficiary.

Noridian further explains the additional criteria for Group 3 powered wheelchairs with either single or multiple power options:

- The beneficiary must require a drive control interface other than a hand or chin-operated standard proportional joystick (examples include but are not limited to head control, sip and puff, switch control); or

[81]See CMS (2005a, Part VII.B.8) ("CMS would like to reassure the community that the DME benefit category does not prevent beneficiaries from using their wheelchairs outside of the home.").

- The beneficiary must meet coverage criteria for a power tilt or a power recline seating system and the system is being used on the wheelchair; or
- The beneficiary will use a ventilator which is mounted on the wheelchair.

Finally, Noridian states that Group 3 wheelchairs are reserved for "the severely impaired patient," with diseases such as ALS or late-stage multiple sclerosis or spinal cord injuries resulting in quadriplegia. While a beneficiary must meet the threshold criteria discussed above (i.e., MAE needed to accomplish MRADLs in the home), a Group 3 powered wheelchair can greatly enhance one's ability to get to and from work and to move about during the workday.

Under L33789, Group 4 wheelchairs are not covered as they "have added capabilities that are not needed in the home. Therefore . . . they will be denied as not reasonable and necessary." Generally, a Group 4 wheelchair base is needed to support an integrated standing feature, making a standing powered wheelchair unavailable through Medicare. Although Group 5 pediatric wheelchairs are covered by Medicare, they are not commonly used by adult Medicare beneficiaries.

In summary, Medicare will pay only for wheelchairs that are required for an individual to accomplish MRADLs within the home. If an individual can navigate his or her home sufficiently to accomplish MRADLs without the use of a wheelchair, whether manual or powered, Medicare will not pay for one regardless of whether the individual requires one to participate in work or other activities outside of the home.[82]

Myoelectric upper-extremity prostheses Medicare regulations authorize Part B payment for certain equipment categorized as prosthetic devices, including

> (2) Prosthetic devices, other than dental, that replace all or part of an internal body organ, including colostomy bags and supplies directly related to colostomy care, including—
> (i) Replacement of prosthetic devices; and
> (3) Leg, arm, back, and neck braces and artificial legs, arms, and eyes, including replacements if required because of a change in the individual's physical condition.[83]

[82]The discussion in this section does not include the Medicare competitive bidding process for wheelchair coverage, legislated by Congress with a phase-in period beginning in 2008. A thorough discussion of this requirement appears in GAO (2016).

[83]42 CFR §§ 410.36(a), 414.202.

CMS policy also lists artificial limbs as an example of prosthetic devices (CMS, 2016b, Section 10.1.2; CMS, 2016d, Section 120A).

Presently, no NCD or LCD governing upper-body prostheses generally or myoelectric devices specifically appears to exist.[84] Absent a specific policy, CMS must take a case-by-case approach to approving specific devices. In general, Medicare coverage and payment are contingent on a determination that

- A service is in a covered benefit category;
- A service is not specifically excluded from Medicare coverage by the Act; and
- The item or service is "reasonable and necessary" for the diagnosis or treatment of an illness or injury, to improve functioning of a malformed body member, or is a covered preventive service. (CMS, 2016c, Section 10.2)[85]

Because a myoelectric arm or hand is listed as a covered prosthetic device and is not specifically excluded by the Medicare Act, Medicare funding theoretically will depend on whether the item is deemed medically necessary, that is, reasonable and necessary to improve functioning of the malformed or missing limb. In the absence of prior authorization in original Medicare, a prosthetics supplier likely would not deliver this item and accept assignment unless there was a track record of adequate payment for such devices.

If the Medicare beneficiary is enrolled in a Medicare Advantage plan, the supplier must work with the beneficiary and his or her physician to fully document medical necessity for the device (CMS, 2016c, Section 10.12.3).[86] In such cases in which there is no NCD or LCD to guide the decision-making process, CMS guidelines allow Medicare Advantage plans to make coverage determinations by applying an objective process based on authoritative evidence (CMS, 2016c, Section 90.5). For example, Regence Medicare Advantage Plan, covering Oregon, Utah, Idaho, and parts of Washington State, provides specific criteria for determining medical necessity for a myoelectric upper-limb prosthesis. Key criteria include the following:

[84]Billing codes do exist for several myoelectric limb replacements. See, for example, billing codes L6935, L6955, and L6967 on the Noridian DME-MAC website (Noridian Healthcare Solutions, 2017).

[85]Although this manual is specific to Medicare Advantage plans, the policy applies to original Medicare as well.

[86]Notably, Medicare policy does require that a "[Medicare Advantage] plan . . . provide all brands and manufacturers of Prosthetics and Orthotics without limitation."

- The patient has an amputation or missing limb at the wrist or above (forearm, elbow, etc.); AND
- Standard body-powered prosthetic devices cannot be used or are insufficient to meet the functional needs of the individual in performing activities of daily living; AND
- The remaining musculature of the arm(s) contains the minimum microvolt threshold to allow operation of a myoelectric prosthetic device, as demonstrated by functional testing using a physical or computer model prosthesis; AND
- The patient has demonstrated sufficient neurological and cognitive function to operate the prosthesis effectively; AND
- The patient is free of comorbidities that could interfere with the functioning of the prosthesis (neuromuscular disease, etc.); AND
- Functional evaluation by a qualified professional (e.g., prosthetist) indicates that with training, use of a myoelectric prosthesis and associated components is necessary to meet the functional needs of the individual (e.g., automatic grasp features; microprocessor control features; or other components to aid gripping, releasing, holding, and coordinating movement of the prosthesis) when performing activities of daily living. This evaluation should consider the patient's needs for control, durability (maintenance), function (speed, work capability), and usability. Both of the following criteria must be met:
  - The device is necessary for the patient to perform instrumental activities of daily living, including job functioning.
  - The device is *not* primarily for the purpose of allowing the patient to perform leisure or recreational activities. (Regence, 2016, pp. 3-4)

Similar policies have been established by other Medicare Advantage plans and other insurers (see Aetna, 2016b; BlueCross BlueShield of Tennessee, 2016). Although original Medicare has not developed detailed guidance for these devices, the guidance used by Medicare Advantage plans provides a good model. This is particularly important given that Medicare covers these devices when medically necessary, including when necessary for "job functioning."

Hearing aids Unlike Medicaid, original Medicare has express coverage exclusions, with the noncoverage of hearing aids being incorporated in the Medicare Act.[87] Although Medicare Part B covers diagnostic hearing and balance exams if ordered by a physician or other medical provider, it does not cover "hearing exams, hearing aids, or exams for fitting hearing aids" (CMS, n.d.-d). In addition, aside from hearing exams ordered by a physician

[87] 42 USC § 1395y(a)(7).

or nonphysician medical practitioner, Medicare does not cover services provided by audiologists (CMS, 2016a), "such as counseling about hearing test results, conducting a functional communication assessment, management planning, or auditory rehabilitation, even though these services are within the scope of practice for audiologists" (NASEM, 2016, p. 210). Although many have urged Congress to revisit Medicare's exclusion of hearing aids in light of the high incidence of hearing loss among older Americans, combined with their underutilization of hearing aids (NASEM, 2016; Richtman, n.d.; Whitson and Lin, 2014), original Medicare continues to deny coverage of this DME. Lack of access to hearing aids is a barrier to independent living and successful employment (Dalton et al., 2003; Kochkin, 2010). As discussed earlier, Medicare Advantage plans may cover hearing aids, depending on the plan selected.

Speech-generating devices Medicare has covered SGDs since 2001 (CMS, 2015a). NCD 50.1 describes SGDs as "speech aids that provide an individual who has a severe speech impairment with the ability to meet his functional speaking needs." As published in 2001, the policy states that an SGD can include devices with "software that allows a laptop computer, desktop computer or personal digital assistant (PDA) to function as a speech generating device," but it notes that nondedicated laptops or other devices that can be used for personal computing are not covered because they are not primarily medical in nature—a policy similar to that of some state Medicaid programs, as discussed above.

This allowance for use of a laptop or PDA, or more recently a tablet computer, combined with the policy precluding the funding of nondedicated devices, resulted in the long-standing strategy discussed above by which the supplier delivered the laptop or tablet with the personal computing functions locked. In fact, CMS confirmed that computer- and PDA-based SGDs were covered when they had been modified to run only SGD software (see Hoyer, 2001). As with some state Medicaid programs, however, nothing in the original CMS policy or its follow-up letter prohibited the Medicare beneficiary from paying to unlock or activate personal computing functions after receiving the device.

Effective July 29, 2015, CMS revised NCD 50.1 to support Medicare coverage of both purpose-built and off-the-shelf computer-based SGDs (CMS, 2014b). As a result, the personal computing functions do not have to be locked when the item is delivered. However, the revised policy makes clear that Medicare will not fund a laptop or tablet from any commercial source and separately purchased SGD software. The SGDs provided under this revised policy still must be provided for the primary purpose of speech generation, and SGD manufacturers and suppliers remain responsible for ensuring that their products meet CMS's expectations.[88] In particular, an SGD must meet Medicare's DME criteria, including the requirement that it be "suitable for use in the home." This requirement should not create a barrier to device acquisition as any individual who needed an SGD to achieve functional communication outside the home would also have a need for in-home communication. Thus, Medicare is a viable funding option for beneficiaries who require SGDs to maximize their employability.

Appealing Medicare Decisions

The appeal process for Medicare DME denials may vary depending on whether an individual receives original Medicare or is enrolled in a Medicare Advantage plan. The time periods for requesting an appeal also vary depending on the level at which the most recent decision was made. Notably, there are potentially five levels of appeal available to Medicare beneficiaries: redetermination by the DME-MAC, reconsideration by a qualified independent contractor, hearing before an administrative law judge, review by the Medicare Appeals Council, and judicial review in a United States District Court (CMS, 2016e). As with other benefit programs, a beneficiary's best chance of prevailing is if he or she is represented by an attorney or advocate who is experienced in health law (Tergesen, 2012).

Veterans Health Administration

The VHA is a comprehensive, integrated health care system that serves more than 8.9 million veterans each year (VA, n.d.-d). Its mission is to "honor America's Veterans by providing exceptional health care that improves their health and well-being" (VA, n.d.-d).

Eligibility for VHA Benefits

Any active duty service member who is "separated under any condition other than dishonorable" potentially qualifies for U.S. Department of Veterans Affairs (VA) health care benefits (VA, n.d.-a).[89] A minimum duty requirement applies to "most Veterans who enlisted after September 7, 1980, or entered active duty after October 16, 1981" (VA, n.d.-a). These veterans "must have served 24 continuous months or the full period for which they were called to active duty in order to be eligible"; however,

---

[88]For a more detailed discussion of the implications of the revised NCD 50.1, see Golinker (2015).

[89]Active duty service members typically receive health benefits from the U.S. Department of Defense through TRICARE.

there are a number of exceptions to this requirement, leading the VA to encourage "all Veterans to apply so that [it] may determine their enrollment eligibility" (VA, n.d.-a). For example, combat veterans from Operation Enduring Freedom, Operation Iraqi Freedom, and Operation New Dawn "can receive cost free medical care for any condition related to their service in the Iraq/Afghanistan theater for five years after the date of their discharge or release" (VA, n.d.-b).

Rehabilitation and Prosthetic Services

The VA's Rehabilitation and Prosthetic Services "is responsible for the national policies and programs for medical rehabilitation, prosthetic and sensory aids services that promote the health, independence and quality of life for Veterans with disabilities" (VA, 2016a). Rehabilitation and Prosthetic Services encompasses a number of national programs relevant to the categories of assistive products and technologies discussed in this report, including physical medicine and rehabilitation, prosthetics and sensory aids service, and audiology and speech pathology. "Rehabilitation and Prosthetic Services is committed to providing the highest quality, comprehensive, interdisciplinary care; the most advanced medical devices and products that are commercially available; and, promoting advancements in rehabilitative care and evidence-based treatment" (VA, 2016a).

Coverage of Selected AT Devices

Wheeled and seated mobility devices Wheelchairs and accessories represented the fifth-largest category of prosthetics and sensory aids provided to veterans in FY 2015. In that year, wheelchair accessories (e.g., custom seats, cushions, back rests, batteries) accounted for the largest set of expenditures within the wheeled mobility category. Lifts that include the wheelchair and scooter lifts represent the next-largest category of expenditure. The VA provides motorized wheelchairs when indicated, as well as manual and customized manual chairs. The VA system can provide wheelchair or scooter lifts to help ensure that veterans can get to their medical appointments and participate in their own health care (Nechanicky, 2016).

The VHA Handbook provides updates on VHA procedures for providing wheelchairs and special mobility devices to veteran beneficiaries. A basic or stock wheelchair is provided to VA beneficiaries who need a wheelchair but have the ability to stand and transfer, or have a disability that is temporary (VA, 2008). Lightweight or ultra-light wheelchairs may be considered for beneficiaries who meet the criteria for normal wheelchairs. However, modifications in the height of the seat and back; in the angle of the seat, back, and footrests; and in the wheel chamber must be considered for ultralight wheelchair users (VA, 2008). Sport model wheelchairs are considered for beneficiaries who have disabilities "resulting in anatomical loss, or loss of use, of at least one lower extremity which prohibits their participation in normal sports activities" (VA, 2008, p. 3).

Wheelchair replacements may be authorized for a variety of reasons, although not solely because a new model has been manufactured. Replacement wheelchairs may be authorized if loss or destruction occurs that is beyond the control of the veteran, when a wheelchair no longer meets the patient's needs because of change in his or her medical condition, or when the wheelchair prescription has changed (VA, 2008).

If a wheelchair requires repair, a prosthetic representative or designee will determine whether it is more cost-effective to repair or replace the wheelchair. Repair rather than replacement is required if the cost of repair is less than half that of replacement (VA, 2008, p. 5). Various sources may be used to obtain wheelchair repairs, such as VA Form 10-2501, a Prosthetic Service Card, a Purchase Card, or local VA repair facilities. The Prosthetic Service Card lists preauthorized repairs, and if repairs exceed this limitation, they must be approved by the VA beneficiary's prosthetic representative (VA, 2008). The cost of wheelchair repair without prior authorization for a veteran will be paid if "obtaining the repairs locally was necessary, expedient, and not a matter of preference over using authorized sources" and if "it is determined that the costs were not excessive or unreasonable" (VA, 2008, p. 5). If damage to the wheelchair was intentional or caused by negligence, the beneficiary will be responsible for the cost of repair.

Upper-extremity prostheses More than 50,000 individuals with major limb loss receive care through the VA (Office of Rehabilitation Services, 2016). The Amputation System of Care (ASoC) is a special program that provides comprehensive, lifelong care and care coordination to eligible veterans and, in partnership with the U.S. Department of Defense, service members with limb loss due to injury or disease. The program is designed to provide specialized expertise and the most up-to-date clinical care, prosthetic technology, and rehabilitation. The Commission on Accreditation of Rehabilitation Facilities (CARF) offers specialty accreditations to programs providing distinguished amputation care and expertise; approximately 38 percent of programs recognized by CARF (24 programs) are VA Medical Centers.

Access to care is based on such factors as level of services required to maximize function, health of the residual and contralateral limb, geographic proximity to the patient's home, and the patient's personal preference (Office of Rehabilitation Services, 2016). Telehealth amputation clinics and other measures are aimed at ensuring access to appropriate clinical care and prosthetic devices regardless of the patient's geographic location (Office of Rehabilitation Services, 2016).

Hearing aids Hearing loss, most commonly high-frequency sensorineural, is among the top three service-connected disabilities (Office of Rehabilitation Services, 2015a). All veterans with VHA benefits are eligible to receive comprehensive audiology services, including hearing screenings, diagnostic hearing evaluations, hearing aid fittings (where applicable), and aural rehabilitation, along with other services (Office of Rehabilitation Services, 2015a). The VA employs more than 1,100 audiologists and is the largest employer of audiologists in the United States. Veterans who are eligible for VA health care are eligible for a hearing aid(s) if it "assists them in their ability to participate in their own health care," regardless of whether their hearing loss is service-connected (Nechanicky, 2016). In particular, the VA will provide hearing aids to veterans "with a hearing impairment resulting from diseases or the existence of another medical condition; those with significant functional or cognitive impairment evidenced by deficiencies in the ability to perform activities of daily living; those who have hearing impairment or combined visual and hearing impairments severe enough that it interferes with their ability to participate actively in their own medical treatment; and veterans who have a service-connected hearing disability that contributes to loss of communication ability" (VA, n.d.-e).

Augmentative and alternative communication devices The VA provides comprehensive speech and language pathology services, including "the screening, evaluation, and treatment of a broad range of communication and swallowing disorders" (Office of Rehabilitation Services, 2015b). Examples of available assistive technologies include picture boards coupled with a pointer, applications for tablets or smartphones, and SGDs that can be accessed by an eye gaze switch (Office of Rehabilitation Services, 2015b).

VA speech-language pathologists provide services to veterans and service members of all ages who have speech, language, and swallowing disorders resulting from numerous medical conditions, including brain injury, progressive neurological disorders, oral and laryngeal cancer, and spinal cord injury and dysfunction. The VA employs more than 400 speech-language pathologists (Office of Rehabilitation Services, 2015b). Nearly 356,000 patient encounters involving VA speech-language pathologists were reported in FY 2014 (Office of Rehabilitation Services, 2015b). These pathologists provide services in outpatient and inpatient settings as well as in patients' homes. Telehealth services are also provided to patients.

Geographic Barriers to Care

The VA recognizes geographically based disparities in access to health care services that affect veterans living in rural communities in particular, such as lack of providers and longer travel distances. In an effort to improve access to care, it has implemented Veterans Transportation Services in more than 80 rural communities nationwide (VA, n.d.-c). The program provides free transportation to and from VA-authorized medical care facilities. As noted above, the VA also provides telehealth options, for example, within its ASoC, audiology, and speech-language pathology programs (Office of Rehabilitation Services, 2015a,b, 2016).

Generally, VA health care is delivered within VA facilities. However, exceptions are made to allow veterans to receive care in non-VA facilities, "such as when VA facilities/services are not feasibly available or cannot be economically provided to the Veteran" (VA, 2016b). In these circumstances, the VA may purchase non-VA care provided that "eligibility and other program criteria are met" (VA, 2016b).

Additionally, the Veteran's Choice program is a new temporary benefits program that allows eligible veterans to receive care outside of the VA if they live more than 40 miles from the closest VA medical facility; if they need to travel to that facility by plane or boat; if travel is excessively burdensome for other reasons; or, for veterans from states without full-service VA medical centers, if they live more than 20 miles from a full-service VA medical facility in another state (VA, 2015). Eligible veterans may also utilize the Veteran's Choice program if they are told that they must wait more than 30 days for a needed appointment.

Special Education Programs as an AT Funding Source for Transition-Aged Youth

The Individuals with Disabilities Education Act (IDEA) guarantees, in every state, that all eligible children receive a free appropriate public education—at no cost to the child or the child's parents—designed to meet their unique needs.[90] IDEA applies to eligible children aged 3 to 21, or until the child receives a regular high school diploma.[91] Since the focus of this report is on the use of AT to achieve employment outcomes, the discussion in this section addresses the AT available to "transition-aged students"—in particular, AT that will support education, training, and/or the ultimate employment goal. IDEA requires that transition services begin no later than age 16.[92]

[90] 20 USC § 1400(d)(1)(A).
[91] 34 CFR §§ 300.101, 300.102.
[92] 20 USC § 1414(d)(1)(A)(viii).

Eligibility for Special Education Services and AT

To qualify for special education services, a child must have a disability, such as a speech, mobility, orthopedic, health, hearing or visual, intellectual, learning, or emotional disability, that requires the child to receive special education and related services.[93] Prior to the start-up of a child's special education program, an individualized education plan (IEP) must be developed for that student, with the input of the student and parent(s). Any item or service the student will receive, including any AT device or service, must be included in the IEP.[94]

Special education is defined as instruction specially designed to meet the unique needs of the child. Related services are defined as developmental, corrective, and other support services required to assist a student with a disability in benefiting from an education; they include occupational therapy, physical therapy, speech pathology, counseling, health services, and parent training.[95]

IDEA[96] fully adopts the definitions of AT devices and services that first appeared in the Technology Related Assistance for Individuals with Disabilities Act in 1988,[97] known by many as the Tech Act and more recently as the AT Act[98]:

> The term "assistive technology device" means any item, piece of equipment, or product system, whether acquired commercially off the shelf, modified, or customized, that is used to increase, maintain, or improve functional capabilities of individuals with disabilities.
>
> The term "assistive technology service" means any service that directly assists an individual with a disability in the selection, acquisition, or use of an assistive technology device.[99]

The IDEA legislation and regulations require that the need for AT be considered for all students in developing their IEP.[100] All of the selected equipment referenced above and discussed below should meet the definition of an AT device as each is a piece of equipment, in some cases modified or customized, used to increase or maintain the functional capabilities of

[93] 34 CFR § 300.8.

[94] 20 USC § 1414(d).

[95] 34 CFR § 300.34 & 39.

[96] 34 CFR §§ 300.5, 300.6.

[97] Public Law 100-407, former 29 USC §§ 2201 *et seq.*

[98] Congress reauthorized this legislation as the Assistive Technology Act of 1998 and later as the Assistive Technology Act of 2004, both codified at 29 U.S.C. §§ 3001 *et seq.*

[99] 29 USC §§ 3002(4) & (5).

[100] 20 USC § 1414(d)(3)(B)(v); 34 CFR § 300.324(a)(2)(v).

an individual with a disability. Importantly, even if the special education system does not purchase the AT in question, the availability of AT services will be important while the student remains in the public school program, particularly for training of the student and school staff, as noted below.

The AT used in schools ranges from low- to high-tech. Examples of the former include simple communication boards, highlighters, modified eating utensils, splints, and graphic organizers (Cook and Polgar, 2008). Examples of the latter include wheelchairs, electronic communication devices, and computers. Applying the principles of universal design for learning, secondary students with disabilities can benefit from various forms of educational technology to improve their academic outcomes. Universal design for learning is a framework used to remove barriers in teaching methods and curriculum materials (Rose and Meyer, 2002). Its central premise is that "curriculum should include alternatives to make it accessible and appropriate for individuals with different backgrounds, learning styles, abilities, and disabilities in widely varied learning contexts" (Rose and Meyer, 2002).

Izzo and colleagues (2009), for example, designed a study to examine the effects of using a text-to-speech support program on the achievement of seven high school students with a variety of disabilities (high-functioning autism, cognitive disability, emotional disability, learning disabilities) within an online transition curriculum in their resource room. All students in the study were reading below grade level according to the AIMSweb Maze reading assessment. A reversal design was used to measure the effects of the text-to-speech program in a 10-unit transition curriculum. Study results indicate that most students improved their reading comprehension and all improved their mean unit quiz scores on the transition curriculum with the use of the text-to-speech program. Importantly, the definition of AT services is very broad and encompasses an AT evaluation, "including a functional evaluation in the individual's customary environment"; "selecting, designing, fitting, customizing, adapting, applying, maintaining, repairing, or replacing of assistive technology devices"; "training or technical assistance for an individual with disabilities, or, where appropriate, the family members, guardians, advocates, or authorized representatives of such an individual"; and "training or technical assistance for professionals (including individuals providing education and rehabilitation services), employers, or other individuals who provide services to, employ, or are otherwise substantially involved in the major life functions of individuals with disabilities."[101]

IDEA also requires that students receive their special education assistance in the least restrictive environment appropriate to their needs.[102]

[101] 29 USC § 3002(5).
[102] 20 USC § 1412(a)(5).

This means that removal from regular education classes occurs only when a student cannot receive a free appropriate public education in regular classes even with "supplemental aids and services,"[103] which could include AT devices or services. When a student is removed from the regular educational environment for part of the day, he or she must still be educated with nondisabled peers to the extent possible.

Transition Services Requirement

No later than age 16, a child's IEP must include a transition services plan.[104] Transition planning requires that schools develop long-range plans for students to prepare them for postschool life; begin to make connections with adult service providers while students are still in school; and look to others, such as the state VR agency, to provide services.

When a Special Education Program Is Required to Provide AT Devices and Services

In determining whether a special education program is likely to pay for an AT device or service, the key question is whether the AT is needed to ensure that the student receives a free appropriate public education. The decision must always be based on the individual needs of the student as determined by the participants in the IEP team meeting. AT can be approved if it is needed to assist the child in achieving meaningful educational progress, remaining in the least restrictive setting, or being prepared for the transition to adult life. AT should always be considered before a decision is made to place a student in a more restrictive setting.

Which of the Selected AT Devices Can Be Funded by the Special Education System

The U.S. Department of Education has made clear that there is no "approved list" of AT devices and services covered by IDEA.[105] Historically, the department had ruled that school districts were not required to provide a personal device that a student would require regardless of whether he or she were in school.[106] Because the definition of an AT device does not include this limitation, however, the department changed its position. It has

[103]20 USC § 1412(a)(5)(A).

[104]20 USC § 1414(d)(1)(A)(viii).

[105]Office for Special Education Programs (OSEP) Policy Letter to D. Naon, 22 Individuals with Disabilities Education Law Report (IDELR) 888 (January 26, 1995).

[106]Policy Letter to Minsky, Education for the Handicapped Law Report (EHLR) 211:19 (April 7, 1978).

stated, for example, that a hearing aid is covered under the definition of an AT device. Therefore, if the child requires a hearing aid to receive a free appropriate public education, the district must provide it at no cost to the child or the child's parents.[107]

A number of practical matters need to be considered for each of the selected AT devices in the four categories discussed here. For example, the special education system need only fund AT required to achieve a free appropriate public education. This means it must fund not necessarily the most expensive AT, just that which works for the intended purpose. Should the school system deny a more expensive item, the student/family can appeal; however, time becomes a major factor for a transition-aged youth who may be graduating or otherwise leaving the public school system in the near future. Finally, the issue of school ownership can become the ultimate barrier to use of an AT device after the student leaves the public school system, since the school owns the device (see the section on ownership below).

A powered wheelchair with seat elevator, tilt-in-space, and integrated standing system meets the definition of an AT device. The use of a wheelchair could also meet the definition of related services, which encompasses transportation in and around school buildings and can involve specialized equipment.[108] Based on this definition, the U.S. Department of Education issued an opinion that if a wheelchair is required, the school district must provide the service at public expense and without charge, regardless of whether the parents possess a wheelchair or can obtain one through private insurance. However, the district is not required to provide the wheelchair for personal use while the student is not in school.[109] The reality, however, is that a school district would likely fund only the most basic manual wheelchair that would allow someone to push the child around the school. While a strong case could be made for a wheelchair the student could operate independently, thus enabling the child to acquire independent living skills as part of a transition services plan,[110] at best a school might provide a very basic powered wheelchair. A special education program is unlikely to fund a powered wheelchair with expensive custom items such as those noted above.

A myoelectric prosthesis would meet the definition of an AT device. Since the prosthesis is attached to the limb through a prosthetic socket and is not a surgically implanted device (which is an exclusion), it would not

[107]OSEP Policy Letter to P. Seiler, 20 IDELR 1216 (November 19, 1993); OSEP Policy Letter to J. Galloway, 22 IDELR 373 (December 22, 1994).

[108]34 CFR § 300.34(c)(16).

[109]OSEP Policy Letter to J. Stohrer, 13 EHLR 213:211, 212 (April 20, 1989).

[110]See 34 CFR § 300.43(a)(2).

be barred based on that exclusion.[111] Without this intervention, a child would be left to participate in school activities with a missing arm or hand, arguably needing this AT to achieve a free appropriate public education. However, the U.S. Department of Education does not appear to have addressed the issue of a child's needing this kind of upper-body prosthesis.

There appears to be only one court case, a 2011 decision of the U.S District Court in Connecticut, that addresses whether a child is entitled to a myoelectric arm funded through the special education program.[112] That case involved the parents of a 3-year-old girl (at the time of the due process hearing) who sought reimbursement for a myoelectric arm they had purchased. The parents appealed an adverse hearing decision to the court, which ruled for the school district. The case involved many unrelated issues, but on the issue of the right to funding of the myoelectric arm, the court held that it was not needed to achieve a free appropriate public education: "J.C. can obtain a meaningful benefit and appropriate educational services without such technology. The video of J.C. and testimony regarding J.C.'s ability to perform tasks with or without the myoelectric arm, demonstrates that the myoelectric arm is not necessary to provide a [free appropriate public education]."

This decision reinforces an important principle of special education law. Even if an item meets the definition of an AT device, it need be funded by the school district only if necessary to achieve a free appropriate public education. With different facts, the court might have reached a different conclusion. Still, any AT device a school might provide to address the child's missing arm or hand might not be in the class of devices of an expensive myoelectric prosthesis.

Binaural hearing aids also meet the definition of an AT device. As noted above, the U.S. Department of Education has stated that a school district must provide a hearing aid, at no cost to the student or parents, if needed to receive a free appropriate public education. This policy would help a student obtain a basic hearing aid in order to benefit from his or her education. However, it is unlikely that a school would fund the more expensive binaural hearing aids to enable the student to communicate fully in a range of other environments outside of school. A case could be made for a child to receive the more expensive binaural hearing aids if this would ensure that the child could hear enough of the content from lectures and classroom discussions to benefit from his or her education.

SGDs are particularly important in the special education context. They

[111]See 34 CFR § 300.34(b), providing that related services do not include surgically implanted devices, such as cochlear implants.

[112]See *J.C. ex rel. C. v. New Fairfield Board of Education*, 2011 Westlaw 1322563 (D. Conn. 2011).

meet the definition of an AT device as a supplementary aid or a special education or related service.[113] If such a device is a student's only effective means of communicating with teachers and peers, it will ensure that he or she can participate effectively in the regular classroom.[114] If specialized software or training in how to use the SGD is necessary, it would represent an AT device or service, respectively, and could also be approved by the special education system.[115] Finally, to fully learn to use the device, benefit from its use, and develop communication abilities, the student should be allowed to take the device home, despite any increased chances of damage to this expensive item.[116] A dual-purpose laptop or tablet that is used as an SGD would become particularly important if the student were transitioning to higher education, and it could be funded by the special education system to ensure that the student would benefit from the special education program and could prepare for the transition to college.

The Right to an Administrative Hearing If an AT Device or Service Is Denied

Under IDEA, parents have the right to request an impartial hearing to appeal actions taken by a school district.[117] At the hearing, the parents have the right to be represented by an attorney or other person with specialized training to compel the attendance of witnesses, to present evidence, and to cross-examine witnesses.[118] The decision of the hearing officer is final unless there is an appeal. States have the option to create a second, state level of administrative review.[119] In that case, either the family or the school district has the right to file an appeal to the state.[120] Following the hearing decision or state-level decision, if applicable, either the family or the school district has the right to appeal to state or federal court.[121]

---

[113] 34 CFR § 300.105(a).

[114] See *School Board of Independent School District No. 11, Anoka-Hennepin v. Pachl*, 36 IDELR 263 (D. Minn. 2002) (in awarding compensatory education for delays in providing an SGD, the court noted that the student did not receive a free appropriate public education because she was "bereft of the ability to communicate").

[115] 34 CFR §§ 300.5 & 300.6.

[116] See 34 CFR § 300.105(b) (allowing special education students to take AT devices home when doing so is necessary to ensure that they benefit from their education).

[117] 20 USC § 1415(b)(6).

[118] 20 USC § 1415(f).

[119] 20 USC § 1415(i)(1)(B).

[120] 20 USC § 1415(g).

[121] 20 USC § 1415(i)(2).

The Issue of Ownership

The question of who owns an AT device is a major one for the transition-aged student. Ordinarily, when a school special education program purchases equipment, it retains ownership. This means that when a student graduates or otherwise completes his or her special education studies and leaves the public school program, an AT device provided to that student will be returned to the school. For this reason, it is important that the student and family consider one of the following strategies if the AT will be important during the transition to higher education, postschool vocational training, or employment:

- Focus on another funding source, such as Medicaid or the state VR program, for purchase of the device or any replacement device that is needed during the last few years of school.
- Determine whether the school has a policy that provides for selling the used AT device, at a discounted rate, either to the student or to the state VR agency to support the student.

Neither IDEA nor the federal VR laws prohibit a VR agency from purchasing an AT device outright for a student who is still enrolled in high school or from purchasing it from the school at graduation. In fact, the U.S. Department of Education has indicated that it is permissible for a school district to transfer an AT device costing more than $5,000 to a state VR agency if the school district will no longer need the device for other students. The department envisions that most such devices will have been modified for the individual student and therefore will no longer be needed by the district when that student graduates. For devices costing less than $5,000, this limitation does not apply, meaning a district could transfer such a device to a VR agency regardless of whether it was needed for other students. The department agrees that coordination between school districts and state VR agencies to enable students with disabilities to continue using AT devices as they move from one program to another is an efficient, cost-effective means of facilitating the transition from school- to work-related services and fully supports this type of cooperation.[122]

The Importance of AT Services for Evaluation, Education, and Training

As a practical matter, it is unlikely that transitioning students can rely on a special education program to fund AT devices they can retain after leaving school. This is particularly true for the very expensive custom

[122]OSEP Policy Letter to S. Goodman, 30 IDELR 611 (June 21, 1998).

powered wheelchairs, binaural hearing aids, and myoelectric prostheses discussed above. However, a special education program could still fund a comprehensive AT evaluation, for example, to determine which SGD system would work best for a student as he or she transitioned to college. If that system could be purchased, such as through Medicaid or a VR agency, training could be implemented through the student's IEP to ensure that he or she would learn to use the device before going on to college. In fact, it is critical that any AT services be spelled out in the student's IEP. The special education system also could be required to provide training, as an AT service, to the student and in some cases to school staff to allow the student to adapt to using an item such as a powered wheelchair with specialty features or a myoelectric prosthesis. To the extent that this AT service allowed the transitioning student to benefit fully from a recent AT acquisition, it would increase the likelihood of success in postschool training, higher education, and ultimately employment.

Transition from High School to the Workplace

According to a recent national survey of service providers conducted by researchers from the Aspen Institute Workforce Strategies Initiative (Jain et al., 2015), nearly 6.7 million young adults aged 16 to 24 are out of school and out of work. The July 2015 unemployment rate among young adults was 12.2 percent, more than double the national average of 5.3 percent (DOL and BLS, 2015). Unemployment is even more severe for young adults of minority groups, particularly African Americans, who have an unemployment rate of 20.7 percent. Moreover, the likelihood of poor employment outcomes tends to increase with severity of disability (Crisp, 2005; Meade et al., 2004; Ozawa and Yeo, 2006; Wagner et al., 2005), with being less well educated (Krause and Terza, 2006; Randolph and Andresen, 2004), and with living in a rural area (Kusmin, 2006). Nationally, almost half of youth who are African American, Hispanic, and Native American drop out of public schools each year (Bridgeland et al., 2006).

An additional challenge is that those who qualify often enroll in benefit programs and are more likely to become lifelong recipients of such programs. As studies of the SSA database indicate, the probability of young adults with disabilities aged 18 to 25 leaving the SSI or SSDI system to go to work is less than 0.1 percent (SSA, 2001). Given the challenges faced by youth with disabilities, successful transitions as well as supports for successful employment and/or vocational preparation are essential.

Overall, successful transition outcomes for ethnic minority youth with disabilities who live in poverty are very limited (Hasnain and Balcazar, 2009; Wells et al., 2003). The social needs of these youth, including limited English proficiency, high rates of mobility and dropout, and teenage parenthood, challenge educators (Taylor-Ritzler, 2007). In fact, many graduating students with disabilities who lack the appropriate training and preparation have a very low likelihood of finding a job that would offer them career advancement opportunities, which in turn translates into fewer opportunities for social mobility (Center for Mental Health in Schools at UCLA, 2008).

Evidence also suggests that environmental barriers may prevent successful transition outcomes. Among these are attitudinal barriers toward youth with disabilities, including low family expectations regarding work and independence and limited opportunities for making choices in childhood through adolescence (Stewart et al., 2010). These barriers make improving transition outcomes even more critical.

Studies of promising practices for transition-aged youth with disabilities suggest that facilitators of successful employment outcomes include, but are not limited to, increasing collaboration and coordination among providers serving these youth (Oertle and Trach, 2007), encouraging youth participation in the workforce during the high school years (Wittenburg and Maag, 2002), encouraging participation in postsecondary education (Weathers et al., 2007), providing work-specific and community participation support (Balcazar et al., 2004), and involving employers in transition programs (Fabian, 2007). Some of these practices, such as youth participation in the workplace during high school and employer participation in transition programs, have been developed primarily for particularly high-risk groups, such as minority youth from urban areas (e.g., Garcia-Iriarte et al., 2007).

Awsumb and colleagues (2016) conducted a study examining VR transition outcomes in youth with disabilities aged 14 to 22. The results showed relationships between race and the chances of being rehabilitated, with white participants being more likely than their African American counterparts to be rehabilitated [χ^2 [1, n = 5,492] = 15.52, $p < 0.001$) and experience successful closure (Awsumb et al., 2016). Overall, African American participants had a higher chance of being nonrehabilitated, while Hispanic participants had the highest percentage of rehabilitation closure and were significantly more likely to be rehabilitated (χ^2 [3, n = 6,252] = 18.17, $p < 0.001$) (Awsumb et al., 2016). Although the number of Hispanics in the sample was relatively small, this finding is important, as it indicates that certain minority groups may have better chances of being rehabilitated than others in the VR system. In addition, participants living in small towns were more likely than those living in large urban areas to have successful outcomes. One possible explanation for this finding is that students living in small towns are likely to find farm jobs, especially during the summer when there is greater demand for labor, and to face less competition for employment compared with students in urban areas, who are competing with many other potential workers.

Summary

In summary, transition-aged youth with disabilities experience many disparities compared with their peers without disabilities in terms of education, employment, and independent living outcomes (Employment and Disability Institute, 2013; Stewart et al., 2010). These disparities may include early dropout, low educational attainment, welfare dependency, and youth unemployment (Ayres, 2013). Ensuring services for successful employment and/or vocational preparation and continued access to appropriate assistive products and technologies is vital to promoting a successful transition from high school to pathways to employment.

State Vocational Rehabilitation Agencies

States are given money to provide VR services to persons with disabilities under Title I of the Rehabilitation Act.[123] Each state must designate a single state agency to administer the VR program unless it designates a second agency to serve individuals who are legally blind.[124]

VR agencies can fund a wide range of goods and services that are connected to a person's vocational goal. Congress has stated that VR services are intended to empower individuals to maximize employability, economic self-sufficiency, independence, and integration into the workplace and the community through "comprehensive and coordinated state-of-the-art programs."[125]

Eligibility for VR Services and the Individualized Plan of Employment

To receive VR services, an individual must be disabled and require such services "to prepare for, secure, retain or regain employment."[126] Any approved service must be connected to the individual's employment goal. Employment goals include full- or part-time competitive employment in an integrated setting; supported employment; or other employment, such as self-employment, telecommuting, and business ownership.[127]

To be eligible for VR services, an individual also must have a mental, physical, or learning disability that interferes with the ability to work. The disability need only be a substantial impediment to employment; it need not be so severe as to qualify the individual for SSDI or SSI benefits.[128] An SSDI

[123] 29 USC § 701 *et seq.*; 34 CFR Part 361.
[124] 29 USC § 722(a)(2).
[125] 29 USC § 701(b)(1).
[126] 29 USC § 722(a)(1).
[127] 34 CFR § 361.5(b)(16).
[128] 29 USC § 705(20)(A).

or SSI beneficiary is presumed eligible for VR services as an individual with a significant disability provided he or she intends to achieve an employment outcome.[129] VR services may be denied to those who cannot benefit from them. However, applicants are presumed capable of employment, despite the severity of a disability, unless the VR agency shows by "clear and convincing" evidence that they cannot benefit.[130]

Many may think of the state VR agency as an adult services program, a concept that is changing as new mandates of the Workforce Innovation and Opportunity Act (WIOA) of 2014 are implemented. WIOA and the federal regulations of 2016 that implement it now require a state VR agency to provide "pre-employment transition services,"[131] serving students with disabilities aged 16 to 21 unless the state decides to provide such services to a different age range under IDEA.[132] Coupled with the new WIOA mandate to serve "youth with disabilities" up to age 24[133] and the continuing mandate for special education programs to serve this population through age 21 or when they exit the public school program (as previously discussed), this requirement theoretically should enhance the ability of youth and young adults with disabilities to acquire AT that will enable them to benefit fully from employment opportunities as well as adult training and education programs, including higher education that will lead to employment.

The state VR agency delivers services pursuant to a written Individualized Plan for Employment.[134] The Individualized Plan for Employment is developed following a required comprehensive assessment that is performed as necessary to determine the employment goal and objectives and the necessary nature and scope of VR services. The assessment entails evaluating the unique strengths, resources, priorities, abilities, and interests of the individual.[135] It may also include a referral for the provision of rehabilitation technology (i.e., AT) services "to assess and develop the capacities of the individual to perform in a work environment."[136]

If a state lacks the resources to provide VR services to all eligible individuals who seek them, it must establish an "order of selection" to be followed in determining which individuals will receive services. The order of selection must ensure that individuals with the most significant disabilities are selected first to receive VR services.[137] The VR agency may not use

[129] 29 USC § 722(a)(3).
[130] 29 USC § 722(a)(2); 34 CFR § 361.42(a)(2).
[131] 34 CFR § 361.65(a)(3).
[132] 34 CFR § 361.5(c)(51).
[133] 34 CFR § 361.5(c)(59).
[134] 29 USC § 722(b)(2)(A).
[135] 29 USC § 705(2)(B).
[136] 29 USC § 705(2)(c).
[137] 36 CFR § 361.43.

any of the following factors in establishing an order of selection: duration of residency; type of disability; age, gender, race, color, or national origin; source of referral; type of expected employment outcome; need for specific services or anticipated cost of services; or individual or family income.[138]

Funding for a Range of AT Devices and Services to Support an Employment Goal

Available VR services include any that are necessary to assist an individual with a disability in "preparing for, securing, retaining, or regaining an employment outcome."[139] The VR agency must ensure that all necessary services are provided and cannot choose to provide only some services to save costs. In fact, the "severity of an individual's disability or the cost of services [including expensive AT] can have no bearing on the scope of services the individual receives."[140] Once an individual has been determined eligible for services, the VR agency must provide funding for all services reasonably necessary to meet the person's approved employment goal subject to his or her obligation to first seek any "similar benefits" that may be available, as discussed below. The VR agency may not place "any arbitrary limits on the nature and scope of VR services to be provided to achieve an employment outcome."[141]

The VR regulations, published by the federal Rehabilitation Services Administration (RSA), provide an extensive list of categories within which services can be provided to support an employment goal.[142] This list includes counseling, guidance, and job placement services provided by the VR agency's staff or through an outside entity. It encompasses, for example, funding for vocational and other training, including higher education; personal assistance while receiving VR services; interpreter services for individuals who are deaf; readers and orientation/mobility services for individuals who are blind; tools, equipment, initial stock, and supplies to support a self-employment goal; other goods and services determined necessary to achieve an employment goal; and postemployment services necessary to retain, regain, or advance in employment.

AT devices and services are clearly available through state VR agencies to support an employment goal. Title I of the Rehabilitation Act and RSA's VR regulations use the definitions of AT devices and services contained in the AT Act[143] and in IDEA. Importantly, the definition of AT services is very

[138] 34 CFR § 361.36(d)(2).
[139] 29 USC § 723(a).
[140] Comments to 2001 regulations, 66 Fed. Reg. 4426.
[141] 34 CFR § 361.50(a).
[142] 34 CFR § 361.48.
[143] See 29 USC § 3001 *et seq.* (AT Act).

broad and includes evaluation to determine the need for a device, customizing or adapting the device for the user, repairs, maintenance, and training in use of the device. Available VR devices and services that may meet these definitions include prosthetic and orthotic devices; eyeglasses; orientation and mobility services, which can include AT; rehabilitation technology services; telecommunications; sensory devices; and other technological aids and devices.[144]

Requirement to Seek "Similar Benefits" Through Other Funding Sources

VR agencies will not pay for a service if a similar or comparable benefit is available through another provider.[145] For example, if an applicant qualifies for personal assistance services through Medicaid, the VR agency will not fund that service. However, the agency cannot deny payment for college tuition because a student loan is available, as loans, which must be repaid, are not similar benefits (U.S. Department of Education, 1991). Comments to the 2001 VR regulations also make it clear that SSI's PASS, discussed below, is not a similar benefit.[146] Additionally, diagnostic services, counseling, referral services, job placement, and rehabilitation technology (i.e., AT) are exempt from the similar benefit requirement.[147]

The VR agency may ask an individual to apply to either Medicaid or Medicare (if eligible for one of those programs) to fund, for example, a powered wheelchair or an SGD, even though those items are exempt from the similar benefit requirement if classified as rehabilitation technology. Both Medicaid and Medicare may be expected to fund such items when they are medically necessary. Advocates often encourage individuals to foster good will with the VR agency by first seeking Medicaid or Medicare funding for these items (Sheldon and Hager, 2011).

Financial Need Criteria for VR Agency Services

A state is not required to consider financial need when providing VR services. However, if a state VR agency chooses to use a financial needs test, it must establish written policies that govern the determination of financial need and that identify the specific VR services that are subject to the test.[148]

The VR agency's financial needs test must consider the individual's

---

[144] 29 USC § 723(a).
[145] 29 USC § 721(a)(8).
[146] 66 Fed. Reg. 4419.
[147] 34 CFR § 361.53(b).
[148] 34 CFR § 361.54(a) and (b)(2)(i).

disability-related expenses. Although the individual may be required to contribute to the cost of a service, the level of that contribution must not be so high as to "effectively deny the individual a necessary service."[149] The following services must be provided without regard to financial need: diagnostic services; counseling, guidance, and referral services; job placement; and personal assistance services. The regulations also exempt from a financial needs test "any auxiliary aid or service," such as interpreter or reader services, that the individual needs to participate in the VR program and that are mandated under Section 504 of the Rehabilitation Act or the ADA.[150]

Additionally, individuals "determined eligible for Social Security benefits under Titles II [SSDI] and XVI [SSI] of the Social Security Act" must be exempt from the financial needs test.[151] This definition applies not only to cash beneficiaries of SSDI and SSI but also to former SSI cash beneficiaries who lost SSI benefits because of work and wages and who continue to receive Medicaid under section 1619(b). Section 1619(b), contained in Title XVI of the Social Security Act, states that for purposes of Medicaid eligibility, a 1619(b) recipient "shall be considered to be receiving [SSI] benefits under" Title XVI.[152]

AT Devices and Services a VR Agency Can Fund

All the items discussed above should meet a VR agency's definition of an AT device as they are all designed to allow an individual to overcome the effects of a disability, provided that a device will allow an individual to benefit from another VR service (such as education or training) and/or achieve a vocational goal. As noted above, many individuals may seek Medicaid or Medicare payment for items under the four device categories discussed herein as an act of goodwill, allowing the VR agency to pay for items and services only it can fund.

A separate challenge is the need to establish that an individual is seeking the least costly device within a category that will meet his or her need to benefit from education or training and/or to succeed in a job. In some cases, the device sought may serve both a medical and a vocational purpose. The result may be the possibility of different funding sources each suggesting it is the other funder's obligation to pay for the device. In such cases, an advocate may seek to negotiate a resolution in which two

---

[149]34 CFR § 361.52(b)(2)(iv).
[150]34 CFR § 361.54(b)(3)(i).
[151]34 CFR 361.54(b)(3)(ii).
[152]42 USC § 1382h.

funding sources, such as Medicaid and the VR agency, each agree to pay a portion of the cost.

Listed below is a sample of devices that could support individuals as they receive VR services or allow them to work after receiving those services. For each, the theory that might support funding the item is described:

- *Powered wheelchair with tilt-in-space, seat elevator, and integrated standing feature*—As discussed earlier, although the power function and other features can all be medically justified in many cases, Medicaid agencies have been known to deny funding for the standing feature, often claiming both that the medical benefit of "passive standing" is not proven through medical research and that the standing feature serves primarily a vocational function. Similarly, VR agencies, which can fund a wheelchair as rehabilitation technology, may claim that one or more of the special features is medical in nature and does not contribute to the person's vocational goal. As noted above, in this situation, an advocate may be able to negotiate a resolution in which Medicaid and the VR agency agree to share the funding to allow the individual to receive the needed wheelchair.
- *Myoelectric upper-extremity prostheses*—Medicaid may agree that a prosthetic device is needed but claim that a less costly prosthesis will be adequate to allow the individual to function in most environments. While Medicaid's decision might be challenged through an appeal, a good case can be made that this cutting-edge prosthesis should be funded by the VR agency to allow the individual to benefit fully from education or training and/or to function fully in the expected work environment.
- *Hearing aids*—As noted above, original Medicare does not cover hearing aids. If the individual has original Medicare coverage only, with neither Medicaid nor a private insurance plan that would cover hearing aids, the VR agency will likely be the only possible payer.
- *Dual-purpose tablet or laptop serving as an SGD and personal computing device*—In the case of individuals who are supported by the VR agency in a college or community college program as a step toward their vocational goals, funding for a personal computing device (laptop or tablet) can be justified to allow them to complete assignments. If the SGD is needed to communicate with teachers and peers, it, too, could be funded by the VR agency to allow the student to benefit from the education program. If the need for the personal computing device and the SGD can be justified, payment for a dual-purpose device should also be justifiable. Such a device

will allow the individual to accomplish both the computing and the speech functions more efficiently than would be possible with two separate devices and likely would cost a fraction of what the two items purchased separately would cost.

Social Security's VR Cost Reimbursement Program

The U.S. Social Security Administration's (SSA's) Cost Reimbursement (CR) program allows for full reimbursement of costs if an SSDI or SSI beneficiary served by a VR agency is employed successfully at the "substantial gainful activity" (SGA) level (in 2017, $1,170 per month for the nonblind and $1,950 for the "statutorily blind") for 9 consecutive months.[153] A beneficiary can meet the "9 consecutive months" criterion by working 9 of 10 consecutive months at the SGA level if "statutorily blind," or by working any 9 of 12 consecutive months at the SGA level if the non-SGA months are for reasons beyond the individual's control and unrelated to his or her disability.[154] The CR provisions allow a VR agency to fully recoup the cost of very expensive AT, such as a powered wheelchair with an integrated standing feature or a myoelectric arm or hand, as long as these earnings requirements are met. The CR program allows for payment to the VR agency with no need to show that the SGA-level work resulted in a termination of benefits.

The state VR agency may also elect to serve an individual under SSA's Ticket to Work program as an "employment network" (EN). The Ticket to Work program's two alternative payment systems each pay the EN flat dollar amounts as the beneficiary progresses toward self-supporting employment and elimination of dependence on benefits.[155] Since these are flat-rate payment systems, the EN, or the VR agency acting as an EN, has no extra incentive to pay for expensive AT to enable the beneficiary to succeed in employment at the highest earnings levels.

When an SSDI or SSI beneficiary has expensive AT needs, it makes the most sense for the VR agency to opt for the CR payment system. The CR system guarantees full reimbursement for AT purchases as long as the beneficiary achieves the more modest earnings outcome, i.e., 9 months of SGA-level work.

---

[153] 20 CFR Part 404, Subpart V; 20 CFR Part 416, Subpart V.

[154] 20 CFR § 404.2110; 20 CFR § 416.2110.

[155] 20 CFR § 411.350; see Ticket to Work (2017) and links to payment charts for both the Outcome Payment System and the Milestone/Outcome Payment System.

Appeal Rights and the Client Assistance Program

If an individual is dissatisfied with a decision by the VR agency, he or she has the right to appeal. Appeals can be pursued through mediation or an administrative hearing before an impartial hearing officer.[156] The Client Assistance Program is available in every state to assist individuals who have questions or who are appealing a VR decision.[157] The individual may also seek assistance from a protection and advocacy (P&A) agency. A P&A agency is available in every state to advocate for individuals with disabilities on a range of issues.[158] Many P&A agencies house the Client Assistance Program.

State Workers' Compensation Programs

Workers' compensation is a system of insurance designed to compensate employees injured within the normal course of their employment. Each state has its own workers' compensation law, which provides for the rules and benefits in its state, while the federal government administers workers' compensation programs for federal employees and certain other federal programs. Under workers' compensation, employees give up their right to sue their employers for negligence, and are exempt from the requirement to prove the employer was negligent, in exchange for receiving medical care and other benefits to compensate for injuries and illnesses sustained in the normal course of employment and to restore their level of functioning to their preinjury status. While the benefits vary by state, several states cover the cost of AT and the services of professionals, clinicians, and teams that can evaluate the need for appropriate assistive devices and train individuals in their use to restore their function. Depending on state law and the extent of advocacy available to the injured worker, these benefits may include the four categories of devices discussed in this report. For example, Iowa's law provides for the payment of all "reasonable and necessary medical care" and "appliances" to treat injuries that are compensable. The word "appliances" has been interpreted to "include many types of medical equipment, also called Assistive Technology" (Iowa Compass, Center for Developmental Disabilities, 2016).

Depending on state law, however, workers' compensation cases often involve a hearing process of some kind by which an injury or illness is declared covered or "compensable." Once an illness or injury has been declared compensable, the employee may have to go through additional

[156] 34 CFR § 361.57(b)(1)(i) & (ii).
[157] 34 CFR § 361.57(b)(1)(v).
[158] See National Disability Rights Network (2017) to link to state P&A agencies.

hearing processes to "convince" the employer or workers' compensation carrier to pay for expensive AT devices.

Some states allow for reimbursement for attorney's fees incurred in contesting these matters, but such reimbursement is not guaranteed. In *Zuback v. Worker's Compensation Appeals Board*, 892 A.2d 41, 48 (2006), for example, Mr. Zuback sought repair or replacement of two stair glides that allowed him to move from floor to floor in his home following a compensable work-related injury that caused him to lose his left leg, his left arm, and two toes on his right foot. A Pennsylvania court held that an employer had a reasonable basis for contesting the benefits the injured worker sought if the suit "was brought to resolve a genuinely disputed issue, not merely to harass the claimant." The court reasoned that since the stair glide issue was a case of first impression, attorney's fees for the injured employee were not required.

Since workers' compensation laws vary from state to state, it is difficult to generalize about what is covered. Yet, since most workers' compensation covers some form of wage replacement—usually a percentage of the injured worker's salary—workers' compensation carriers and employers have an incentive to pay for AT and related services that will help return injured workers to work. These decisions are made on a case-by-case basis, depending on state law and the costs involved, and not all devices will be available uniformly from vendors across the country, nor will professionals trained to evaluate injured workers to determine their need for such a device and teach them how to use it.

PRIVATE FUNDING SOURCES

Self-Pay

Purchasing AT on one's own is always an option. However, many assistive products and technologies cost thousands of dollars, eliminating self-pay as a full payment option for many individuals. Private health insurance (discussed later in the chapter), for individuals who have access to it, is one mechanism for covering at least a portion of the cost of required products and technologies. Private disability insurance also may serve as a source of funding for some work-related AT. Current beneficiaries of SSI and SSDI are generally on fixed incomes with high medical expenses, putting self-pay for expensive AT out of reach for most without assistance from Medicare, Medicaid, or a VR agency. In addition, several programs, including SSI's PASS, state financing of low-cost loans, and ABLE accounts, may assist individuals in financing the acquisition of needed AT, as described below.

Supplemental Security Income's Plan to Achieve Self-Support

SSI is a means-tested program administered by SSA. An SSI beneficiary must have limited income and resources.[159] SSI can be an individual's only source of income, or it can supplement another source of income, such as SSDI or wages.

The maximum SSI federal benefit rate (FBR) is $735 per month in 2017. States have the option of supplementing the FBR. The example below uses the FBR with no state supplement. The SSI payment is determined by subtracting countable income from the state's maximum SSI rate or base rate (i.e., the FBR plus optional state supplement).

The SSI program allows many income exclusions; for example, the first $65 plus 50 percent of any remaining earned income in a month is excluded and not part of countable income. The SSI program also allows up to $2,000 in countable resources. Many items are excluded from countable resources; for example, a vehicle used as transportation by the SSI beneficiary or another household member is excluded and not counted against the $2,000 resource limit (SSA, 2016c).

Eligibility for a PASS

SSI's PASS allows an individual with a disability to exclude income and/or resources that otherwise would be countable when they will be used to support an occupational objective.[160] By doing so, the person retains SSI, becomes eligible for more SSI, or becomes eligible for SSI as a new applicant. The PASS enables the individual to achieve an occupational objective, i.e., self-support, through use of this excluded income and resources. For example, the PASS may enable a person to pay for education or training needed to become self-supporting or for items related to setting up a business, such as an accessible food truck.

People with disabilities receiving SSI must submit their proposed PASS to SSA in writing, preferably using SSA Form 545.[161] Anyone, including the SSI applicant or beneficiary, can write a PASS. Given the detail required to complete the PASS form, however, individuals may want to seek assistance with its completion. Staff at SSA-funded Work Incentives Planning and

---

[159]See 20 CFR § 416.1100 *et seq.* (income) and § 416.1201 *et seq.* (resources).

[160]42 USC §§ 1382a(b)(4)(A)(iii) and (B)(iv), 1382b(a)(4); 20 CFR § 416.1180 *et seq.*; POMS SI 00870.001 *et seq.* For a more detailed discussion of the PASS, see Sheldon and Lopez-Soto (n.d.).

[161]SSA's Form 545, although not mandatory, should be used by individuals and their advocates to submit PASS proposals. This form is available at www.ssa.gov/online/ssa-545.pdf (accessed January 22, 2017).

Assistance projects, which are funded in every state,[162] may be able to assist with drafting a PASS proposal.

Several items must be included in the written PASS proposal, including[163]

- a specific occupational objective,
- specific savings and planned disbursement goals related to the objective,
- a list of goods and services requiring savings or payments and anticipated amounts,
- a specific time frame for achieving the objective,
- identification and segregation of any money or other resources being accumulated, and
- a detailed business plan when self-employment is a goal.

The PASS proposal can be approved for as long a period as necessary, with a beginning date and reasonable ending date as necessary to meet the occupational objective.[164] If the PASS will pay for items related to an undergraduate program, for example, a reasonable time frame might be 4 or 5 years and possibly longer if the objective requires a master's degree.

Items That Can Be Funded Through a PASS

Money set aside through a PASS can be used for anything that is related to achieving the individual's approved occupational objective. The following is a representative list of goods and services that can be purchased with the income or resources set aside in the PASS if reasonable and necessary to achieve this objective (SSA, 2012a):

- tuition, books, supplies, fees, and costs connected to education or occupational training
- costs for room and board when attending educational, training, employment, trade, or business activities
- equipment, supplies, operating capital, and inventory required to establish and carry on a trade or business
- equipment/tools either specific to the individual's condition or designed for general use
- medically related items, including specialized equipment (i.e., AT)

---

[162]See SSA (2017) and follow links to locate the Work Incentives Planning and Assistance project for a state or region of a state.

[163]20 CFR § 416.1181; POMS SI 00870.006.

[164]20 CFR § 416.1181.

- operational or access modifications to buildings, vehicles, etc., to accommodate disabilities
- transportation costs, including lease/rental or purchase of a vehicle, public transportation and common carriers, fuel costs, registration fees, and initial cost of insurance premiums
- job search or relocation services
- taxes and government-imposed user fees (e.g., permits, licenses) connected with obtaining any of the above
- finance and service charges and/or maintenance costs for any of the above

The PASS can also include any other costs that are reasonable and necessary to attain the occupational objective.

As discussed in the section on public funding above, some of the selected items in each of the four AT categories could potentially be funded through Medicaid, Medicare, a special education program, or a state VR agency. All of the AT devices selected for discussion in each of the four categories could be funded with money deposited into a PASS account as long as they had a demonstrated connection to the chosen occupational objective. Since a PASS is a short-term funding source and an individual is allowed only one PASS for the same occupational objective, a PASS should be viewed as a source of supplemental funding for an item, as the source of funding for an item that cannot be funded through other means, or as an alternative to a loan that must be repaid. For example, even though strategies are available for obtaining Medicaid or Medicare funding for a dual-purpose laptop or tablet, an individual may have a reason to obtain a specific laptop or tablet to meet school-related personal computing needs, with the purchase of SGD software to follow. This requirement could make Medicaid or Medicare funding a challenge.

Hypothetical Example: Use of a PASS to Fund an AT Device to Support an Occupational Objective

This example involves an individual who receives \$620 in SSDI and \$135 in SSI per month. The person uses a powered wheelchair and has a single hearing aid to address his severe hearing deficit. He attends college with the objective of becoming a math teacher and is completing the first year of an expected 6-year program leading to the bachelor's and master's degrees needed to achieve this objective. The state VR agency is paying for tuition, related costs to attend college, and specialized transportation to and from the campus in his powered wheelchair.

In addition, the individual seeks PASS funding for a modified van (\$29,000 for the van, \$40,000 for van modifications) that will allow him to travel to student teaching assignments, then employment as a teacher following graduation; a second, lightweight wheelchair ($2,800) that will serve as a back-up when his powered wheelchair is undergoing predictable repairs and can be used for work-related mobility in places where a powered wheelchair is not easily used; and binaural hearing aids ($4,200), which will allow him to achieve a higher degree of functional hearing in a classroom setting when he becomes a teacher. This scenario assumes that the person's state VR agency will pay for the vehicle modifications but not the vehicle itself; that neither Medicaid nor Medicare will pay for the second wheelchair, each claiming that his needs are met through the powered wheelchair; and that neither Medicaid nor Medicare will pay for the binaural hearing aids, each claiming that his needs are met by the current single hearing aid he uses.

The individual submits a PASS proposal to save for all three items at a total cost of $36,000. For purposes of this scenario, starting in July and continuing for 5 years (60 months), he will put $600 per month into a designated bank account to save for these items. His plan, as approved by SSA, provides that he will purchase the lightweight wheelchair and binaural hearing aids during his final year of undergraduate school, allowing him to begin using both items prior to his required student teaching. He will purchase the van during the same year, using savings to make a large down payment and using PASS funds to make installment payments through the end of the PASS approval period. SSA's PASS policy is flexible and will permit amendments as needed, for example, to allow the individual to pay for 1 or more years of van insurance or to purchase needed software or apps for his laptop or tablet. This is how the individual's SSI payment would be calculated:

- *Total income*—$620 unearned (SSDI), $0 unearned
- *Total expenses for PASS:* $600 per month; $0 earned
- *SSI calculation*—total countable income = $0 ($620 – $600 PASS expense = $20 – $20 unearned income exclusion = $0); new SSI payment amount = $735 ($735 SSI FBR – $0 countable income after PASS exclusions = $735)

Thus, the PASS would enable this individual to achieve

- accumulation of $36,000 toward the purchase of a vehicle, a lightweight wheelchair, and binaural hearing aids;
- the leveraging of $40,000 from his state VR agency to pay for van modifications (allowing him to travel with his wheelchair);

- maintenance of monthly income, for living expenses, at the same level; and
- retention of automatic eligibility for Medicaid in most states (ensuring a continued funding source for AT and many other items).

Appeal if a PASS Proposal Is Denied

The denial of a PASS proposal, or any part of the proposal, is considered a decision affecting the right to SSI benefits and is subject to the SSI appeals process. This process involves three potential appeals before SSA (reconsideration, administrative law judge hearing, and Appeals Council) and a potential appeal to the federal district court.[165] Following any adverse decision (i.e., denial of the proposal or denial following a reconsideration or hearing), the PASS applicant is allowed 60 days from receipt of that decision to request an appeal or review of the most recent decision. Similarly, if the SSI beneficiary loses an appeal at the reconsideration, administrative law judge hearing, or Appeals Council stage, he or she has 60 days to appeal to the next level.

State Alternative Financing Programs: A Source of Low-Cost Loans

The federally funded Alternative Financing Program (AFP) exists in more than 30 states.[166] AFPs provide loan financing for AT, with low or reduced interest rates for persons with disabilities who meet the program criteria. Additionally, several states have AFP-like AT loan programs that are funded differently (CATADA, 2017a,b). This section describes all such programs as AFPs.

An AFP may be a source of funding for AT when no other funding source exists. It may be able to extend or arrange for credit when the individual with a disability or his or her family would not ordinarily meet the standards of creditworthiness. Every AT device discussed herein could be funded through an AFP loan.

Typical Operation of AFPs

Generally, AFPs may use three different methods: a revolving loan, a loan guarantee, or an interest rate buy-down. Some programs offer one or two of these methods, some all three. Key aspects of the loan program may include the following:

---

[165] See 20 CFR § 416.1400 *et seq*.

[166] See CATADA (2017a) for information on participation in state financing and other state-level activities.

- Dollar ranges for loans—For federal FY 2010, the national average of loans made was $10,498, with a range of under $1,000 to more than $50,000 (see U.S. Department of Education, 2014).
- Interest rates—For federal FY 2010, reported rates varied from 0 percent to 10.24 percent (RESNA Catalyst Project, 2017).
- Term for repayment—The term typically ranges from 2 to 7 years, but some programs offer a longer repayment period for home equity loans.
- Creditworthiness issues—Although a loan program will want to have reasonable assurance that loans will be repaid, some programs, unlike traditional lenders, will offer loans to individuals without a good credit rating.

Items Purchased with Loan Funds

The items commonly purchased with loan funds include many that are not easily funded through traditional funding sources, such as Medicaid, Medicare, a state VR agency, or special education programs. In some cases, another funding source will pay up to a funding limit or provide funding subject to a copayment, and an AFP loan can be used to pay for the balance. The following are the common categories for loans, along with one or more examples of a non-loan funding source:

- *Vehicle modifications and transportation*—State VR agencies can fund vehicle modifications to support an occupational objective.
- *Computers and related equipment*—iPADs and similar devices have become popular items funded through a loan program and could include a dual-purpose laptop or tablet that would be used as an SGD. State VR agencies may fund these costs if related to an occupational objective, and both Medicaid and Medicare can be funding sources for dual-purpose laptops or tablets that also serve as SGDs.
- *Mobility, seating, and positioning equipment*—These items can often be funded through Medicaid, Medicare, or a private insurance plan. Both Medicare and private insurance may require a significant copayment that could be financed through an AFP loan.
- *Environmental adaptations and home modifications*—If the item in question is considered outside the scope of traditional Medicaid, a Medicaid waiver program, if available, may be able to cover this cost. Waiver programs, however, typically have dollar limits on what they will pay for each year, making an AFP loan an attractive supplement.

- *Hearing*—Medicaid may be a funding source. As discussed earlier, Medicare by law excludes funding for hearing aids. Many private insurance plans may also specifically exclude coverage of hearing aids.

For FY 2010, the four most common categories of AT purchased through AFP loans were vehicle modifications and transportation; hearing; environmental adaptations and home modifications; and mobility, seating, and positioning in that order (U.S. Department of Education, 2014, Table 30).

A state AFP can be an important source of funding for AT when no other funding is readily available. An AFP loan can also be used to fund AT pending an appeal to another funding source, such as Medicaid or a state VR agency. An AFP loan can be used as well to pay for vocationally related items not available through the state VR agency but written into an approved SSI PASS. The money to be set aside in the PASS would then be used later to pay off the loan after the individual had already purchased and received the equipment. In the PASS example described earlier, for example, the individual might not have good credit scores and could use an AFP loan to purchase the van. He would use PASS savings for a down payment, then use the PASS savings to make payments on the loan.

Achieving a Better Life Experience Accounts

The Stephen Beck, Jr., Achieving a Better Life Experience Act was signed into law on December 19, 2014, with an effective date of December 18, 2015. This law, Internal Revenue Code 529A, creates a tax-advantaged account that can be used to save funds for the disability-related expenses of a "designated beneficiary," who must be blind or disabled by a condition that began before the individual's 26th birthday.[167] ABLE accounts can be established and maintained by a state or a state agency directly, or by contract with a private company as an instrument of the state.

During 2016, the first ABLE accounts were authorized in seven states: Florida, Kentucky, Michigan, Nebraska, Ohio, Oregon, and Tennessee.[168] The Florida accounts are available only to Florida residents, while the other states operate what are known as national ABLE accounts. An eligible individual can open an ABLE account through a national ABLE program in any state.

[167]26 USC § 529A; 80 Fed. Reg. 35602-35620 (proposed regulations, dated June 22, 2015); POMS SI 01130.740.

[168]The ABLE National Resource Center (2017) homepage includes a regularly updated U.S. map that provides links to active state ABLE account programs.

Disability Criteria for the Designated Beneficiary

To qualify as a designated beneficiary, the individual must

- be eligible for SSDI or SSI disability benefits, based on a disability or blindness that began before age 26; or
- be an individual who has certified, or have a parent or guardian that has certified, that he or she has a medically determinable impairment—i.e., disability or blindness occurring before age 26—"which results in marked and severe functional limitations" that have lasted or are expected to last 12 consecutive months, or are likely to result in death.[169]

The law provides that the certification of disability must be filed with the secretary of the treasury.[170] Interim guidance issued by the Internal Revenue Service (IRS) on November 20, 2015, pending final regulations, provides that the disability certification is deemed to have been filed with the secretary of the treasury once the state ABLE program has received the certification (IRS, 2015a). This guidance goes on to provide that the certification requirements are met if the individual, the individual's agent under power of attorney, or his/her parent or guardian certifies, under penalty of perjury, that he or she has a "signed physician's diagnosis" and that the signed diagnosis will be retained and provided to the ABLE program or the IRS upon request (IRS, 2015b, pp. 8-9).

Contributions to an ABLE Account

Any "person" can contribute to an individual's ABLE account, including the designated beneficiary. A person, as defined by IRS rules, includes a trust or an estate. The maximum combined contributions cannot exceed the current year's IRS gift tax-exempt amount—$14,000 in 2016.[171]

Use of Funds in an ABLE Account for Qualified Disability Expenses

The designated beneficiary is permitted to withdraw money from the ABLE account to meet qualified disability expenses (QDEs). Although the law characterizes these as expenses "related to the blindness or disability of the designated beneficiary and for the benefit of the designated beneficiary," comments to the proposed regulations note that "the Treasury Department and the IRS conclude that the term 'qualified disability expenses' should

---

[169]26 USC § 529A(e).
[170]26 USC § 529A(e)(1).
[171]See proposed regulations, 26 CFR § 1.529A-2.

be broadly construed to permit the inclusion of basic living expenses and should not be limited to items for which there is a medical necessity or which provide no benefits to others in addition to the benefit to the eligible individual."[172]

Section 529A(e)(5) of the law provides a list of expenses that would be considered QDEs, including

- education and employment training and support,
- housing and transportation,
- AT and personal support services,
- health and prevention and wellness,
- financial management and administrative services and expenses for ABLE account oversight and monitoring,
- legal fees, and
- funeral and burial.

The law then goes on to add "other expenses" approved by the treasury secretary,[173] interpreted by the interim guidance and proposed regulations to include basic living expenses.[174]

Clearly, ABLE account funds can be used to purchase or contribute to the cost of any of the AT devices that fit into the four categories discussed herein. As with a PASS, the individual with a disability or designated beneficiary of the ABLE account should always look to other funding sources first, relying on ABLE funds to pay for those items that cannot be funded, for example, through Medicaid or Medicare. Since medical necessity need not be demonstrated for an ABLE account QDE, the use of ABLE funds would be appropriate, for example, when a funder such as Medicaid did not find the requested AT to be medically necessary.

Examples of how ABLE funds could be used to fund AT devices include the following:

- *Powered wheelchair with integrated standing feature*—If the Medicaid agency would pay for the powered wheelchair and other features but not the standing feature, the individual could arrange with Medicaid and the equipment supplier for the extra cost of the standing feature to be paid through the ABLE account.
- *Binaural hearing aids*—If the individual's only insurance coverage were through Medicare, which excludes hearing aids from coverage, the ABLE account could be the best way to fund the item.

[172] 80 Fed. Reg. 35608.
[173] 26 USC § 529A(e)(5).
[174] 80 Fed. Reg. 35614-15, proposed 26 CFR § 1529A-2(h).

- *A dedicated SGD*—If the individual's only insurance coverage was Medicare and the individual was not eligible for the Qualified Medicare Beneficiaries Program (which would pay for the Part B 20 percent copayment [see the Medicare discussion above]), the ABLE account could fund the copayment (e.g., $1,200 if the cost of the device were $6,000).

How ABLE Accounts Affect Continued SSI Eligibility

The SSI program has issued policy provisions governing the treatment of money placed in ABLE accounts, the funds held in those accounts, the status of SSI and Medicaid when the total value of an ABLE account exceeds $100,000, and the use of ABLE funds to meet designated disability expenses (SSA, 2016d). These provisions provide that

- contributions of the designated beneficiary still count as income for SSI, while contributions from all other sources are excluded and not counted as income;
- earnings from the ABLE account are excluded by SSI; and
- up to $100,000 of the account balance is excluded by SSI and not counted toward the $2,000 SSI resource limit.

ABLE account distributions The SSI policy provides that ABLE account distributions are not income of the designated beneficiary for SSI purposes but a "conversion of a resource from one form to another . . . regardless of whether the distributions are for non-housing QDEs, housing QDEs, or non-qualified expenses" (SSA, 2016d).[175] The exclusion of housing-related QDEs from income is extremely important, as the payment of housing expenses (e.g., rent, mortgage, utility costs) by a third party, including a trust, would ordinarily be considered in-kind income and could reduce the SSI payment by up to one-third of the SSI FBR (i.e., $245 per month in 2017) (SSA, 2012b).

When the ABLE account balance exceeds $100,000 As noted, SSI eligibility is not affected as long as the ABLE account balance does not exceed $100,000. No designated beneficiary is expected to exceed the $100,000 limit in the near future because of the yearly $14,000 cumulative limit on contributions. However, individuals with disabilities need to understand these provisions for future planning purposes.

When the ABLE account balance exceeds $100,000, the SSI program

---

[175]Readers must keep in mind, however, that the use of ABLE funds for nonqualified expenses may have tax consequences.

will count any of the excess money toward the $2,000 resource limit. SSI policy calls for an indefinite benefit suspension and continuing eligibility for Medicaid during periods of excess resources attributable to an ABLE account (SSA, 2016d). Ordinarily, if an individual exceeded SSI's $2,000 resource limit for 12 consecutive months, the person would be terminated from benefits and would need to submit a new application if his or her resources fell below $2,000 in a future month (SSA, 2016e). This special provision allows SSI to be suspended for 12 months or longer, allowing the designated beneficiary to return to payment status in any future months in which his or her countable resources, including ABLE account funding in excess of $100,000, are within the $2,000 limit.

The retention of Medicaid during the period of indefinite suspension is very important to any individual who will need continuing Medicaid to cover a range of expenses, including AT devices. This provision is particularly important for individuals who are no longer dependent on the modest SSI payment they were receiving but need Medicaid for AT and other health-related costs. It is also important for individuals who are no longer receiving SSI payments because of the budgeting of earnings and retain Medicaid through the 1619(b) work incentive discussed in the section on Medicaid above.

Impact of the ABLE Account on Other Key Federally Authorized Benefits

The U.S. Department of the Treasury has said that "[in] general, neither the ABLE account nor distributions from the account are treated as income or resources of a designated beneficiary . . . in determining that designated beneficiary's qualification for federal benefits [other than SSI and Medicaid]."[176] However, no provision in the law or the proposed regulations references how any specific federal benefit program will implement this provision. The discussion here is limited to the interrelationship between ABLE accounts and four other AT funding sources discussed herein: Medicaid's Buy-In Programs for working individuals, Medicare Savings Programs (MSPs), the state VR agencies, and SSI's PASS.

Medicaid Buy-In Programs This powerful work incentive, discussed earlier in the section on Medicaid, allows individuals with disabilities to qualify for Medicaid at countable earnings levels set by individual states. For example, a number of states set their countable income standard at 250 percent of the federal poverty level. Federal criteria governing Medicaid Buy-In Programs require that SSI rules be applied for counting of income and resources unless specific provisions enacted by a state provide for more liberal rules.

[176] Interim Guidance, IR-2015-130, p. 2.

Since the ABLE-related SSI rules discussed above are now a part of SSI's income and resource rules, a Medicaid Buy-In Program is required, for example, to follow the rules that allow for exclusion of ABLE accounts even if they total more than $100,000 to allow an individual to retain Medicaid.

MSPs As outlined earlier in the section on Medicare, MSPs provide for Medicaid agencies to pay Medicare Part B premiums and, in some cases, copayments if a financial needs test is met. As noted, in determining countable income and assets for MSP eligibility, states must follow all SSI income and resource exclusion rules. Since ABLE account resources up to $100,000 are now exempt in the SSI program, they are also exempt in determining MSP eligibility. This means that a Medicare beneficiary can retain a significant balance of his or her ABLE account and still qualify for the Qualified Medicare Beneficiaries program, which will pay for both Part B premiums and the 20 percent copayment on any AT device covered by Medicare as DME.

State VR agencies As noted earlier in the section on state VR agencies, an SSI or SSDI beneficiary automatically meets the VR agency's financial need criteria for receipt of funding for a range of services, including AT devices and services. Since individuals can now retain SSI cash payment status notwithstanding ABLE account resources up to $100,000, financial eligibility for VR agency funding will continue as well.

SSI's PASS The PASS, as explained above, allows for exclusion of both income and resources to be used in support of an approved occupational objective. Since up to $100,000 in an ABLE account is an exempt resource for SSI purposes, there is no requirement that an individual exhaust his or her ABLE funds before using the PASS to purchase needed AT, for example. To the extent that the PASS savings are insufficient to support the occupational objective in an individual case, an ABLE account distribution can be used to supplement those funds available in the PASS, for example, to pay for needed AT.

Charitable Programs

The ability to find funding for a specific AT device will vary from case to case. It may depend on whether the individual is eligible for one of the funding sources discussed above, such as Medicaid or Medicare. It may also depend on the ability to show that the item is needed to benefit from a child's special education program or the ability to convince the state VR agency that the item is needed to progress toward an occupational objective when the state VR program has enough money remaining in its budget to pay for it. In some cases, one of the public funding sources discussed above may have denied the requested item, which will mean initiating a time-consuming appeal to have even a chance of receiving funding.

When an individual or family cannot identify a public or noncharitable private funding source to pay for needed AT, a charitable organization may be an option. The charity might be a well-known state or national entity or a lesser-known one found through word-of-mouth or Internet research. It might even be a local charity that makes funding available only for residents.

Charities are unlike public funding entities in several respects. For example, a charity may choose to target only one type of disability for assistance, provide funding only for a specific type of equipment, or pay only a percentage of the purchase price of AT. In some cases, a charity may be available to fund a large copayment required to obtain an AT device, such as the 20 percent Medicare Part B copayment required to fund an expensive wheelchair or SGD.

The item(s) a charity is willing to fund may vary from year to year depending on its updated priorities or the amount of donations it has received to support its annual activities. Some charities may require proof that the individual seeking assistance has exhausted other sources of funding, such as Medicaid and private insurance, while others may request a written statement of need and allocate their limited resources based on a committee's review of competing applications. If a charity declines to provide funding for an item, an individual may be able to express his or her concerns in writing to the organization's funding manager, but charities are not known to offer formal appeals to challenge their decisions. Over time, charities have been known to change their focus, merge with other charities, or even cease operations. For these reasons, a charity should typically be viewed as a last resort for AT funding.

This section first describes strategies for locating a national charity that could be a funding source for AT devices—strategies that may work at the state and local levels as well. It then provides some examples of national charities that, at the time of this writing, were potential funding sources for the categories of AT that are the focus of this report.

Strategies for Locating a National Charity

Internet searches on any major search engine should lead to information about national, state, or local charities. Sometimes these searches will yield specific organizations that make funds for AT or the AT itself available at little or no cost. The searches may also lead to websites that compile lists of potential charitable funding sources for AT. For example, the United Spinal Association's "Spinal Cord Resource Center Page" provides a range of links to sources of grants and loans and other funding sources, including other funding source compilation sites (United Spinal Association, 2015). As the person searching compiles a list of potential funding sources, it is always best to contact the source directly (by email or phone) to confirm that the information on the site is still current.

Internet searches can be time-consuming and create the challenge of finding a way to deftly sort through what the search yields. One approach is to open a separate word processing document, such as a Word file, making sure to save it for future reference. Each time a useful or apparently useful website is found, "block and paste" can be used to drop the full Internet address or URL into the word processing document, giving it a descriptive name such as "Spinal Cord Resource Center Page." At a later time, this funding source document can be better organized by AT category or type of funding source. This can also be a good way for an individual to retain any lesser-known public funding sources, such as the state-operated crime victims compensation program or workers' compensation program, both of which in some cases could be a fruitful AT funding source.[177]

Examples of National Charities

The examples below are provided by way of illustration. They are representative of the type of assistance that may be available through national charities. In a specific case, a good Internet search may turn up any number of better examples for an AT device that cannot otherwise be funded. Any in-depth research should encompass state and local charities as well. Overall, although charities may never be a substitute for a well-funded public system of funding, they can be a life saver in individual cases.

United Cerebral Palsy (UCP) Elsie S. Bellows Fund This national program, operated by UCP, provides grants for purchasing or repairing AT devices for individuals with disabilities. Individuals with disabilities and their families who are in financial need and lack other funding resources are eligible (United Cerebral Palsy, 2015). Funding is made available through UCP's local affiliates, which directly assess an individual's AT needs and financial qualifications. Examples of allowable AT requests include manual and powered wheelchairs, computer equipment (presumably including the dual-purpose laptop/tablet and SGD), and hearing aids.

Friends of Disabled Adults and Children (FODAC) FODAC provides adults and children with disabilities, nationwide, with free or low-cost

[177]For more information on the crime victims and workers' compensation programs, see NLS (2011b, 2015).

wheelchairs and other DME, vehicle and home adaptations, and more (FODAC, 2017). The organization depends, in part, on donations of new and used DME. Its volunteer-run repair shop cleans and refurbishes the equipment and matches it to the specifications of the new user. Relevant to the discussion herein, FODAC can provide free or low-cost new and used wheelchairs, as well as low-cost repairs, to individuals not otherwise able the cover those costs.

Foundation for Sight and Sound Through its Help America Hear Program, the Foundation for Sight and Sound provides new high-quality hearing aids, nationwide, to men, women, and children with limited financial resources (Foundation for Sight and Sound, 2016). The organization's website asks individuals to exhaust all other financial resources, including but not limited to available credit, family support, money market accounts, mutual funds, 401(k) plans, trust funds, annuities, and savings/checking and state-sponsored programs, before turning to this charity.

Private Health Insurance

Private (or commercial) health insurance encompasses any nongovernmental health insurance. Employers and individuals can contract with private health insurance providers either to administer or to pay specified health care costs for eligible individuals. When employers are "self-insured," they are responsible for health care costs, although their plans typically are administered by an insurance company (Community Health Advocates, 2012). By contrast, "fully insured" employers pay premiums to the insurance company, which is then responsible for the covered costs when an eligible employee needs care (Community Health Advocates, 2012). Fully insured plans must comply with federal and state regulations (Community Health Advocates, 2012; Kubrin, 2016).

Private health insurance varies considerably in price and the benefits offered. Factors affecting what benefits are available, the rights of the client, and the like, include the type of insurance the client has (e.g., health maintenance organization [HMO]), preferred provider organization, point of service), whether the plan is self-insured or fully insured, the state in which the employer is based, whether the employer is covered by the Employee Retirement Income Security Act, and whether the plan is "grandfathered" under federal health care reform (Community Health Advocates, 2012).

Eligibility for coverage and payment of benefits depend on the terms of the plan. As with private disability insurance, employers can specify eligibility criteria for coverage of their employees.

Funding for Selected AT Devices

Fully insured private health insurance plans provide coverage for DME and prostheses and orthotics. Most of the variation in coverage relates to the level of cost sharing rather than the types of devices covered (Kubrin, 2016). For fully insured commercial HMO or deductible HMO plans, deductible levels range from \$250 to \$5,000; coinsurance ranges from zero to 40 percent; and out-of-pocket costs range from around \$500 to \$5,000, with two or three times that for the family deductible (Kubrin, 2016).

Powered wheelchairs and accessories The Tufts Health Plan (2017d) may cover a powered wheelchair when a number of criteria are met, including the individual's being unable to "propel a manual wheelchair more than 50 feet"; "propel a manual wheelchair sufficient distances to manage within the community, including but not limited to attending appointments, working and managing household responsibilities, at least three times per week"; and "meet the criteria for" or safely use a power operated vehicle (i.e, a three- or four-wheeled device with tiller steering and limited seat modification capabilities [Tufts, 2017c]). Tufts (2017d) expressly excludes "coverage of a power wheelchair and/or accessories and components" when used for convenience, primarily for recreation or leisure, or for community mobility only. In addition, it excludes coverage when the powered wheelchair is requested in addition to the individual's "primary mobility device (e.g., manual wheelchair, power operated vehicle)." It also does not cover certain wheelchair modifications or accessories, including any type of powered seat elevation system, any type of powered standing system, a powered wheelchair seat cushion, or an environmental control unit (Tufts, 2017d).

Likewise, Aetna may cover powered wheelchairs if they are considered medically necessary under specified conditions. Powered wheelchairs expressly are not considered medically necessary if needed only for use outside of the home, and Group 4 wheelchairs are not considered to be medically necessary because they have added capabilities that are not needed for use in the home (Aetna, 2016d).

Myoelectric upper-extremity prostheses A review of general coverage of myoelectric upper-extremity prostheses among several private health insurance carriers indicates a number of common criteria for the medical necessity of such a device (Aetna, 2016b; Amerigroup, 2016; Tufts, 2016). Several of the criteria relate to the ability to use the device, for example, having (1) "sufficient neurological, myocutaneous, and cognitive function to operate the prosthesis effectively," (2) "sustained a minimum of a wrist or above partial limb amputation," and (3) "sufficient microvolt threshold in the residual limb to allow proper function of the prosthesis" (Tufts, 2016;

see also Aetna, 2016b; Amerigroup, 2016). Aetna (2016b) and Amerigroup (2016) also include a requirement that there be no comorbidities, such as neuromuscular disease, "that could interfere with maintaining function of the prosthesis." Amerigroup (2016) and Tufts Health Plan (2016) each stipulate as well that the individual not function "in an environment that would inhibit function of the prosthesis," such as wet environments or situations involving electrical discharges. Notably, all three carriers also require as a criterion for medical necessity that a "standard body powered prosthetic device cannot be used" or is "insufficient to meet the functional needs" of the person (Aetna, 2016b; Amerigroup, 2016; Tufts, 2016) "in performing activities of daily living" (Aetna, 2016b; Tufts, 2016).

Hearing aids Hearing aids often are not covered under private health insurance, or coverage may be sold as an optional rider (unless state mandated) (Andrews, 2012; Calderone, 2017b). Aetna, for example, excludes coverage of hearing aids from most of its benefit plans. Such exclusions apply to "air conduction hearing aids, implantable hearing aids and semi-implantable hearing aids" (Aetna, 2016a). Individuals who are covered must satisfy the criteria for medical necessity (Aetna, 2016a). However, the Tufts Health Plan covers "medically necessary audiology evaluations and related services for hearing disorders" as specified in its policies, including coverage for hearing aids for members aged 21 and younger in Massachusetts and adults in New Hampshire and Rhode Island in accordance with state requirements (Tufts, 2017a). New Hampshire and Rhode Island are two of four states that require hearing aid coverage for adults; Arkansas and Connecticut are the other two (ASHA,2017). Twenty states, including Massachusetts, require hearing aid coverage for children (ASHA, 2017). Although approximately 60 percent of respondents to *Consumer Reports'* survey of 131,686 readers with hearing challenges found that "none of the initial hearing-aid costs were covered by health insurance," 37 percent indicated that they saved some money on hearing aids through their private health insurance plans (Calderone, 2017a,b). Some insurers, such as Aetna, offer discounts on hearing aids through arrangements with outside companies (Calderone, 2017a). And United Healthcare now offers lower-cost hearing aids through a collaboration with hi HealthInnovations, an Optum business, and UnitedHealth Group (UnitedHealth Group, 2017).

Speech-generating devices The Tufts Health Plan covers SGDs as DME when medically necessary, subject to a copay of up to 30 percent (Tufts, 2017b). The plan "does not compensate for devices, accessories or software programs that are considered to be not the least intensive level of services (E2508, E2510, E2511, E2512)" (Tufts, 2017b, p. 9). Aetna (2016c) considers SGDs to be medically necessary DME and will cover them for individuals who meet all of the requisite criteria. Provided the SGD is used only by "a person with a severe speech impairment and is primarily used for the purpose of generating speech," it does not have to be dedicated to speech generation for it to be considered DME. Although devices such as computers, tablets, and smartphones are not covered because they are not dedicated SGDs, "software that enables such devices to function as a SGD is considered an SGD; however, installation of the program or technical support is not separately reimbursable" (Aetna, 2016c). For a given individual, Aetna (2016c) considers only one SGD or speech-generating software program at a time to be medically necessary.

Private Disability Insurance

As part of the information gathering for the committee's review of selected disability compensation programs, representatives from two private disability insurance providers, Unum and Prudential Financial, addressed the committee during open session. Since private disability insurance is a potential source of funding for certain assistive products and technologies, a brief discussion is included in this chapter. Greater detail on private disability programs is provided in Chapter 8.

Eligibility for Private Disability Insurance Benefits

Employers and individuals can contract with private disability insurance providers to pay monetary benefits when a covered individual becomes disabled and unable to work. Eligibility for coverage and payment of benefits depend on the terms of the contract between the employer or individual and the insurance provider. Employers can specify eligibility criteria for coverage of their employees based, for example, on the number of hours they work (Jackson, 2016).

Funding for Selected AT Devices

Notably, private disability insurers typically define disability "based on the essential functions of the occupation" (Jackson, 2016). When deciding a claim, the insurer must determine whether the claimant's medical condition supports the inability to perform the occupation (Jackson, 2016; see also Tugman and Kramschuster, 2016). For claimants who may be able to return to work with reasonable accommodations, including AT, the insurer may provide certain products or technologies or reimburse the employer for at least a portion of the cost of work site modifications "that will assist the employee in performing the substantial and material duties of the occupation" (Jackson, 2016; see also Tugman and Kramschuster, 2016).

Private disability insurers utilize assistive products and technologies in support of occupational functioning, which is different from supporting activities of daily living (ADLs) or instrumental activities of daily living (IADLs) (Jackson, 2016).

This focus on returning the claimant to work with his or her employer has implications for the types of assistive products and technologies private insurers provide. Musculoskeletal conditions are among the most common for both short- and long-term disability claims. Common assistive devices provided include sit/stand workstations; antifatigue mats; ergonomic workstations, chairs, and keyboards; special shoes, gloves, and belts; transfer devices (scissor lift, pivot disc); speech-to-text software; and the like (Jackson, 2016; Tugman and Kramschuster, 2016). Private disability insurers may provide scooters or other wheeled mobility devices if required to restore or maintain occupational functioning, although the provision of such devices is less common (on the order of 5 percent) (Jackson, 2016). Other commonly provided products and technologies address visual and auditory conditions: text-to-speech software, magnification, and closed-caption television for visual impairments; amplification, text telephone, and vibrating pagers for notification for hearing impairments; and white noise machines for tinnitus (Jackson, 2016; Tugman and Kramschuster, 2016). Private disability insurers do not provide assistive products and technologies unless the devices directly support occupational functioning (Jackson, 2016; Tugman and Kramschuster, 2016). Thus, the types of assistive products and technologies required by individuals to engage in ADLs and IADLs, including those described in this report, typically are not covered by private disability insurers.

WORKPLACE REASONABLE ACCOMMODATIONS

Americans with Disabilities Act

Congress passed the ADA in 1990 to end discrimination in the form of, among other things, the "failure to make modifications to existing facilities and practices, [and] exclusionary qualification standards and criteria" for people with disabilities.[178] After a series of Supreme Court cases narrowed the application of the ADA in employment cases, Congress passed the ADA Amendments Act of 2008 (Public Law 110-325) to restore its original intent for a broad interpretation of ADA protections.

The ADA prohibits discrimination against individuals with disabilities in the areas of employment in Title I, state and local government services in Title II, places of public accommodations in Title III, and transportation

[178] 42 USC § 12101(a)(5).

and other areas not relevant to employment. As summarized in Chapter 1, it provides three definitions of disability, only one of which an individual must meet to qualify as a person with a disability. The first definition requires having a physical or mental impairment that substantially limits one or more major life activities. This definition is often referred to as the "actual disability" prong.[179] Congress prescribed a broad interpretation for all of the terms in this definition. The second definition requires having "a record of a physical or mental impairment that substantially limited a major life activity."[180] Some refer to this as the "record of" prong. This definition applies to someone who, although not currently experiencing a physical or mental impairment that substantially limits a major life activity, met the definition in the past. The third definition applies to people whom others regard as having a substantially limiting impairment.[181] This means that others treat the individual differently, including committing actions prohibited by the ADA, because of an actual or a perceived impairment that is not both "transitory and minor."[182]

Individuals who seek employment fall under Title I's ADA protections if they are "qualified individuals with disabilities." Qualified individuals with disabilities are those who satisfy "the requisite skill, experience, education and other job-related requirements of the employment position" they want and "with or without reasonable accommodation, can perform the essential functions of such position."[183]

The ADA defines reasonable accommodations as modifications to the job application process to allow for access to the process, modifications to the work environment or the way work is usually performed that enable a person to perform the essential functions of the job, and/or other modifications that allow an individual to enjoy all of the privileges of employment.[184] Absent undue hardship, employers must make reasonable accommodations for individuals who meet the "actual disability" and "record of" definitions[185] if requested. The employer also needs to be aware that the individual is a person with a disability, which requires that the employee or potential employee disclose his or her disability.[186,187]

---

[179] 29 CFR § 1630.2(g).

[180] 29 CFR § 1630.2(g)(1)(ii).

[181] 29 CFR § 1630.2(g)(1)(iii).

[182] 29 CFR § 1630.2(g)(1)(iii).

[183] 29 CFR § 1630.2(m).

[184] 29 CFR § 1630.2(o)(1). This section was not affected by the ADA Amendments Act of 2008.

[185] Employers need not make reasonable accommodations for people who only meet the "regarded as" prong for the definition of individuals with disabilities.

[186] 29 CFR § 1630.9.

[187] *Morisky v. Broward County*, 80 F.3d 445 (11th Cir. 1996).

The ADA defines undue hardship as "an action requiring significant difficulty or expense" when viewed in the context of four factors[188]: the nature and cost of the accommodations, the overall financial resources of the facility or facilities and the business entity itself, the potential impact of the accommodations on operations, and the type of operation of the business. Thus, while cost may be an issue for a small business, other circumstances may render accommodations an undue hardship for larger businesses for other reasons, such as the accommodations' interfering with the ability of other employees to perform their jobs.

For example, the Equal Economic Opportunity Commission's (2002) *Enforcement Guidance on Reasonable Accommodation and Undue Hardship under the Americans with Disabilities Act* explains that as a reasonable accommodation, employers are not required to lower production rates or quality standards, nor are they required to eliminate essential functions. Further, employers are not required to provide personal-use items such as eyeglasses, wheelchairs, and hearing aids for use outside the workplace. As the guidance states:

> An employer does not have to provide as reasonable accommodations personal use items needed in accomplishing daily activities both on and off the job. Thus, an employer is not required to provide an employee with a prosthetic limb, a wheelchair, eyeglasses, hearing aids, or similar devices if they are also needed off the job.[189] (EEOC, 2002)

Thus, reasonable accommodations are limited to enabling the performance of a specific job for which an applicant with a disability applies, and the legal obligation to make reasonable accommodations applies only to work site and workplace accommodations that are not an undue hardship. Employers are not required to provide items considered personal items, such as wheelchairs, hearing aids, augmentative communication devices, and prosthetic devices, that are specifically excluded from the definition of reasonable accommodations under the ADA.

It is important to note as well that air carriers are exempt from the ADA, although the act covers airports and the services provided within them. The Air Carrier Transportation Act (ACTA) provides guidelines for the transport of people with disabilities within aircraft,[190] but while an important piece of legislation, it has significant shortcomings. Some jobs require periodic air travel, especially as one advances within an organization. Unfortunately, ACTA does not require and most airlines do not provide

---

[188]42 USC § 12111 (10)(A)(B).

[189]The section referenced was not affected by the ADA Amendments Act of 2008.

[190]Air Carrier Access Act, codified at 14 CFR § 382.1 *et seq.* (2009).

adequate seating for individuals with severe disabilities, especially in coach. In addition, such individuals often find bathrooms on aircraft inaccessible, and onboard wheelchairs are inadequate.

Employer Accommodations

Subject to the limitations concerning undue hardship and personal-use items, the ADA provides that "reasonable accommodations" made by employers

> may include—(A) making existing facilities used by employees readily accessible to and usable by individuals with disabilities; and (B) job restructuring, part-time or modified work schedules, reassignment to a vacant position, acquisition or modification of equipment or devices, appropriate adjustment or modifications of examinations, training materials or policies, the provision of qualified readers or interpreters, and other similar accommodations for individuals with disabilities.[191,192]

The Job Accommodation Network (JAN) is a service of the U.S. Department of Labor's Office of Disability Employment Policy (JAN, 2016). In 2004, JAN initiated an ongoing study based on interviews of employers, representing a variety of sizes and industries, who had contacted JAN with questions about workplace accommodations and/or the ADA.[193] Employers consistently report that most accommodations they make are at no or low cost (JAN, 2016). Of the 700 employers who provided cost information related to accommodations, 410 (59 percent) reported that accommodations needed by employees were provided at no cost; 36 percent (n = 256) provided the accommodations for a one-time cost; only 4 percent (n = 25) reported that providing accommodations "resulted in an ongoing, annual cost to the company"; and 1 percent (n = 9) reported that accommodations resulted in a combination of one-time and annual costs (JAN, 2016). Available employer cost data show that "the typical one-time expenditure by employers was $500" (JAN, 2016, p. 4).

At the federal level, section 504 of the Rehabilitation Act of 1973 protects "qualified individual[s]" who have a disability from exclusion from, denial of benefits of, or discrimination under any program that receives federal monies or any federal employer. Although each federal agency develops its own section 504 regulations, common requirements include "reasonable accommodation for employees with disabilities; program

[191]42 USC § 12111(9) (1994); 29 CFR § 1630.2(o)(2)(i-ii) (1997).

[192]The section referenced was not affected by the ADA Amendments Act of 2008.

[193] Between January 2004 and December 2006, 1,182 employers were interviewed, and between June 28, 2008, and July 31, 2016, 1,157 were interviewed.

accessibility; effective communication with people who have hearing or vision disabilities; and accessible new construction and alterations" (U.S. Department of Justice, 2009, Rehabilitation Act). The Computer/Electronic Accommodations Program (CAP), for example, is a centrally funded program that provides reasonable accommodations for Department of Defense employees with disabilities. The program's mission "is to provide assistive technology and accommodations to support individuals with disabilities and wounded, ill and injured Service members throughout the Federal Government in accessing information and communication technology" (CAP, 2017). In 2000, CAP was granted "the authority to provide assistive technology, devices and support services free of charge to Federal agencies that have a partnership agreement with CAP" (CAP, 2017).

Among states, employment of people with disabilities is addressed in different ways. In 2009, for example, Massachusetts developed and adopted its Strategic Plan to Make Massachusetts a Model Employer for People with Disabilities (Commonwealth of Massachusetts, 2009). In 2010, as part of this plan, the state began to collect data on the reasonable accommodations it provided to its own employees. Data for three quarters of 2010 showed that the state had made a total of 1,319 reasonable accommodations "ranging from duty and schedule modifications to furniture and equipment acquisition" (AT Program News, 2011):

- The most common type of accommodation made was in the category of furniture and equipment (from specialized seating to computers), at an average cost of $262.00.
- The most expensive category tracked was telecommunications, with an average cost of $530.00.
- The average cost of all reasonable accommodations made during these quarters was $170.00.

Several global and national employers have targeted hiring for people in certain disability groups. For example, Walgreens and CVS target people with developmental disabilities and autism in their targeted hiring program. SAP, Microsoft, and AT&T target autistic adults. Ernst and Young has won awards for its diversity hiring; it has also targeted autistic adults to fill 1 percent of its workforce. These employers often go above and beyond what the ADA requires, providing special training, such as assistance with time management, communication, and workplace rules and etiquette. While there is no standard set of AT that autistic people use, the assumption is that these exemplar employers provide some AT to meet each individual's needs for an accessible workplace.

JAN is "the leading source of free, expert and confidential guidance on workplace accommodations and disability employment issues" (ODEP, n.d.). "Working toward practical solutions that benefit both employer and employee, JAN helps people with disabilities enhance their employability, and shows employers how to capitalize on the value and talent that people with disabilities add to the workplace" (JAN, n.d.). JAN offers free one-to-one consultation on workplace accommodations and the ADA via phone and online (JAN, n.d.). Common reasonable accommodations include physical alterations to buildings and/or equipment to provide access for someone with mobility issues, flexible scheduling of work hours, purchase/installation of AT that is not a personal-use item, and allowing employees to work from home (Balser, 2007). Most of the accommodations provided are low-cost solutions that do not include the AT that is the subject of this report.

HEALTH LITERACY, EDUCATION, AND KNOWLEDGE OF ASSISTIVE PRODUCTS AND TECHNOLOGIES

Health literacy is defined as "the degree to which individuals have the capacity to obtain, process, and understand basic health information and services needed to make appropriate health decisions" (HHS, 2000b, 2007, p. 2.1). A variety of personal and systemic factors affect individuals' health literacy, including the knowledge of health topics and communication skills of professionals as well as lay persons, culture, and situational demands (HHS, 2007). People's health literacy affects their ability to

- Navigate the health care system, including filling out complex forms and locating providers and services
- Share personal information, such as health history, with providers
- Engage in self-care and chronic disease management
- Understand mathematical concepts such as probability and risk. (HHS, 2007, p. 2.1)

The 2003 National Assessment of Adult Literacy (NAAL), which included a component on health literacy, examined the English literacy of more than 19,000 adults (aged 16 and older) in the United States (Kutner et al., 2006). The health literacy measures focused on three domains: clinical, prevention, and navigation of the health care system. Tasks typically associated with a provider–patient encounter were represented in the clinical domain. Prevention involved tasks associated with "maintaining and improving" one's health, including disease prevention, early intervention, and managing chronic illness (Kutner et al., 2006, p. 3). "Activities related to understanding how the health care system works and individual rights and responsibilities" were included in the domain of navigating the health care system (Kutner et al., 2006, p. 3).

The materials presented were "selected to be representative of real-world health-related information, including insurance information, medicine directions, and preventive care information" (Kutner et al., 2006, p. 3). There were 28 health literacy tasks "designed to elicit respondents' skills for locating and understanding health-related information and services and to represent the three general literacy scales—prose, document, and quantitative—developed to report NAAL results" (Kutner et al., 2006, p. 3).

Overall, 53 percent of respondents demonstrated intermediate health literacy, 12 percent demonstrated proficient health literacy, 22 percent demonstrated basic health literacy, and 14 percent demonstrated below basic health literacy (Kutner et al., 2006). Notably, women demonstrated a higher average health literacy than men, and adults aged 65 and older demonstrated lower average health literacy than those in younger age groups. White and Asian/Pacific Islander adults demonstrated higher average health literacy than black, Hispanic, American Indian/Alaska Native, and multiracial adults. Hispanic respondents demonstrated the lowest average health literacy among the different racial/ethnic groups. English language proficiency and education level also were associated with health literacy. Individuals who spoke English only prior to high school demonstrated higher average health literacy than those who were non-English speakers or who spoke other languages in addition to English. Average health literacy increased with educational level, beginning with high school: 49 percent of individuals who "never attended or did not complete high school" demonstrated below basic health literacy, while just 15 percent of high school graduates and 3 percent of college graduates (bachelor's degree) demonstrated below basic health literacy. Poverty level also was associated with health literacy, with individuals living below the poverty level demonstrating lower average health literacy than those living above it (Kutner et al., 2006).

The complexity of health information may contribute to lower health literacy than one might expect even among individuals with higher levels of educational achievement (HHS, 2007). In addition, differences in language and culture may affect health literacy. Not only is limited proficiency in English a potential barrier to understanding health information; health care specialties also have their own languages that are acquired by practitioners, which may complicate communication with the lay public (HHS, 2007). Culture (i.e., medical culture as well as different world cultures) also plays a role in health literacy. Different cultures may demonstrate different approaches to matters of health, disease, disability, and authority (e.g., health care providers, insurance programs and providers), which can affect how individuals respond to health information they receive. Cultural and linguistic competency among health professionals can facilitate health literacy.

As in all areas of health care, consideration of health literacy is important when thinking about the use of assistive products and technologies. One study looking at a sample of written materials available to amputees containing information about preoperative care, the surgical procedure, and postoperative prosthetic care concluded that "more than one-third to half of the general population would have difficulty understanding the written information" in the materials (Hrnack et al., 2009). Several studies examining health literacy and hearing health care indicate a similar mismatch between the language used in written materials and by providers and the literacy levels of the individuals receiving care (Atcherson et al., 2013; Caposecco et al., 2014; Nair and Cienkowski, 2010; NASEM, 2016, p. 239ff.).

Education of professionals with respect to health literacy and cultural and linguistic competency is a first step toward increasing the health literacy of their clients in terms of understanding their health challenges and options for addressing them (AAA, 2012; Smith and Gutman, 2011). Education of the public with respect to disability, impairments, and the variety of assistive products and technologies available is important as well. Such education not only may provide a basis on which health care providers could build when interacting with patients but also could help inform users and potential users of assistive products and technologies about the range of options available to them. Individuals' acquisition of assistive devices may be promoted by their knowledge of their device options, their needs, their coverage options, and their means of pursuing the device(s) they need.

Community-based education as well as education campaigns targeted toward employers may help dispel myths, misperceptions, stereotypes, and fears often associated with disability (Lengnick-Hall et al., n.d.; McNaughton et al., 2003; Shinohara and Wobbrock, 2011). Employers and others unfamiliar with AT and disabilities may place barriers on the pathway to employment for individuals who use AT based on misperceptions about their ability to perform the job (Lengnick-Hall et al., n.d.; Shinohara and Wobbrock, 2011). Dissemination of publicly available, evidence-based information on assistive products and technologies and their use by individuals in the workplace may help reduce barriers to employment.

FINDINGS AND CONCLUSIONS

Findings

7-1. Financial access to assistive products and technologies and qualified providers varies significantly across reimbursement and funding sources in the United States.

7-2. Numerous pathways exist to access assistive products and technologies and related services based on eligibility for coverage.

7-3. Different coverage sources vary with respect to their mission, their eligibility requirements, and the types of assistive products and technologies and related services they cover:
   - Medicaid programs vary from state to state with respect to both the individuals who are eligible to enroll and the health care services that are covered.
   - Medicare funds only wheelchairs that are required for an individual to accomplish mobility-related activities of daily living within the home.
   - Original Medicare (Part B) does not cover hearing aids.
   - Medicare Advantage plans may cover hearing aids, depending on the plan selected.
   - Private health insurance coverage for assistive products and technologies varies depending on the plan and, in some cases (e.g., hearing aids), the state in which the beneficiary resides.
   - Some coverage options are designed specifically to provide pathways to employment or return to work, while others focus on medical necessity.
   - The Veterans Health Administration (VHA) is an integrated health care system that provides high-quality, comprehensive, interdisciplinary care and assistive products and technologies to veterans.

7-4. Thorough documentation by qualified medical professionals of an individual's medical and functional need for specific assistive products and technologies is often critical to obtaining Medicaid approval and funding.

7-5. Accurate assessment and selection of assistive products and technologies are critical for users as many Medicaid programs and other sources of coverage maintain an expected duration of use for particular devices and will not provide a replacement until this time period has elapsed.

7-6. Individuals' acquisition of assistive devices may be promoted by their knowledge of their device options, their needs, their coverage options, and their means of pursuing the device(s) they need.

7-7. Representation by an attorney or advocate who is experienced in health law could help individuals secure Medicaid or Medicare coverage and approval of various medical supplies, equipment, and assistive devices.

7-8. The distribution of funds varies among state vocational rehabilitation agencies and school districts.

7-9. Loss of coverage of and access to assistive products and technologies and related services among youth of transition age is a significant impediment to their successful transition to work, vocational readiness, or further education.

7-10. Workplace reasonable accommodations are limited to enabling the performance of specific jobs for which an applicant with a disability applies, and the legal obligation to make reasonable accommodations applies only to work site and workplace accommodations that are not an undue hardship. Employers are not required to provide items considered personal, such as wheelchairs, hearing aids, augmentative communication devices, and prosthetic devices, which are specifically excluded from the definition of reasonable accommodations under the Americans with Disabilities Act.

7-11. Health literacy, which may include knowledge about assistive products and technologies, varies greatly among adults in the United States, although individuals at lower socioeconomic levels generally demonstrate lower average health literacy.

Conclusions

7-1. Coverage generally is quite limited for assistive products and technologies and for the services of qualified providers and teams with the knowledge, skill, and expertise to properly evaluate, fit, train, and monitor people in the use of those products and technologies. Coverage varies considerably from case to case, state to state, district to district, urban to rural and frontier areas, and funding source to funding source. [Findings 7-1, 7-2, 7-3]

7-2. Although coverage for the cost of assistive products and technologies may be available, considerable variation exists from case to case, state to state, district to district, urban to rural and frontier areas, and funding source to funding source in the availability of the devices themselves and of the services of qualified providers and teams with the knowledge, skill, and expertise to properly evaluate, fit, train, and monitor people in their use. [Findings 7-4, 7-5, 7-8]

7-3. Individuals of low socioeconomic status are limited in their access to coverage for assistive products and technologies and related services, as well as in their ability to obtain the devices and services when they are covered. [Findings 7-6, 7-8]

7-4. A variety of personal factors, including ethnic, cultural, and language barriers, may affect access to assistive products and technologies and related services when they are covered. [Findings 7-1, 7-2, 7-6, 7-8, 7-9, 7-10]

7-5. Salient regulations and coverage policies do not appear to be keeping pace with advances in assistive products and technologies and their potential to enhance activities and participation for individuals with impairments. [Findings 7-3, 7-8, 7-9]

7-6. Some coverage models, such as those of the VHA, vocational rehabilitation agencies, private disability carriers (e.g., Unum and Prudential), and some private health insurers, are more holistic than others, providing access to a greater range of assistive products and technologies and related services that are appropriate to meeting individuals' needs and facilitating their ability to work. [Finding 7-3]

7-7. Ensuring continued access to appropriate assistive products and technologies and related services is vital to promoting a successful transition from high school to pathways to employment. [Finding 7-10]

7-8. Knowledge and training that empower users to self-advocate or have a significant other (e.g., family member, friend, or professional) advocate for them can lead to successful access to appropriate assistive products and technologies and related services. [Findings 7-6, 7-7, 7-11]

REFERENCES

AAA (American Academy of Audiology). 2012. *Standards of practice for audiology*. http://www.audiology.org/sites/default/files/documents/StandardsofPractice.pdf (accessed July 18, 2017).

ABLE National Resource Center. 2017. *What we're about*. http://ablenrc.org (accessed April 7, 2017).

Aetna. 2016a. *Hearing aids*. Policy no. 0612. http://www.aetna.com/cpb/medical/data/600_699/0612.html (accessed January 12, 2017).

Aetna. 2016b. *Myoelectric upper limb prostheses*. Policy no. 0399. http://www.aetna.com/cpb/medical/data/300_399/0399.html (accessed January 12, 2017).

Aetna. 2016c. *Speech generating devices*. Policy no. 0437. http://www.aetna.com/cpb/medical/data/400_499/0437.html (accessed January 12, 2017).

Aetna. 2016d. *Wheelchairs and power operated vehicles (scooters)*. Policy no. 0271. http://www.aetna.com/cpb/medical/data/200_299/0271.html (accessed January 12, 2017).

Amerigroup. 2016. *Clinical UM guideline: Myoelectric upper extremity prosthetic devices*. Guideline CG-OR-PR-05. https://medicalpolicies.amerigroup.com/medicalpolicies/guidelines/gl_pw_c169421.htm (accessed January 12, 2017).

Andrews, M. 2012. Unlike most insurers, United Healthcare is offering big discounts on hearing aids. *The Washington Post*, April 9. https://www.washingtonpost.com/national/health-science/unlike-mostinsurers-unitedhealthcare-is-offering-big-discounts-on-hearingaids/2012/04/09/gIQA8I0Z6S_story.html?utm_term=.41e62d96906d (accessed January 13, 2017).

Arva, J., G. Paleg, M. Lange, J. Lieberman, M. Schmeler, B. Dicianno, M. Babince, and L. Rosen. 2009. RESNA position on the application of wheelchair standing devices. *Assistive Technology* 21(3):161-168.

ASHA (American Speech-Language-Hearing Association). 2017. *State insurance mandates for hearing aids.* http://www.asha.org/advocacy/state/issues/ha_reimbursement (accessed February 9, 2017).

AT Program News. 2011. The average cost of a reasonable accommodation for a Massachusetts state employee is . . . *AT Program News*, March 28. http://www.atprogramnews.com/2011/03/the-average-cost-of-a-reasonable-accommodation-for-a-massachusetts-state-employee-is-.html (accessed January 23, 2017).

Atcherson, S. R., R. I. Zraick, and K. Hadden. 2013. A need for health literacy curriculum: Knowledge of health literacy among U.S. audiologists and speech-language pathologists in Arkansas. *Education for Health* 26(2):85-88.

Awsumb, J. M., F. E. Balcazar, and F. Alvarado. 2016. Vocational rehabilitation transition outcomes of youth with disabilities from a Midwestern state. *Rehabilitation Research, Policy, and Education* 30(1):48-64.

Ayres, S. 2013. America's 10 million unemployed youth spell danger for future economic growth. *Center for American Progress*, June 5. http://www.americanprogress.org/issues/economy/report/2013/06/05/65373/americas-10-million-unemployed-youth-spell-danger-for-future-economic-growth (accessed January 18, 2017).

Balcazar, F. E., T. Garate-Serafini, and C. B. Keys. 2004. The need for action when conducting intervention research: The multiple roles of community psychologist. *American Journal of Community Psychology* 33(3-4):243-252.

Balser, D. 2007. Predictors of workplace accommodations for employees with mobility-related disabilities. *Administration & Society* 39(5):656-683.

BlueCross BlueShield of Tennessee. 2016. *BlueCross BlueShield of Tennessee medical policy manual: Myoelectric prosthetic components for the upper limb.* https://www.bcbst.com/mpmanual/Myoelectric_Prosthetic_Components_for_the_Upper_Limb.htm (accessed January 23, 2017).

Bridgeland, J. M., J. J. DiIulio, and K. B. Morrison. 2006. *The silent epidemic: Perspectives of high school dropouts.* Washington, DC: Civic Enterprises.

Calderone, J. 2017a. 5 ways to cut hearing aid costs. *Consumer Reports.* http://www.consumerreports.org/hearing-aids/save-on-cost-of-prescription-hearing-aids (accessed April 7, 2017).

Calderone, J. 2017b. What you need to know when buying a hearing aid. *Consumer Reports.* http://www.consumerreports.org/hearing-aids/what-you-need-to-know-when-buying-a-hearing-aid (accessed April 7, 2017).

CAP (Computer/Electronic Accommodations Program). 2017. *About CAP.* http://www.cap.mil/AboutCAP/AboutCAP.aspx (accessed January 10, 2017).

Caposecco, A., L. Hickson, and C. Meyer. 2014. Hearing aid user guides: Suitability for older adults. *International Journal of Audiology* 53(Suppl 1):S43-S51.

CATADA (Center for Assistive Technology Act Data Assistance). 2017a. *AT Program Activity Participation.* http://www.catada.info/content/program-activity-participation (accessed May 31, 2017).

CATADA. 2017b. *State AT Program Information.* http://www.catada.info/content/state-program-information (accessed May 31, 2017).

Center for Medicare Advocacy. n.d.-a. *Durable Medical Equipment (DME).* http://www.medicareadvocacy.org/medicare-info/medicare-part-b/durable-medical-equipment (accessed January 22, 2017).

Center for Medicare Advocacy. n.d.-b. *Medicare savings programs.* http://www.medicareadvocacy.org/medicare-info/medicare-savings-programs (accessed January 18, 2017).

Center for Mental Health in Schools at UCLA (University of California, Los Angeles). 2008. *Frameworks for systematic transformation of students and learning supports.* http://smhp.psych.ucla.edu/pdfdocs/systemic/frameworksforsystemictransformation.pdf (accessed January 23, 2017).

Center for Workers with Disabilities/American Public Human Services Administration. n.d. *Fact sheet #15 Medicaid buy-in*. http://www.nationaldisabilitynavigator.org/ndnrc-materials/fact-sheets/fact-sheet-15 (accessed January 17, 2017).

CMS (Centers for Medicare & Medicaid Services). 2005a. *Decision memo for mobility assistive equipment (CAG-00274N)*. https://www.cms.gov/medicare-coverage-database/details/nca-decision-memo.aspx?NCAId=143&DocID=CAG-00274N&bc=gAAAABAACAAAAA%3d%3d& (accessed January 23, 2017).

CMS. 2005b. *National Coverage Determination (NCD) for Durable Medical Equipment reference list (280.1)*. https://www.cms.gov/medicare-coverage-database/details/ncd-details.aspx?NCDId=190&bc=AgAAQAAAAAAA&ncdver=2 (accessed January 23, 2017).

CMS. 2005c. *National Coverage Determination (NCD) for Mobility Assistive Equipment (MAE)*. https://www.cms.gov/medicare-coverage-database/details/ncd-details.aspx?NCDId=219&ncdver=2&bc=AgAAgAAAAAAA& (accessed January 17, 2017).

CMS. 2013. *CMS letter to Texas Health and Human Services Commission, May 21, 2013*. http://www.nls.org/files/Disability%20Law%20Hotlines/National%20AT%20Advocacy/TXDMEfinal05212013.pdf (accessed January 22, 2017).

CMS. 2014a. *EPSDT—A guide for state coverage in the Medicaid benefit for children and adolescents*. http://www.medicaid.gov/Medicaid-CHIP-Program-Information/By-Topics/Benefits/Early-and-Periodic-Screening-Diagnostic-and-Treatment.html (accessed January 23, 2017).

CMS. 2014b. *Speech generating devices*. https://www.cms.gov/medicare-coverage-database/details/medicare-coverage-document-details.aspx?MCDId=26&mcdtypename=National+Benefit+Category+Analyses&MCDIndexType=3&bc=AgAEAAAAAAAAAA%3d%3d&#final (accessed January 17, 2017).

CMS. 2015a. *National Coverage Determination (NCD) for speech generating devices*. https://www.cms.gov/medicare-coverage-database/details/ncd-details.aspx?NCDId=274&ncdver=1&DocID=50.1&SearchType=Advanced&bc=IAAAABAAAAAA& (accessed January 17, 2017).

CMS. 2015b. *On its 50th anniversary, more than 55 million Americans covered by Medicare*. https://www.cms.gov/Newsroom/MediaReleaseDatabase/Press-releases/2015-Press-releases-items/2015-07-28.html (accessed January 17, 2017).

CMS. 2015c. *Prior authorization of Power Mobility Devices (PMDs) demonstration*. https://www.cms.gov/Research-Statistics-Data-and-Systems/Monitoring-Programs/Medicare-FFS-Compliance-Programs/Medical-Review/PADemo.html (accessed January 22, 2017).

CMS. 2016a. *Audiology services*. https://www.cms.gov/Medicare/Medicare-Fee-For-Service-Payment/PhysicianFeeSched/audiology.html (accessed March 12, 2017).

CMS. 2016b. *Medicare claims processing manual: Chapter 20—Durable Medical Equipment, Prosthetics, Orthotics, and Supplies (DMEPOS)*. https://www.cms.gov/Regulations-and-Guidance/Guidance/Manuals/downloads/clm104c20.pdf (accessed January 23, 2017).

CMS. 2016c. *Medicare managed care manual: Chapter 4—Benefits and beneficiary protections*. https://www.cms.gov/Regulations-and-Guidance/Guidance/Manuals/Downloads/mc86c04.pdf (accessed January 22, 2017).

CMS. 2016d. *Medicare managed care manual: Chapter 15—Covered medical and other health services*. https://www.cms.gov/Regulations-and-Guidance/Guidance/Manuals/downloads/bp102c15.pdf (accessed January 22, 2017).

CMS. 2016e. *Medicare parts A & B appeals process*. ICN 006562. https://www.cms.gov/Outreach-and-Education/Medicare-Learning-Network-MLN/MLNProducts/downloads/MedicareAppealsprocess.pdf (accessed January 23, 2017).

CMS. 2016f. *Medicare program integrity manual: Chapter 5—Items and services having special DME review considerations*. https://www.cms.gov/Regulations-and-Guidance/Guidance/Manuals/downloads/pim83c05.pdf (accessed January 23, 2017).

CMS. 2016g. *Who are the MACs.* https://www.cms.gov/Medicare/Medicare-Contracting/Medicare-Administrative-Contractors/Who-are-the-MACs.html (accessed January 23, 2017).

CMS. 2017. *What's Medicare supplemental insurance (Medigap)?* https://www.medicare.gov/supplement-other-insurance/medigap/whats-medigap.html (accessed March 10, 2017).

CMS. n.d.-a. *Competitive Bidding Program.* https://www.medicare.gov/what-medicare-covers/part-b/competitive-bidding-program.html (accessed January 17, 2017).

CMS. n.d.-b. *License agreements.* https://www.cms.gov/medicare-coverage-database/details/lcd-details.aspx?LCDId=33789&ver=11&Date=&DocID=L33789&bc=iAAAABAAAAAAA%3d%3d& (accessed February 21, 2017).

CMS. n.d.-c. *List of Medicaid benefits.* https://www.medicaid.gov/medicaid/benefits/list-of-benefits/index.html (accessed February 21, 2017).

CMS. n.d.-d. *Your Medicare coverage: Hearing & balance exams & hearing aids.* https://www.medicare.gov/coverage/hearing-and-balance-exam-and-hearing-aids.html (accessed March 12, 2017).

Commonwealth of Massachusetts. 2009. *Strategic plan to make Massachusetts a model employer for people with disabilities report of the Disability Task Force on Employment.* http://www.mass.gov/anf/employment-equal-access-disability/diversity-access-and-opportunity/model-employer/model-employer-for-people-with-disabilities.html (accessed January 23, 2017).

Community Health Advocates. 2012. *Section 9A.1—What is commercial insurance?* http://www.communityhealthadvocates.org/publications/advocates-guide/section-9a1-%E2%80%93-what-commercial-insurance (accessed January 12, 2017).

Cook, A., and J. Polgar. 2008. *Cook & Hussey's assistive technologies: Principles and practices*, 3rd ed. St. Louis, MO: Mosby Elsevier Publisher.

Crisp, R. 2005. Key factors related to vocational outcome: Trends for six disability groups. *Journal of Rehabilitation* 71(4):30-37.

Dalton, D. S., K. J. Cruickshanks, B. E. Klein, R. Klein, T. L. Wiley, and D. M. Nondahl. 2003. The impact of hearing loss on quality of life in older adults. *Gerontologist* 43(5):661-668.

Dicianno, B. E., A. Morgan, J. Lieberman, and L. Rosen. 2016. Rehabilitation Engineering & Assistive Technology Society (RESNA) position on the application of wheelchair standing devices: 2013 current state of the literature. *Assistive Technology* 28(1):57-62.

DOL (U.S. Department of Labor) and BLS (U.S. Bureau of Labor Statistics). 2015. *Employment and unemployment among youth summary.* www.bls.gov/news.release/youth.nr0.htm (accessed January 23, 2017).

Domin, D., D. Golden, and F. A. Smith. 2016. *A national data summary of state assistive technology programs: Fiscal year 2015.* http://www.catada.info/sites/catada.info/files/files/AT_nationalreport2016_accessible.pdf (accessed January 23, 2017).

EEOC (U.S. Equal Employment Opportunity Commission). 2002. *EEOC enforcement guidance on reasonable accommodation and undue hardship under the Americans with Disabilities Act.* https://www.eeoc.gov/policy/docs/accommodation.html (accessed September 15, 2016).

Employment and Disability Institute. 2013. *Absence and disability management practices for an aging workforce.* http://digitalcommons.ilr.cornell.edu/cgi/viewcontent.cgi?article=1320&context=edicollect (accessed January 23, 2017).

Fabian, E. S. 2007. Urban youth with disabilities: Factors affecting transition employment. *Rehabilitation Counseling Bulletin* 50(3):130-138.

FODAC (Friends of Disabled Adults and Children). 2017. *About our programs.* http://www.fodac.org/programs (accessed April 7, 2017).

Foundation for Sight and Sound. 2016. *Help America Hear Program.* https://www.foundationforsightandsound.org/help_america_hear.php?gclid=CMHv3u3BgNECFQdWDQodd3wCyA (accessed January 17, 2017).

GAO (U.S. General Accountability Office). 2016. *Medicare: Utilization and expenditures for complex wheelchair accessories.* http://www.gao.gov/assets/680/677602.pdf (accessed January 22, 2017).

Garcia-Iriarte, E., F. Balcazar, and T. Taylor-Ritzler. 2007. Analysis of case managers' support of youth with disabilities transitioning from school to work. *Journal of Vocational Rehabilitation* 26(3):129-140.

Golinker, L. 2015. *SGD Medicare developments, August 2015: Frequently asked questions.* https://www.resna.org/sites/default/files/legacy/resources/2015%2008%2006%20FAQ%20re%202015%20NCD%20and%20Gleason%20Act%20Final.pdf (accessed January 22, 2017).

Hoyer, T. E. 2001. *CMS letter to Lewis Golinker, May 4, 2001.* http://aacfundinghelp.com/funding_programs/01.%20Medicare/A2.%20Computer%20and%20PDA%20Based%20Device%20Coverage/Letter%20dated%20May%204,2001%20to%20Lewis%20Golinker.pdf (accessed January 22, 2017).

Hasnain, R., and F. Balcazar. 2009. Predicting community- versus facility-based employment for transition-aged, young adults with disabilities: The role of race, ethnicity, and support systems. *Journal of Vocational Rehabilitation* 31(3):175-188.

HHS (U.S. Department of Health and Human Services). 2000a. *Olmstead update no. 3.* http://www.nasddds.org/uploads/documents/Olmstead_letter_31.pdf (accessed February 21, 2017).

HHS. 2000b. *Healthy People 2010.* Washington, DC: U.S. Government Printing Office.

HHS. 2007. *Quick guide to health literacy.* https://health.gov/communication/literacy/quickguide/Quickguide.pdf (accessed March 14, 2017).

HLAA (Hearing Loss Association of America). 2015. *Medicaid regulations.* http://www.hearingloss.org/content/medicaid-regulations (accessed February 9, 2017).

Hrnack, S. A., S. P. Elmore, and G. W. Brindley 2009. Literacy and patient information in the amputee population. *Journal of Prosthetics and Orthotics* 21(4):223-226.

Iowa Compass, Center for Developmental Disabilities. 2016. *Workers' compensation as a source for assistive technology funding.* http://www.iowacompass.org/workerscomptipsheet.htm (accessed January 23, 2017).

IRS (Internal Revenue Service). 2015a. *New IRS guidance to simplify ABLE program administration.* https://www.irs.gov/uac/newsroom/new-irs-guidance-to-simplify-able-program-administration (accessed April 7, 2017).

IRS. 2015b. *Notice 2015-81: Section 529A interim guidance regarding certain provisions of proposed regulations relating to qualified ABLE programs.* https://www.irs.gov/pub/irs-drop/n-15-81.pdf (accessed April 7, 2017).

Izzo, M., A. Yurick, and B. McArrell. 2009. Supported eText: Effects of text-to-speech on access and achievement for high school students with disabilities. *Journal of Special Education Technology* 24(3):9-20.

Jackson, M. 2016. *Utilization of assistive products and technology.* Presentation to the NASEM Committee on the Use of Selected Assistive Products and Technologies in Eliminating or Reducing the Effects of Impairments, Washington, DC, May 16.

Jain, R., M. Conway, and V. Choitz. 2015. *Connecting young adults to employment: Results from a national survey of service providers.* Washington, DC: The Aspen Institute. http://www.aspenwsi.org/wordpress/wp-content/uploads/YAemploy.pdf (accessed January 23, 2017).

JAN (Job Accommodation Network). 2016. *Workplace accommodations: Low cost, high impact.* http://askjan.org/media/lowcosthighimpact.html (accessed January 23, 2017).

JAN. n.d. *Frequently asked questions*. http://askjan.org/links/faqs.htm#1 (accessed January 23, 2017).

Justice in Aging. 2016. *Durable Medical Equipment: CMS request for information*. http://www.justiceinaging.org/wp-content/uploads/2016/07/DME_Comments_July2016.pdf (accessed February 21, 2017).

Kaiser Family Foundation. n.d. *Medicaid managed care market tracker*. http://kff.org/data-collection/medicaid-managed-care-market-tracker (accessed January 17, 2017).

Kehn, M. 2013. *Enrollment, employment, and earnings in the Medicaid Buy-In program, 2011*. https://www.mathematica-mpr.com/our-publications-and-findings/publications/enrollment-employment-and-earnings-in-the-medicaid-buyin-program-2011 (accessed January 17, 2017).

Kochkin, S. 2010. MarkeTrak VIII: The efficacy of hearing aids in achieving compensation equity in the workplace. *The Hearing Journal* 63(10):19-24.

Krause, J. S., and J. V. Terza. 2006. Injury and demographic factors predictive of disparities in earnings after spinal cord injury. *Archives of Physical Medicine and Rehabilitation* 87(10):1318-1326.

Kubrin, D. 2016. *Durable Medical Equipment (DME) coverage: Fully insured commercial insurance perspective*. Presentation to the Committee on the Use of Selected Assistive Products and Technologies in Eliminating or Reducing the Effects of Impairments, Washington, DC, July 18.

Kusmin, L. D. 2006. *Rural America at a glance, 2006 edition*. Economic Information Bulletin Number 18. Washington, DC: U.S. Department of Agriculture, Economic Research Service. https://www.ers.usda.gov/webdocs/publications/eib18/29299_eib18_002.pdf (accessed January 23, 2017).

Kutner, M., E. Greenberg, Y. Jin, and C. Paulsen. 2006. *The health literacy of America's adults: Results from the 2003 National Assessment of Adult Literacy* (NCES 2006-483). U.S. Department of Education. Washington, DC: National Center for Education Statistics.

Lengnick-Hall, M. L., P. M. Gaunt, and A. A. R. Brooks. n.d. *Why employers don't hire people with disabilities: A survey of the literature*. Wichita, KS: CPRF. http://www.cprf.org/studies/why-employers-dont-hire-people-with-disabilities-a-survey-of-the-literature (accessed March 14, 2017).

McNaughton, D., J. Light, and S. Gulla. 2003. Opening up a "whole new world": Employer and co-worker perspectives on working with individuals who use augmentative and alternative communication. *Augmentative and Alternative Communication* 19(4):235-253.

Meade, M. A., A. Lewis, M. Njeri Jackson, and D. W. Hess. 2004. Race, employment, and spinal cord injury. *Archives of Physical Medicine and Rehabilitation* 85(11):1782-1792.

Nair, E. L., and K. M. Cienkowski. 2010. The impact of health literacy on patient understanding of counseling and education materials. *International Journal of Audiology* 49(2):71-75.

NASEM (National Academies of Sciences, Engineering, and Medicine). 2016. *Hearing health care for older adults: Priorities for improving access and affordability*. Washington, DC: The National Academies Press.

National Disability Rights Network. 2017. *NDRN member agencies*. http://ndrn.org/en/ndrn-member-agencies.html (accessed April 7, 2017).

Nechanicky, P. L. 2016. *Veterans Health Administration: Prosthetic and sensory aids service*. Presentation to the Committee on the Use of Selected Assistive Products and Technologies in Eliminating or Reducing the Effects of Impairments, Washington, DC, March 16.

New York State Department of Health. 2016. *Medicaid Buy-In program for working people with disabilities*. https://www.health.ny.gov/health_care/medicaid/program/buy_in (accessed January 17, 2017).

NLS (Neighborhood Legal Services, Inc.). 2011a. *Letters of medical justification: A checklist for health care providers.* http://nls.org/Disability/NationalAssistiveTechnologyProject/DidYouKnow/Medicaid/LettersofMedicalJustification (accessed January 22, 2017).

NLS. 2011b. *Workers' compensation and AT.* http://www.nls.org/Disability/National AssistiveTechnologyProject/DidYouKnow/WorkersComp (accessed January 23, 2017).

NLS. 2015. *The crime victims compensation fund—a little known funding source for AT in some cases.* http://www.nls.org/files/Disability%20Law%20Hotlines/Did%20You%20Know/Crime%20Victims%20Compensation%20Fund.pdf (accessed January 23, 2017).

Noridian Healthcare Solutions. 2016. *Group 3 power wheelchair requirements.* https://med.noridianmedicare.com/web/jddme/dmepos/pmds/group-3-power-wheelchair-requirements (accessed January 17, 2017).

Noridian Healthcare Solutions. 2017. *Correct coding—billing of powered L-coded items.* https://med.noridianmedicare.com/web/jddme/article-detail/-/view/2230703/correct-coding-billing-of-powered-l-coded-items (April 7, 2017).

ODEP (Office of Disability Employment Policy). n.d. *Disability employment policy resources by topic.* https://www.dol.gov/odep/resources/jan.htm (accessed January 23, 2017).

Oertle, K. M., and J. S. Trach. 2007. Interagency collaboration: The importance of rehabilitation professionals' involvement in transition. *Journal of Rehabilitation* 73(3):36-44.

Office of Rehabilitation Services. 2015a. *Fact sheet for audiology services.* http://www.prosthetics.va.gov/factsheet/Audiology-FactSheet.pdf (accessed January 11, 2017).

Office of Rehabilitation Services. 2015b. *Speech-language pathology fact sheet.* Washington, DC: VA. http://www.prosthetics.va.gov/factsheet/SLP-FactSheet.pdf (accessed January 11, 2017).

Office of Rehabilitation Services. 2016. *Fact sheet for amputation system of care.* Washington, DC: VA. http://www.prosthetics.va.gov/factsheet/ASoC-FactSheet.pdf (accessed January 11, 2017).

Ozawa, M. N., and Y. H. Yeo. 2006. Work status and work performance of people with disabilities. *Journal of Disability Policy Studies* 17(3):180-190.

Paleg, G., and R. Livingstone. 2015. Systematic review and clinical recommendations for dosage of supported home-based standing programs for adults with stroke, spinal cord injury and other neurological conditions. *BMC Musculoskeletal Disorders* 16(1):358.

Paradise, J. 2015. *Medicaid moving forward.* http://kff.org/health-reform/issue-brief/medicaid-moving-forward (accessed January 17, 2017).

Randolph, D. W., and E. M. Andresen. 2004. Disability, gender, and unemployment relationships in the United States from the Behavioral Risk Factor Surveillance System. *Disability & Society* 19(4):403-414.

Regence. 2016. *Regence medical policy manual: Myoelectric prosthetic components for the upper limb.* Policy no. 80. http://blue.regence.com/trgmedpol/dme/dme80.pdf (accessed January 23, 2017).

RESNA Catalyst Project. 2017. *AFP Information Center.* http://resnaprojects.org/afp/info center/index.html (accessed January 22, 2017).

Richardson, S. K. 1998. *Letter from Director of the Centers for Medicaid and State Operations to State Medical Director, September 4, 1998.* http://www.medicaid.gov/Federal-Policy-Guidance/downloads/SMD090498.pdf (accessed January 23, 2017).

Richtman, M. n.d. *Medicare must continue to evolve—add coverage for hearing aids.* http://www.medicareadvocacy.org/46-medicare-must-continue-to-evolve-add-coverage-for-hearing-aids (accessed January 23, 2017).

Rose, D. H., and A. Meyer. 2002. *Teaching every student in the Digital Age: Universal design for learning.* Alexandria, VA: Association for Supervision and Curriculum Development.

Sheldon, J. R., and R. M. Hager. 2011. *Work, assistive technology and transition-aged youth: Funding for work-related assistive technology through special education programs, state vocational rehabilitation agencies, Medicaid, Medicare and SSI's plan for achieving self support.* http://nls.org/files/What's%20New/WorkATandTAY.pdf (accessed January 22, 2017).

Sheldon, J. R., and E. Lopez-Soto. n.d. *Plan for achieving self-support: An SSI work incentive and approach to self-directing vocational rehabilitation to support a range of work goals.* http://digitalcommons.ilr.cornell.edu/cgi/viewcontent.cgi?article=1267&context=edicollect (accessed January 22, 2017).

Sheldon, J. R., and M. O'Connell. 2016 (unpublished). *Analysis of financial access to committee-selected assistive products and technologies: Discussion of funding sources for wheeled/seated mobility devices, upper extremity prostheses, and products and technologies that pertain to hearing and to communication and speech.* Paper commissioned by the Committee on the Use of Selected Assistive Products and Technologies, National Academies of Sciences, Engineering, and Medicine, Washington, DC.

Shinohara, K., and J. O. Wobbrock. 2011. *In the shadow of misperception: Assistive technology use and social interactions.* Presented at CHI 2011, Vancouver, BC, Canada, May 7-12.

Smith, D. L., and Gutman, S. A. 2011. Health literacy in occupational therapy practice and research. *American Journal of Occupational Therapy* 65(July/August):367-369.

SSA (U.S. Social Security Administration). 2001. *Income of disabled worker beneficiaries.* No. 13-11706. Washington, DC: Office of Policy, Research, Evaluation and Statistics, SSA.

SSA. 2011. *SI 01715.005 Medicaid groups.* https://secure.ssa.gov/poms.nsf/lnx/0501715005 (accessed January 17, 2017).

SSA. 2012a. *SI 00870.025 Documenting and reviewing a PASS-PASS expert.* https://secure.ssa.gov/poms.nsf/lnx/0500870025 (accessed January 17, 2017).

SSA. 2012b. *SI 00835.300 Presumed Maximum Value (PMV) Rule.* https://secure.ssa.gov/poms.nsf/lnx/0500835300 (accessed January 17, 2017).

SSA. 2014a. *SI 01715.010 Medicaid and Supplemental Security Income (SSI) program.* https://secure.ssa.gov/poms.nsf/lnx/0501715010 (accessed January 17, 2017).

SSA. 2014b. *SI 02302.050 Individualized threshold calculation.* https://secure.ssa.gov/poms.nsf/lnx/0502302050 (accessed January 17, 2017).

SSA. 2014c. *HI 00610.001 Scope of benefits (SMI).* https://secure.ssa.gov/poms.nsf/lnx/0600610001 (accessed January 17, 2017).

SSA. 2015a. *SI 02302.010 1619 Policy principles.* https://secure.ssa.gov/poms.nsf/lnx/0502302010 (accessed January 17, 2017).

SSA. 2015b. *HI 00801.170 Premium-HI for the working disabled.* https://secure.ssa.gov/poms.nsf/lnx/0600801170 (accessed January 17, 2017).

SSA. 2015c. *HI 00805.005 Eligibility for SMI.* https://secure.ssa.gov/poms.nsf/lnx/0600805005 (accessed January 17, 2017).

SSA. 2015d. *HI 00601.001 Scope of benefits.* https://secure.ssa.gov/poms.nsf/lnx/0600601001 (accessed January 17, 2017).

SSA. 2015e. *HI 00208.066 The Medicare Advantage (MA) program.* https://secure.ssa.gov/apps10/poms.nsf/lnx/0600208066 (accessed January 17, 2017).

SSA. 2016a. *SI 0175.020 List of state Medicaid programs for the aged, blind, and disabled.* https://secure.ssa.gov/poms.NSF/lnx/0501715020 (accessed January 17, 2017).

SSA. 2016b. *SI 02302.200 Charted threshold amounts.* https://secure.ssa.gov/poms.nsf/lnx/0502302200 (accessed January 17, 2017).

SSA. 2016c. *SI 01130.200 Automobiles and other vehicles used for transportation.* https://secure.ssa.gov/apps10/poms.nsf/lnx/0501130200 (accessed January 17, 2017).

SSA. 2016d. *SI 01130.740 Achieving a Better Life Experience (ABLE) account*. https://secure.ssa.gov/poms.nsf/lnx/0501130740 (accessed January 17, 2017).

SSA. 2016e. *SI 02301.201 Description of SSI posteligibility (PE) events*. https://secure.ssa.gov/poms.nsf/lnx/0502301201 (accessed January 17, 2017).

SSA. 2017. *Ticket to work: Find help*. https://www.choosework.net/findhelp (accessed April 7, 2017).

Stewart, D., M. Freeman, M. Law, H. Healy, J. Burke-Gaffney, M. Forhan, N. Young, and S. Guenther. 2010. Transition to adulthood for youth with disabilities: Evidence from the literature. In *International encyclopedia of rehabilitation*, edited by J. H. Stone and M. Blouin. http://cirrie.buffalo.edu/encyclopedia/en/article/110 (accessed January 23, 2017).

Taylor-Ritzler, T. 2007. A grounded theory of first high school dropout for urban, ethnic minority teenage mothers with learning disabilities. *The Community Psychologist* 40(2):18-20.

Tergesen, A. 2012. If Medicare tells you "no." *Wall Street Journal*, October 18. http://www.wsj.com/articles/SB10000872396390443890304578006274005071746 (accessed January 22, 2017).

Ticket to Work. 2017. *Payments under the Ticket program*. https://yourtickettowork.com/web/ttw/payments (accessed April 7, 2017).

TMHP (Texas Medicaid & Health Partnership). 2016. *Texas Medicaid provider procedures manual,* Vol. 2. http://www.tmhp.com/tmppm/2016/Vol2_Durable_Medical_Equipment_and_Supplies_Handbook.pdf (accessed February 21, 2017).

Tufts (Tufts Health Plan). 2016. *Medical necessity guidelines: Upper limb prostheses*. https://tuftshealthplan.com/documents/providers/guidelines/medical-necessity-guidelines/upper-limb-prostheses-mng (accessed April 6, 2017).

Tufts. 2017a. *Audiology professional payment policy*. https://tuftshealthplan.com/documents/providers/payment-policies/audiology-professional-payment-policy (accessed April 7, 2017).

Tufts. 2017b. *Durable medical equipment payment policy*. https://tuftshealthplan.com/documents/providers/payment-policies/durable-medical-equipment-payment-poli (accessed April 7, 2017).

Tufts. 2017c. *Medical necessity guidelines: Power operated vehicles*. https://tuftshealthplan.com/documents/providers/guidelines/medical-necessity-guidelines/power-operated-vehicle (accessed April 7, 2017).

Tufts. 2017d. *Medical necessity guidelines: Power wheelchairs*. https://tuftshealthplan.com/documents/providers/guidelines/medical-necessity-guidelines/power-wheelchairs (accessed April 7, 2017).

Tugman, K., and J. Kramschuster. 2016. *The use of assistive technology in return-to-work*. Presentation to the NASEM Committee on the Use of Selected Assistive Devices in Eliminating or Reducing the Effects of Impairments, Washington, DC, September 27.

United Cerebral Palsy. 2015. *The UCP Elsie S. Bellows Fund*. http://ucp.org/resources/assistive-technology/the-ucp-elsie-s-bellows-fund (accessed January 17, 2017).

United Spinal Association. 2015. *Financial assistance for individuals with disabilities*. http://www.spinalcord.org/resource-center/askus/index.php?pg=kb.printer.friendly&id=10 (accessed January 17, 2017).

UnitedHealth Group. 2017. *Affordable hearing aids now available to UnitedHealthcare vision plan customers nationwide*. http://www.unitedhealthgroup.com/newsroom/articles/feed/unitedhealthcare/2013/0724affordablehearingaids.aspx (accessed April 5, 2017).

U.S. Department of Education. 1991. *Policy Directive: RSA-PD-92-02*. https://www2.ed.gov/policy/speced/guid/rsa/pd-92-02.pdf (accessed April 7, 2017).

U.S. Department of Education. 2014. *Annual report to Congress on the Assistive Technology Act of 1998, as amended, for fiscal years 2009 and 2010*. https://www2.ed.gov/about/reports/annual/rsa/atsg/2009-10/at-act-report-2009-10.pdf (accessed January 17, 2017).

U.S. Department of Justice. 2009. *A guide to disability rights laws*. https://www.ada.gov/cguide.htm#anchor65610 (accessed January 10, 2017).

VA (U.S. Department of Veterans Affairs). 2008. *Wheelchairs and special mobility aids*. https://www.va.gov/vhapublications/ViewPublication.asp?pub_ID=1634 (accessed March 13, 2017).

VA. 2015. *Veterans Health Administration: Ten things to know about the Choice Program*. https://www.va.gov/HEALTH/NewsFeatures/2015/July/10-Things-to-Know-About-Choice-Program.asp (accessed January 17, 2017).

VA. 2016a. *Rehabilitation and prosthetic services*. http://www.prosthetics.va.gov (accessed January 17, 2017).

VA. 2016b. *VHA Office of Community Care*. https://www.va.gov/PURCHASEDCARE/programs/providerinfo/provider_info_NVC.asp#sthash.FpKU9r5P.dpuf (accessed January 17, 2017).

VA. n.d.-a. *Health benefits: Veterans eligibility*. https://www.va.gov/HEALTHBENEFITS/apply/veterans.asp (accessed January 10, 2017).

V.A. n.d.-b. *Returning service members (OEF/OIF/OND)*. http://www.oefoif.va.gov (accessed January 23, 2017).

VA. n.d.-c. *Veterans Benefits Administration*. http://www.benefits.va.gov/benefits (accessed January 23, 2017).

VA. n.d.-d. *Veterans Health Administration: About VHA*. https://www.va.gov/health/aboutVHA.asp (accessed January 23, 2017).

VA. n.d.-e. *Federal benefits for veterans, dependents and survivors: Chapter 1 health care benefits*. https://www.va.gov/opa/publications/benefits_book/benefits_chap01.asp (accessed March 13, 2017).

Wagner, M., L. Newman, R. Cameto, and P. Levine. 2005. *Changes over time in the early post school outcomes of youth with disabilities. A report of findings from the National Longitudinal Transition Study (NLTS) and the National Longitudinal Transition Study-2 (NLTS2)*. Washington, DC: National Center for Special Education Research.

Weathers, R. R., G. Walter, S. Schley, J. Hennessey, J. Hemmeter, and R. V. Burkhauser. 2007. How postsecondary education improves adult outcomes for Supplemental Security Income children with severe hearing impairments. *Social Security Bulletin* 67(2):101-131.

Wells, T., G. Sandefur, and D. Hogan. 2003. What happens after the high school years among young person with disabilities? *Social Forces* 82(2):803-832.

Whitson, H. E., and F. R. Lin. 2014. Hearing and vision care for older adults: sensing a need to update Medicare policy. *JAMA* 312(17):1739-1740.

Wittenburg, D. C., and E. Maag. 2002. School to where? A literature review on economic outcomes of youth with disabilities. *Journal of Vocational Rehabilitation* 17(4):265-280.

ANNEX TABLE 7-1
Summary of Payer or Coverage Options for Assistive Devices

Standard	Relevant Coverage or Payer	Coverage Parameters	
Educationally relevant	School system	Must promote educationally relevant goals in the student's individualized education plan (IEP)	
Medically necessary	Private insurance	Devices must be required because of a medical condition	
	Medicare/Medicaid		

	Limitations: Policy-Related	Limitations: Device-Related	Limitations: Geographic
	Devices are taken away when students graduate	May not be the most effective device	High-tech devices may not be available in rural and frontier areas and equally across the country Individuals trained in assessment of the need for appropriate assistive devices and/or the use of high-tech devices are not available nationwide
	Policies specifically exclude devices designed to perform work tasks	Private insurance and Medicaid may not cover the cost of clinicians able to train people to use the devices	Trained clinicians may not be available nationwide to assess the need for appropriate assistive devices and/or teach people to use the devices
	Medicare limits devices to those used in the home	May limit the type of device covered (e.g., standard rather than custom wheelchair; low-tech prosthetic devices rather than devices that meet the person's need to be able to return to work) Medicare and private insurance do not pay for hearing aids or communication devices	

continued

ANNEX TABLE 7-1
Continued

Standard	Relevant Coverage or Payer	Coverage Parameters
Vocationally relevant	Vocational rehabilitation (VR) service	Depends on the budget and the VR counselor and must be related to a vocational goal
	Disability insurance	Depends on the policy
	Workers' compensation	States require employers to cover employees and will pay for home modifications, medical devices, assistive technology (AT), personal care services, and workplace modifications and accommodations, especially if needed to return to work
	Supplemental Security Income (SSI) Plan to Achieve Self-Support (PASS)	Allows a person who is eligible for SSI to set money aside for any purpose tied to achieving the person's occupational objective from a specific approved plan

	Limitations: Policy-Related	Limitations: Device-Related	Limitations: Geographic
	No guarantee of devices; availability can vary geographic-ally and from VR counselor to VR counselor		Devices and access to trained clinicians who can assess the need for appropriate assistive devices and train users are not available nationwide
	Usually covers devices that will facilitate the individual's return to work		
	No guarantee of these benefits; may require extensive advocacy, hiring an attorney, etc.	Can cover hearing aids, custom wheelchairs, prosthetic devices	
	Short-term funding; a person is allowed only one PASS for the same occupational objective	Can cover devices, AT, making buildings accessible, etc. related to an occupational objective; good when other funding sources are not available	

continued

ANNEX TABLE 7-1
Continued

Standard	Relevant Coverage or Payer	Coverage Parameters	
Service-related	Veterans Health Administration (VHA)	Promote health, independence, and quality of life for eligible U.S. military veterans with disabilities	
Job-Specific Workplace Reasonable Accommodations	Employers	Designed to enable a person to perform his or her job; not necessarily a device	
Qualified Disability Expenses	Achieving a Better Life Experience (ABLE) Accounts	Covers AT and personal support services	
Assistive Technology Act	Statewide programs but not necessarily a payer or provider	Equipment used to "increase, maintain, or improve functional capabilities of individuals with disabilities" (29 USC Sec 3002(4))	

	Limitations: Policy-Related	Limitations: Device-Related	Limitations: Geographic
	All veterans enrolled in the U.S. Department of Veterans Affairs (VA) health care system are eligible for all needed prosthetics, medical equipment, and supplies; two significant groups of veterans are eligible even if not enrolled: (1) veterans needing prosthetics, medical equipment, and supplies for a service-connected disability, and (2) veterans with a service-connected disability rated at least 50 percent	Replacement of devices still considered to be experimental requires specific VHA Headquarters approval	Care delivered within VHA facilities, although programs are available to address geographic barriers to care: Veterans Transportation Services, telehealth, Veterans Choice program
	No guarantee of reasonable accommodations; may require significant advocacy and/or litigation to acquire	The Americans with Disabilities Act (ADA) does not require smaller employers to provide expensive devices Employer may require that a device remain in the workplace and not be used outside the workplace	Experts trained to perform worksite assessments and make reasonable accommodations in the workplace are not available nationwide.
	Up to $100,000 in ABLE accounts is an exempt resource for SSI purposes; can be used for items not considered medically necessary by Medicaid and Medicare in the limited number of states that have set up their ABLE account programs to date	Could cover any of the devices considered in this report with a limit of $100,000	Devices and access to trained clinicians who can assess the need for appropriate assistive devices and train users are not available nationwide; not all states participate in ABLE accounts at this time
	"Required state-level activities include: state financing activities, device reutilization programs, device loan programs, and device demonstration programs. Required state leadership activities include: training and technical assistance, public awareness and information and assistance activities, and coordination and collaboration." (Domin et al., 2016)	Generally does not provide actual devices; provides loaner devices for demonstration or temporary use, recycled devices, etc.; may not meet the individual's need to return to work; provides loans to purchase AT items	Devices and access to trained clinicians who can assess the need for appropriate assistive devices and train users are not available nationwide

8

Review of Social Security and Other Selected Disability Compensation Programs

As part of the statement of task for this study, the U.S. Social Security Administration (SSA) asked the committee to "describe the decision-making processes of other government or private monetary disability benefit programs regarding the use of the selected assistive products and technologies." To meet this objective, in addition to reviewing relevant policy and procedural documents, the committee spoke to representatives of the U.S. Department of Veterans Affairs' (VA's) Veterans Benefits Administration (VBA); Service Canada's Canada Pension Plan (CPP) program; and two private disability insurance providers, Unum and Prudential Financial.[1] The committee selected the VBA because it is another large U.S. federal disability program, and some VA disability beneficiaries also receive benefits from SSA. Service Canada's CPP was selected because, like the SSA disability programs, it is a federally administered program funded by worker and employer contributions that provides disability and retirement benefits to

[1]The amount of information provided to or obtained by the committee varied among the programs discussed in this chapter. There is much publicly available information about the programs and overall disability determination processes of SSA, the VA, and the CPP. With respect to specific questions of whether or how these agencies consider the use of assistive products and technologies in their decision-making processes, the committee had to rely more heavily on the written or oral information provided by each entity. There is significantly less publicly available information on the disability determination processes and procedures of private disability insurers. For this reason, the committee had to rely primarily on the information provided by the representatives of the two private disability insurance providers discussed in this chapter.

eligible individuals. Unum and Prudential were selected because they are two of the largest private disability insurance providers in the United States.

This chapter provides a brief overview of each of these programs, along with a description of their general disability determination processes and the evidence they consider in making determinations. The programs, including SSA's disability programs, are then compared with respect to their consideration of relevant assistive products and technologies, the evidence required by adjudicators to make a determination, and the professionals permitted to provide this evidence. Annex Table 8-1 at the end of this chapter summarizes elements of each of the programs, allowing for comparisons among them. Differences among the programs, especially with respect to mission, and variability in the amount and detail of the information available to the committee limit to some extent the comparisons that can be made.

OVERVIEW OF SOCIAL SECURITY ADMINISTRATION AND OTHER SELECTED PROGRAMS

Social Security Administration

As described in Chapter 1, SSA oversees two programs that provide benefits based on disability through the Social Security Act: Social Security Disability Insurance (SSDI) and Supplemental Security Income (SSI). SSDI provides benefits to qualified individuals[2] "who cannot work because they have a severe medical condition expected to last at least one year or result in death" and to certain members of their families (SSA, 2016a, p. 7). SSI provides "monthly payments to people with limited incomes and resources who are aged, blind, or disabled" (SSA, 2016a, p. 8). In 2015, the most recent year for which data are available, 10,806,466 individuals (including dependents) received an average monthly benefit of $1,022.29 through the SSDI program (SSA, 2017a, Table 5.A1). In that same year, 8,309,564 individuals (7,084,221 categorized as disabled and 67,851 as blind) received an average of $541.28 in monthly SSI benefits through federal payments, state supplementation, or both (SSA, 2017a, Table 7.A1).

SSA currently considers assistive devices in the nonmedical and medical areas of its program guidelines. During determinations of substantial gainful activity (SGA)[3] and income eligibility for SSI benefits, the reasonable cost of items, devices, or services needed by applicants to enable work with their impairment is subtracted from eligible earnings, even when those

[2]Qualified individuals include those who have worked long enough and have paid Social Security taxes (SSA, 2016a, p. 7).

[3]20 CFR §§ 404.1510, 416.910.

items or services are used for activities of daily living in addition to work. SSA also considers assistive devices in its medical disability determination process.

Veterans Benefits Administration

The VA provides monetary benefits to eligible veterans and their dependents and spouses through the VBA. The VBA's mission, in cooperation with the other administrations within the VA, is to provide "benefits and services to the veterans and their families in a responsive, timely and compassionate manner in recognition of their service to the Nation" (VBA, 2017). The VBA provides disability compensation and other assistance services, including the Vocational Rehabilitation and Employment (VR&E) program, to veterans, survivors, and their families (VA, 2017). The VA describes disability compensation as "a monthly tax-free benefit paid to Veterans who are at least 10% disabled because of injuries or diseases that were incurred in or aggravated during active duty, active duty for training, or inactive duty training" (VA, 2016d). Veterans also may receive benefits for disabilities related or secondary to those that occurred during service or for disabilities presumed to be related to service, even when they occurred later (VA, 2016c). The VBA's disability rating system and determination of service-related disabilities are discussed later in this chapter. Special monthly compensation can be paid in addition to disability compensation if applicants require aid and assistance by other persons or if they have certain impairments rendering them totally disabled (e.g., loss or loss of use of a hand or leg) (VA, 2016c). In fiscal year (FY) 2015, the VBA processed and completed more than 1.38 million disability compensation claims, with an average processing time of 93.1 days per claim (VA, 2016a). In the same year, 4,168,774 veterans received compensation benefits for service-related disabilities in an average amount of $14,444 per individual, or a total of $60.21 billion (VA, 2016b). Provision of assistive products and technologies to veterans falls under the auspices of the Veterans Health Administration (VHA) (see Chapter 7).

The VR&E program "assists Veterans with service-connected disabilities and an employment handicap and Service members who are in the process of transitioning from military to civilian employment prepare for, find, and keep suitable jobs" (VR&E, 2016). For individuals with service-related disabilities that are sufficiently severe as to preclude work, VR&E provides services to facilitate "their ability to live as independently as possible" (VR&E, 2016).

Canada Pension Plan

Service Canada, which is part of Employment and Social Development Canada, "provides Canadians with a single point of access to a wide range of government services and benefits," including the CPP (Government of Canada, 2017d). Similar to SSA's Old Age, Survivor, and Disability Insurance (i.e., Social Security) in the United States, the CPP is a federal social insurance program, funded by worker and employer contributions, intended to provide benefits when a worker retires, becomes disabled, or dies. The CPP covers residents of all provinces and territories except Quebec, which has its own similar program, the Quebec Pension Plan. Although CPP disability benefits are awarded based on severe and prolonged disabilities, they are "not designed to pay for such things as medications and devices," which fall under the purview of provincial programs (Government of Canada, 2017a). Disability determination guidelines for CPP adjudicators do not take assistive products and technologies into account, although adjudicators may include these items implicitly as "medical treatment" according to a CPP representative who spoke to the committee during a public session (Kidd, 2016). As noted, the provision of assistive devices for personal and/or vocational use falls under the purview of provincial governments, which are responsible for health care delivery through a variety of programs. In FY 2014, approximately 5.3 million CPP beneficiaries, including 329,000 people with disabilities and 83,000 children with disabled parents, received payments (Government of Canada, 2015a). Disability benefits represented $4.2 billion (11 percent) of total CPP benefits paid from $45.0 billion in employee and employer contributions during that year (Government of Canada, 2015a).

Selected Private Disability Insurance Providers

During two of the committee's public sessions, invited speakers from Unum and Prudential Financial provided information about disability determination and consideration or provision of assistive devices in the private insurance sector. Unum is one of the leading providers of employment-based group and individual disability insurance in the United States, with a focus on return-to-work and other work capacity strategies (Jackson, 2016). Unum reports processing nearly 490,000 new claims and paying $5.5 billion in benefits in 2012 (Unum, 2017a). The company served more than 80,000 employers (representing more than 17 million participants) across the United States during the same year (Unum, 2017a). Similarly, Prudential is a group and individual disability insurance provider, with a mission to "enable customers' employees to return to work as soon as possible after a disabling event" (Tugman and Kramschuster, 2016). Prudential reports the provision of disability insurance for 2,500 clients (representing 1.3 million participants) for short-term disability and 3,100 clients (representing 2.1 million participants) for long-term disability (Prudential Financial, 2017).

The committee was unable to obtain specific guidelines on the processes used for consideration of assistive products and technologies in private insurance disability determinations, as details of eligibility for benefits are specified in client contracts. However, Unum "utilizes assistive devices and technology in support of occupational functioning" (Jackson, 2016), and Prudential specified that it covered assistive products and technologies primarily for return-to-work purposes, most commonly musculoskeletal aids such as modified workstations, chairs, or mobility devices (Tugman and Kramschuster, 2016).

DISABILITY DETERMINATION (ADJUDICATION) PROCESSES AND EVIDENCE CONSIDERED

Processes

Social Security Administration

In FY 2014, SSA processed 3,054,900 SSDI claims and 2,395,500 SSI claims, 2,181,700 of which were in the category of blind or disabled (SSA, 2015a, Tables 2.F5, 2.F6). As summarized in Chapter 1, SSA processes adult disability claims using a five-step "sequential evaluation process," which assesses whether an individual may be found disabled (unable to engage in SGA [SSA, 2017b]) under the Social Security Act.

Step 1: Social Security field offices perform financial screens to deny claims for applicants who work and earn income above the SGA limit (Wixon and Strand, 2013). If an applicant is performing SGA, which encompasses "significant physical or mental activities" done (or of a kind usually done) "for pay or profit, whether or not a profit is realized,"[4] then SSA will find the individual not disabled under the act. SGA for 2017 is specified as earnings of $1,170 per month for nonblind individuals and $1,950 for statutorily blind individuals (SSA, 2017b).

Step 2: Applicants receive medical screens to determine whether they have a medically determinable severe impairment (SSA, 2012a). If the applicant does not have a medically determinable severe impairment or combination of impairments that meets the duration requirement,[5] SSA will find the individual not disabled under the act. If the applicant has

[4]20 CFR § 404.1572.
[5]20 CFR § 404.1509.

such an impairment or combination of impairments, SSA will identify the impairment(s) and proceed to Step 3.

Step 3: An applicant's impairment is assessed using the *Listing of Impairments* (SSA, n.d.-b), a regulatory list of medical conditions and criteria created by SSA to assist in disability determination. If an applicant's impairment "meets" or "equals" a listing and meets the duration requirement, the applicant is allowed benefits. To "meet" a listing, a claimant must have a medically determinable impairment that satisfies all of the criteria in the listing. An impairment "equals" a listing if it is "at least equal in severity and duration to the criteria of any listed impairment" (SSA, 2016d). If the applicant does not have an impairment(s) that meets or medically equals an impairment in the Listings or meets the duration requirement, SSA proceeds to Step 4.

Step 4: Residual functional capacity (RFC) is an individual's "maximum capacity for performance taking into account the limitations resulting from their impairment(s)" (SSA, 2016b, p. 2). An RFC assessment includes a written analysis of functional capabilities, both exertional and nonexertional,[6] based on all relevant available evidence. In this step, SSA assesses whether an applicant's RFC allows him or her to perform past work. Specifically, Disability Determination Services (DDS) considers whether the applicant's RFC meets or exceeds the skill requirements for his or her past relevant work (generally in the past 15 years prior to adjudication), based on the person's capacity to perform work-related activities (Wixon and Strand, 2013). If it is determined that the applicant can perform his or her past work with his or her current RFC, the application for benefits is denied. If the applicant cannot still perform his or her past relevant work, SSA proceeds to the fifth and final step.

Step 5: An applicant's RFC and vocational factors such as age, education, and work experience and transferable skills are considered in determining whether the applicant can perform other work in the national economy. Applicants who are determined unable to perform work in the national economy are allowed benefits, while those who are determined to be able to perform such work are denied. SSA uses a set of guidelines that combine medical–vocational patterns into "rules" for decision making, often referred to as "The Grid." When a claim involves nonexertional impairments such as certain mental, sensory, or skin disorders, the analysis may involve consideration of more than one rule.

[6]Assessment of RFC exertional capacity considers sitting, standing, walking, lifting, carrying, pushing, and pulling. Assessment of RFC nonexertional capacity considers "work-related limitations and restrictions that do not depend on a person's physical strength," including stooping, climbing, reaching, handling, fingering, seeing, hearing, understanding and remembering instructions, responding appropriately to supervision, and tolerating temperature extremes (SSA, 2016b).

In addition, SSA includes two options for faster disability determinations. Compassionate Allowances permit faster identification of medical conditions (e.g., acute leukemia, amyotrophic lateral sclerosis [ALS], pancreatic cancer) that are most likely to meet SSA's current definition of disability with minimal but sufficient objective medical evidence, allowing the applicant to receive benefits more quickly (SSA, 2015b). In Quick Disability Determinations, initial applications are screened using a computer-based predictive model to identify cases in which a favorable disability determination is highly likely and medical evidence is easily available. The model allows these high-likelihood claims to receive priority and be expedited in cases involving more serious impairments (SSA, 2015b).

Veterans Benefits Administration

The VBA disability determination process can be divided into two main steps: the development of medical evidence and the rating process (IOM, 2007). Claims are processed by the Veterans Service Centers (VSCs) in VBA regional offices and are handled by six specialized teams: public contact, triage, predetermination, rating, postdetermination, and appeals—before a determination is made. Medical evidence collected by the predetermination team includes information from public and private medical records as well as the applicant's attending physicians regarding the extent of impairment, functional limitations, and disability. This evidence is often supplemented by a compensation and pension (C&P) examination ordered by the rating veterans service representative (RVSR) during the determination process and performed by a VHA clinician or medical contractor. To be evaluated for a disability under VBA guidelines, individuals must have an impairment related to their service. This relationship to service may be a direct connection, an aggravation (existing condition aggravated by service), secondary (illness or injury experienced after service that is related to a different impairment with a service connection), or a presumption (an unproven but likely connection, such as in the case of chronic diseases presumed to be connected to exposure during service).

The VBA disability rating process is based on the VA Schedule for Rating Disabilities (VASRD), consisting of approximately 800 unique diagnostic codes allowing adjudicators to compare an applicant's illness or injury with standardized disability evaluation criteria (Flohr, 2016). VBA disability compensation is paid to beneficiaries on a monthly basis, and the rates of compensation are dependent on the VBA disability rating system in increments of 10 percent, from 10 percent to 100 percent disabling (where a rating of 100 percent is a complete impairment of earning capacity). Thus, in contrast to the binary SSA determination process whereby applicants are found to be either disabled or not disabled, the VBA system allows veterans receiving benefits to be considered partially disabled. In addition, they may work while receiving benefits, with no limit on their earnings (IOM, 2015, p. 70). The RVSR is tasked with considering an applicant's medical evidence in assigning evaluation level(s) for the person's impairment(s) based on VASRD tables, codes, and corresponding percentage levels. Disability ratings are then compiled and used by the VSC postdetermination team to process awards and notify claimants of benefit-related decisions.

Canada Pension Plan

Service Canada uses an adjudication framework to evaluate applications for CPP disability benefits (Government of Canada, 2015b). In a process similar to that of SSDI, applications for benefits in this program are assessed only if applicants have made the required contributions to the CPP through participation in the eligible Canadian labor market for 4 of the last 6 years at or above the minimum earning level ($5,400 in 2016), or for 3 of the last 6 years if the individual has contributed at or above the minimum earning level for at least 25 years (Government of Canada, 2017c). The adjudication framework includes five components used to implement federal policy regarding disability evaluation. As with SSA disability programs, CPP disability determination does not account for a continuum of severity; instead, applicants are deemed eligible or ineligible for benefits based on the outcome of their claim (Kidd, 2016). Two of the framework components do address the severity and duration of the applicant's impairment(s). First the applicant must meet the "severe criterion for the prime indicator," which requires the existence of a medical condition (the prime indicator) that is *severe*, meaning it regularly inhibits any type of work, not just the work usually done. Second, the "severe disability" must be *prolonged*, meaning it is "long term and of indefinite duration, or is likely to result in death" (Government of Canada, 2015b).

A third component of the adjudication process is demonstration by the applicant that he or she is "incapable regularly of pursing any substantially gainful occupation" as a result of the physical or mental impairment. This criterion includes consideration of work activity with respect to performance, productivity, and profitability. A substantially gainful occupation is defined as "an occupation that provides a salary or wages equal to the maximum annual amount a person could receive as a disability pension" (Government of Canada, 2015b).

A fourth component of the CPP adjudication process takes account of personal characteristics, "intrinsic factors that are unique to a particular person" and directly impact an applicant's regular capacity to engage in a substantially gainful occupation (Government of Canada, 2015b). Personal characteristics, which are evaluated on a case-by-case basis in the context of the medical condition, include age, education, and work experience. Personal characteristics alone do not qualify an applicant for disability benefits. Socioeconomic factors such as unemployment rates, access to jobs, or preferred working hours are not considered in making a disability determination (Government of Canada, 2015b).

The fifth component of the adjudication framework is a "reasonably satisfied" standard of proof for making disability determinations, which is synonymous with the term "more likely than not." Adjudicators are instructed to use this standard when assessing eligibility for the CPP. Applying this standard entails considering the listed medical condition, the likely progression of the impairment, the applicant's functional limitations, the impact of treatment, testimony from medical sources, and additional medical issues to determine whether the individual is "more likely than not" incapable of regular pursuit of any substantially gainful occupation (Government of Canada, 2015b).

Selected Private Disability Insurance Providers

Disability determination for private insurance varies by company. Although there are different, policy-specific definitions of disability, a core concept is the inability "to perform the material and substantial duties of [one's] occupation as it is defined in the national economy" as a result of illness or injury (Unum, 2017b; see also Prudential Financial, 2015).

Unum's claims are evaluated by a disability benefits specialist (DBS) who integrates all of the relevant information, including results of clinical tests and medical records. Medical and vocational staff then review all of this information as well as contact the applicant's attending clinicians. The DBS uses the results of this review to compile restrictions and limitations on employment based on the medical condition. Specific eligibility and benefit amounts are based on contracted agreements with Unum clients, either individuals or employers. If these agreements include the potential for work site modification, a vocational rehabilitation consultant evaluates the claimant's current essential job duties and identifies limitations in the ability to perform these duties in accordance with the DBS's findings (Jackson, 2016).

Prudential employs a similar approach, wherein a disability claims manager reviews the claimant's file along with clinician reports to determine the severity of the medical impairment and individual's prognosis. These results are combined with a workplace assessment performed by a vocational rehabilitation specialist detailing physical, environmental, and cognitive occupational demands that may limit or inhibit a claimant's full return to work (Tugman and Kramschuster, 2016).

Evidence Considered

Types of Evidence

Social Security Administration SSA currently defines evidence as any information related to an individual's claim that is submitted to SSA by the claimant or anyone else as well as information that SSA obtains while developing the claim. Evidence generally is categorized as objective medical evidence (signs, laboratory findings, or both), medical opinions, other medical evidence from medical sources, evidence from nonmedical sources, and prior administrative medical findings of the state or federal DDS medical consultants and psychological consultants.

Every SSA disability claim must include evidence that supports the individual's claim that he or she is blind or disabled. Medical evidence may come from individual medical sources and from various health care facilities where the claimant has received health care services. The medical evidence may be in any format, such as paper and electronic medical records. It may reflect a clear length of treatment that provides a longitudinal account of the impairment(s), or it may reflect individual examinations or singular hospitalizations.

Before determining whether an individual is disabled, SSA will develop the individual's complete medical history for at least the 12-month period preceding the month in which the individual files the application unless there is a reason to believe that development for a different period is necessary. SSA will make every reasonable effort (as defined in its regulations) to help the individual obtain his or her medical reports from his or her own medical sources when he or she gives SSA permission to request the reports.

If existing evidence is insufficient to enable a determination, SSA may contact the claimant's medical sources for additional information and/or order a consultative examination. A consultative examination includes additional tests or assessments that provide better understanding of the existence and severity of the claimant's impairment(s), and it produces a written statement describing what the claimant can still perform functionally despite the impairment(s) (unless the disability claim is in relation to statutory blindness). It is preferred that the consultative examination be performed by the claimant's own medical provider unless that clinician prefers not to do so or lacks the requisite equipment; there exist conflicts or inconsistencies that could not feasibly be resolved by the clinician; or SSA's prior experience working with the clinician indicates that this individual may not be a productive source (SSA, n.d.-c).

In addition to medical evidence, an SSA claimant may submit evidence from nonmedical sources. This evidence can help demonstrate the ways in which the assessed impairment impacts the claimant's ability to function in a work setting. Evidence may come from a variety of nonmedical sources, including public/private agencies, schools, parents or other family members, caregivers, social workers, and employers (SSA, n.d.-c).

Veterans Benefits Administration The VBA requires fulfilment of three evidentiary requirements before a disability claim can be adjudicated: evidence of military status (e.g., discharge or separation papers), service treatment records, and additional medical evidence (VA, 2015). VBA protocol designates the evidentiary responsibilities of the claimant as obtaining appropriate records from agencies outside the federal government, such as state or local agencies, private doctors or hospitals, and former employers, as well as providing adequate information to the VBA so information can be obtained. In turn, the VBA is responsible for obtaining appropriate records from federal agencies, such as the military, VBA medical centers, or SSA, as well as providing a medical examination or opinion if necessary.

Evidence included in a VBA disability claim is similar to that required by SSA, encompassing both medical and lay evidence. This evidence must be found to be credible—"inherently believable or [have] been received from a competent source"—and probative—"relevant to the issue in question, and . . . have sufficient weight, either by itself or in combination with other evidence, to persuade the decision-maker about a fact" (VA, 2013).

Canada Pension Plan In the process of making CPP disability determinations, Service Canada adjudicators take into account all pertinent evidence, including medical evidence, work impairments and capacity, claimant interviews, clinician interviews, medical reports from treatment sources, diagnostic tests, reports from employers, and functional capacity assessments. Federal records on past use of social services, such as employment insurance, also are taken into account (Government of Canada, 2015b). Service Canada categorizes medical evidence permitted in a disability determination as either objective or subjective. Objective evidence includes symptoms, deficits, or impairments that can be observed or measured through diagnostic tests, laboratory findings, or functional observations. Subjective evidence, which may be supported by objective information, is evidence that cannot be directly observed or measured, such as physician interviews or descriptions in a medical record.

Selected Private Disability Insurance Providers Prudential and Unum both provided information regarding types of evidence they consider in their disability insurance determinations. Prudential evaluations use medical evidence from medical records and the claimant's attending physician(s) as well as that provided by in-house physicians or registered nurses. Once the claimant has been determined to have a disability preventing total return to work and is receiving disability benefits through his or her employer contract, functional capacity and limitations are assessed. Functional evidence is identified by the claimant's attending physician as well as Prudential clinicians. This evidence is combined with information from the Prudential vocational rehabilitation specialist, who identifies physical, environmental, and cognitive demands of the claimant's current employment, along with potential accommodations or assistive devices. Unum also uses medical and functional evidence to process a disability claim and potentially facilitate a return to work. Medical evidence includes a claimant's medical records as well as evidence from his or her attending physician(s) detailing restrictions and limitations resulting from the specific impairment. Medical evidence is considered along with essential job duties identified by the vocational rehabilitation consultant to identify potential accommodations or assistive devices that may facilitate a safe and successful return to work.

Professionals Providing the Evidence

Social Security Administration According to SSA regulations, all medical sources can provide medical evidence for a disability claim. However, only certain medical sources can provide the objective medical evidence necessary to establish the existence of impairment. These medical sources, called acceptable medical sources, include licensed physicians (medical or osteopathic doctors), licensed or certified psychologists (including school psychologists or licensed/certified individuals performing the same function in a school setting),[7] licensed optometrists,[8] licensed podiatrists,[9] and qualified speech-language pathologists.[10,11] For claims filed on or after March 27, 2017, acceptable medical sources also include advanced practice registered nurses (APRNs), physician assistants (PAs), and audiologists (SSA, 2016e).[12]

[7]Evidence from school psychologists or qualified professionals performing the same function is considered only for claims of intellectual disability, learning disability, or borderline intellectual function.

[8]Evidence from licensed optometrists is considered only for claims regarding visual disorders.

[9]Evidence from licensed podiatrists is considered only for claims regarding impairments of the foot or foot and ankle, as state treatment laws permit.

[10]To be considered qualified, speech-language pathologists must be licensed by a "state professional licensing agency or be fully certified by the state education agency" in that state or "hold a certificate of clinical competence from the American Speech-Language-Hearing Association."

[11]20 CFR § 404.1513.

[12]APRNs and PAs are acceptable medical sources for evaluation of impairments within their licensed scope of practice only. Audiologists are acceptable medical sources for evaluation of impairments related to hearing loss, auditory processing disorders, and balance disorders within their licensed scope of practice only.

Veterans Benefits Administration The VBA defines competent medical evidence as evidence provided by sources with education, training, or experience qualifying them to provide medical diagnoses, statements, or opinions. Medical evidence may additionally include "statements conveying sound medical principles found in medical treatises" or "statements contained in authoritative writings such as medical and scientific articles and research reports or analyses." Conversely, competent lay evidence is defined as evidence provided by a source who lacks specialized education, experience, or training but who has "knowledge of facts or circumstances and conveys matters that can be observed and described by a lay person."[13]

Canada Pension Plan Service Canada designates professionals who are able to provide medical evidence as "qualified family physicians, specialists, and other health professionals." Additional specifications identify professionals able to provide evidence for a claimant's capacity to work, including psychologists, neuropsychologists, physiotherapists, occupational therapists, and vocational rehabilitation professionals (Government of Canada, 2015b).

Selected Private Disability Insurance Providers The committee was unable to obtain specific information regarding the requirements of private insurance companies with respect to sources of evidence. Prudential disability claim forms indicate that medical evidence should be obtained from a primary care physician, supplemented by evidence from "all other physicians [the claimant has] consulted for this condition" (Prudential Financial, 2016). Unum disability claim forms require evidence from attending physicians or other health care providers, without reference to specific provider qualifications or education (Unum, 2016).

Adjudicator Training/Credentials

Social Security Administration Initial and reconsideration-level SSA disability determinations occur at state DDSs through collaboration among a disability examiner (DE), a medical consultant, and/or a psychological consultant (PC) (SSA, 2016c). DE training requirements are regulated at the state level, but on average, DEs must have 2 years of training, mentorship, and experience with cases to be fully trained in the DDS, with additional experience allowing them to assess increasingly complex claims and vocational issues (Owen, 2009). Essential DE skills include an understanding of medical conditions, vocational factors, medical terminology, and SSA regulatory guidelines. Medical consultants, who must be licensed physicians,

[13] 38 CFR § 3.159.

evaluate physical impairments.[14] PCs, who must be licensed psychiatrists or qualified psychologists, evaluate mental impairments. To be qualified as a PC, a psychologist must be (1) a "licensed or certified psychologist at the independent practice level of psychology" in that state; (2) either in possession of a doctorate degree in psychology from a clinical psychology program[15] or "in a national register of health service providers in psychology which the Commissioner of Social Security deems appropriate"; and (3) possess 2 years of supervised clinical experience as a psychologist, at least one of which is after a master's degree (SSA, 2016c).

Veterans Benefits Administration VBA adjudicators are disability rating specialists identified as veterans service representatives or RVSRs, depending on their VSC team and role. These adjudicators may be health professionals, including nurses or physicians (Flohr, 2016). Medical examiners who are commissioned to perform C&P examinations as part of the disability determination process are VHA employees or medical contractors with certification to perform the required testing or evaluation. VHA examiners who perform these evaluations are monitored by the Compensation and Pension Examination Program, a joint initiative of the VHA and VBA establishing baseline performance for examiners, performance improvement initiatives, performance monitoring, and provision of feedback. These performance requirements also mandate that C&P examiners have full knowledge of the requirements of the disability determination and examination process (IOM, 2007). Non-VHA examiners are medical contractors employed by QTC Medical Group, the "largest provider of government-outsourced occupational health and disability examination services in the nation" (QTC, 2012). These examiners must meet specific QTC requirements and undergo training and performance monitoring through an internal quality assurance program approved by the VBA medical director.

Canada Pension Plan CPP medical adjudicators are health professionals who review applications for benefits. These professionals are trained nurses with additional relevant knowledge of CPP legislation, regulations, policies, and procedures. Nurses who act as disability adjudicators are drawn from a variety of medical specialties (Government of Canada, 2015b).

Selected Private Disability Insurance Providers Training and qualifications for disability adjudicators vary throughout the private disability insurance

---

[14] See Bipartisan Budget Act of 2015, section 832 (H.R. 1314).

[15] Acceptable doctorate degrees in psychology must be received from a medical institution accredited by an organization recognized by the Council for Higher Education Accreditation (formerly known as the Council on Post-Secondary Accreditation).

sector. Prudential employs a team of internal disability claims managers, along with vocational rehabilitation specialists, who are experienced case managers with a master's degree or higher in rehabilitation counseling and national Commission on Rehabilitation Counselor Certification. A vocational rehabilitation specialist works with employers, claimants, and attending physicians to develop and implement return-to-work plans, depending on the claimant's individual impairment. Prudential also employs board-certified physicians and registered nurses to assist in the disability determination and vocational rehabilitation process (Tugman and Kramschuster, 2016). Unum disability claims are processed by a contracted DBS with the help of vocational rehabilitation consultants, who are master's-level rehabilitation specialists with additional training in counseling philosophy. Medical evidence is reviewed and supported by on-site physicians in more than 30 specialties, registered nurses, and behavioral health specialists (Jackson, 2016).

CONSIDERATION OF SELECTED ASSISTIVE PRODUCTS AND TECHNOLOGIES

Wheeled and Seated Mobility Devices

Disability determination for SSA programs does not include use of a wheeled and seated mobility device (WSMD) as a criterion for a successful claim. Instead, SSA considers "most adults who must use a [WSMD] for ambulation to have an impairment that meets or medically equals a Listing generally because of their inability to ambulate effectively" (SSA, 2016b). SSA guidelines define the inability to ambulate effectively as "an extreme limitation of the ability to walk; i.e., an impairment(s) that interferes very seriously with the individual's ability to independently initiate, sustain, or complete activities" (SSA, n.d.-a). Ambulation, in this case, denotes independent mobility without the use of handheld assistive device(s) if the device(s) limits the functional abilities of both upper extremities (SSA, n.d.-a). Accordingly, within the sequential evaluation process, SSA reports that function in the context of WSMD use has never been evaluated beyond Step 3 (meeting or medically equaling a listing) for applicants who must use a WSMD (SSA, 2016b). Listings that are commonly used to allow an application for a person using a WSMD are musculoskeletal system (disorders of the spine, amputation); skin disorders (burns); and neurological (central nervous system vascular accident, cerebral palsy, spinal cord or nerve root lesions, multiple sclerosis, muscular dystrophy). If these claims were to be assessed in Steps 4 and/or 5 of the evaluation process, policy indicates that RFC would be evaluated with a focus on the applicant's ability to "use both hands to manipulate and handle small objects and to see small objects at close range" (SSA, 2016b). These are good examples of nonexertional abilities whose impairment, when combined with the inability to stand or walk for most of the workday, can affect an individual's ability to perform SGA.

Similarly, the VBA adjudication process does not include use of a WSMD as an explicit factor in determining disability. Instead, the impairment is evaluated based on the functional impairment or loss of use that is the underlying cause of the functional inability (Flohr, 2016). This functional assessment criterion requires the RVSR to consider not only medical evidence pertaining to this impairment but also the effects of the impairment requiring the use of a WSMD on the individual's ordinary activity.[16] If an individual requires constant use of a WSMD, the impairment is likely to be considered complete loss of function of both lower extremities and to be rated as such on the disability rating scale. If an individual requires periodic use of a WSMD, the impairment will correspond to a different level on the disability rating scale according to functional assessment criteria (Flohr, 2016).

Service Canada guidelines for the administration of CPP disability benefits do not include specific consideration of WSMD use in the disability determination process. Guidance stipulates that "the CPP disability benefit is not designed to pay for such things as medications and assistive devices" (Government of Canada, 2017b). However, disability adjudicators are instructed to assess the impact of treatment as part of medical evidence for a claim, defined as "what is needed to restore or improve the health and function of a particular person, or what is needed to prevent or delay deterioration" (Government of Canada, 2015b). The use of a WSMD provides "insight and necessary coping mechanisms for adapting to the person's identified limitations" (Government of Canada, 2015b, Section 2.3) and therefore, theoretically, could be considered by medical adjudicators in their assessment of a person's ability to engage in substantially gainful employment in the short term and the future.

With respect to the private disability insurance industry, representatives from Prudential reported that the majority of diagnoses handled by their company are musculoskeletal in origin, resulting in the provision or consideration of assistive devices that will allow the claimant to "return to work," such as sit/stand workstations, ergonomic workstations, mobility aids, or WSMDs (Tugman and Kramschuster, 2016). Representatives from Unum likewise stated that a majority of their company's short- and long-term disability claims (excluding maternity claims) are musculoskeletal in origin. They also said, however, that WSMDs are rarely encountered in the realm of private insurance, being considered for only an estimated 5 percent of claims processed by the company (Jackson, 2016).

[16] 38 CFR § 4.10.

Upper-Extremity Prostheses

As with WSMDs, SSA disability determination guidelines do not include use of upper-extremity prostheses (UEPs) as an explicit criterion for a successful claim. According to SSA, "most people who must use [bilateral] upper extremity prostheses have an impairment(s) that meets or medically equals a listing generally because of their 'inability to perform fine and gross movements effectively'" (SSA, 2016b). SSA defines the inability to perform fine and gross movements effectively as "an extreme loss of function of both upper extremities . . . that interferes very seriously with the person's ability to independently initiate, sustain, or complete activities" (SSA, n.d.-a). It is important to note that SSA guidelines for applicants missing an upper extremity were created when prosthetic technology was less common and "use of such prostheses generally precluded fine manipulative abilities, as they were generally equipped with a hook or pincers" (SSA, 2016b). Most SSA applicants who use bilateral UEPs will have their claim approved at Step 3 of the sequential evaluation process because their impairment typically meets or medically equals a listing (SSA, 2016b). The most common listings used to approve people with these devices are musculoskeletal system listings (disorders of the spine, amputation, soft tissue injury) and skin disorders listings (burns) (SSA, 2016b). If an applicant's RFC is assessed in Steps 4 and/or 5 of the evaluation process, the adjudicator looks for a reduction of strength and nonexertional capacities. If strength and nonexertional limitations are combined with standing and walking limitations, the claim is often approved (SSA, 2016b). For cases of amputation specifically, loss or partial loss of an upper extremity is considered based on "the condition of the remaining stump, the person's ability to use [a] prosthesis, and the person's remaining ability for fine and gross manipulation" (SSA, 2012b).

The disability determination process used by the VBA does not specifically include the use of UEPs; instead, upper-extremity amputation or loss of use is assessed using the disability rating scale. Functional impairment or the potential capacity restored by the use of prostheses is not assessed according to the rating scale, just the existence and severity of the amputation or loss of use. Impairments can be evaluated at 90 percent if the amputation/loss of use occurs at the shoulder and at 60 percent if the impairment occurs lower in the extremity (e.g., elbow). A joint replacement or prosthetic implant is evaluated at 100 percent for 1 year postimplantation and then reevaluated to assess the functional capabilities of that joint. When evaluating function for applicants using UEPs, the functional benefit of the prostheses is not taken into account; evaluations are performed without the prostheses. This contrasts with VBA guidelines for evaluations of lower-limb amputations, which take into account whether a prosthetic device provides a functional benefit for the applicant.[17]

As with WSMDs, Service Canada guidelines for the administration of CPP disability benefits do not include consideration of the use of UEPs in the disability determination process. Rather, these devices are considered indirectly through the impact of treatment (i.e., ability to successfully wear a device and use it for a sustained period of time) on an applicant's ability to perform substantially gainful employment.

Little evidence was available to the committee regarding the details and sucess rates of claims involving use of UEPs submitted to private disability insurers. The Unum representative stated that in 2015, the company processed fewer than 100 amputation-related claims and that this number had remained below 100 for the past 3 years (Jackson, 2016). Both Prudential and Unum rarely encounter such claims, including claimants using UEPs (Jackson, 2016; Tugman and Kramschuster, 2016).

Hearing-Related Products and Technologies

SSA has specific guidelines regarding the use and consideration of hearing-related products and technologies in the disability determination process. In Step 3 of the sequential evaluation process, to determine whether an applicant's impairment meets or medically equals a listing related to hearing impairment (not treated with cochlear implantation), the adjudicator considers only the individual's ability to hear without hearing aids. Past SSA guidelines allowed for Step 3 testing using hearing aids, but this provision was modified in current guidelines because (1) hearing aids could not be used consistently for exams as a result of applicants' forgetting the aids or bringing ones that were malfunctioning; (2) generic hearing aids are now less common because of more customizable technology; (3) clinical practice rarely involves performing aided hearing tests; (4) aided testing does not represent the ability to use the devices in other environments or over the long term; and (5) criteria for listing-level impairments include that a hearing impairment must be severe enough that the use of aids is unlikely to allow significant improvement (SSA, 2016b). If an applicant's hearing loss is treated with cochlear implantation, he or she is eligible to receive disability benefits for 1 year after the initial implantation, at which point the impairment(s) is reassessed using word recognition testing (SSA, n.d.-b). If an applicant's hearing loss does not meet or medically equal a listing in this step, RFC is evaluated using hearing aids (SSA, 2016b). Particular attention is paid in Steps 4 and 5 of the sequential evaluation process to the individual's ability to communicate, which is impacted by an inability to hear.

---

[17]38 CFR § 4.10.

VBA adjudicators are instructed to assess disability applicants based on the results of uncorrected hearing tests. If additional exams are requested, they are conducted by a state-licensed audiologist without the use of hearing aids (Flohr, 2016).

Service Canada guidelines for the administration of CPP disability benefits do not include consideration of hearing-related products and technologies in the disability determination process. These devices are considered indirectly through the impact of treatment (i.e., ability to successfully wear a device and use it for a sustained period of time) on an applicant's ability to perform substantially gainful employment.

Consideration of hearing-related products and technologies in the private disability insurance sector focuses on the provision of these devices to facilitate return-to-work capabilities, as a claimant's impairment will allow. Prudential includes amplified telephones or headsets, teletypewriters, and vibrating pagers for notification as assistive products commonly provided for its clients to assist with return to work (Tugman and Kramschuster, 2016). Unum includes hearing-related computer technology or devices, as well as white noise machines for tinnitus, as assistive technologies commonly provided or subsidized under employer contracts (Jackson, 2016).

Speech-Related Products and Technologies

According to SSA protocol, the ability to produce speech by any means includes the use of "mechanical or electronic devices that improve voice or articulation" (SSA, n.d.-b). It is evaluated on the basis of "(1) audibility—the ability to speak at a level sufficient to be heard; (2) intelligibility—the ability to articulate and link phonetic units of speech with sufficient accuracy to be understood; and (3) functional efficiency—the ability to produce and sustain [a] serviceably fast rate of speech output over a useful period of time" (SSA, 2003). Although the use of speech-related products and technologies is not included as a criterion in SSA guidelines, applicants using these devices are assessed based on an underlying condition(s) that may meet or medically equal listings generally (Step 3). These listings often include special senses and speech systems listings (loss of speech) and neurological disorders listings (central nervous system vascular accident) (SSA, 2016b). If the impairment does not meet or medically equal a listing related to speech impairment, SSA adjudicators are instructed to assess the claimant's speech and communication limitations in the determination of RFC. At Step 4 of the sequential evaluation process, SSA will determine whether the RFC allows the individual to perform his or her past relevant work. At Step 5, SSA considers the RFC together with the individual's vocational factors (e.g., age, education, and work experience) to determine whether the individual can perform other work in the national economy (SSA, 2016b).

According to VBA protocol, speech impairments are not evaluated separately from their underlying conditions. Underlying conditions may include such impairments as traumatic brain injury or ALS; the associated speech impairment is not listed separately from the primary impairment on a VBA disability application. In addition, speech-generating assistive devices and other speech-related technologies are not taken into account when an applicant's impairment is assessed (Flohr, 2016).

Service Canada guidelines for the administration of CPP disability benefits do not include consideration of speech-related products and technologies in the disability determination process. These devices are considered indirectly through the impact of treatment (i.e., ability to successfully wear a device and use it for a sustained period of time) on an applicant's ability to perform substantially gainful employment.

Information regarding consideration or provision of speech-related products and technologies in the private disability insurance industry was not available to the committee. This category of products was not listed by Prudential or Unum as assistive devices commonly provided for employees in return-to-work contracts.

SUMMARY OF POINTS OF COMPARISON AMONG DIFFERENT PROGRAMS

The committee identified a number of general points of comparison among the different disability programs examined: the size of the program as of FY 2015 (if available); whether the program's mission is primarily personal (to improve the well-being of the claimant) or vocational (to facilitate return to work or workplace accommodations); and whether the disability determination system used is binary (disabled versus not disabled) or graduated (degree of disability on a continuum). SSA oversees the largest program the committee examined, with more than 19 million individuals and their dependents receiving disability payments through the SSDI or SSI program in FY 2015. During that same period, the VBA served more than 4 million veterans with disabilities, followed by CPP, with 329,000 beneficiaries (and 83,000 dependents) receiving disability benefits, and the private disability insurance companies, with Unum serving 80,000 and Prudential serving 5,600 employers, respectively. In general, government-sponsored programs (SSA, VBA, and CPP) describe the purpose of their disability benefits programs as supporting and providing living assistance to individuals with disabilities, with a focus on meeting their personal and financial needs. In contrast, representatives from both Unum and Prudential indicated that the focus of their disability determination processes is primarily on facilitating return to work or vocational assistance if possible. It should be noted that the VBA also supports return to work and vocational assistance through its VR&E program.

FINDINGS AND CONCLUSION

Findings

8-1. Unum utilizes assistive products and technologies in support of occupational functioning in its private insurance disability determinations.

8-2. Prudential Financial specified that assistive products and technologies—most commonly musculoskeletal aids such as modified workstations, chairs, or mobility devices—were covered primarily for return-to-work purposes.

8-3. Disability determination guidelines for Canada Pension Plan (CPP) adjudicators do not explicitly take assistive products and technologies into account, although these devices are implicitly considered by adjudicators as being "medical treatment" or "necessary coping mechanisms."

8-4. In both the Social Security Administration (SSA) and Veterans Benefits Administration (VBA) programs, applicants using wheeled and seated mobility devices are evaluated based on loss of function due to the underlying impairment. Adults who must use a wheeled and seated mobility device (WSMD) for ambulation may meet or equal SSA listings generally because of their "inability to ambulate effectively." CPP's assessment of a person's ability to engage in substantial gainful employment in the short term and the future takes WSMDs into account since they provide "insight and necessary coping mechanisms for adapting to the person's identified limitations."

8-5. During functional assessments, SSA adjudicators consider an applicant's ability to use upper-extremity prostheses (UEPs) in the case of amputation(s). With regard to lower-extremity amputations, SSA policy requires that adjudicators consider how an individual ambulates with the prosthesis in place. If the individual is medically capable of wearing a lower-extremity prosthetic device and lacks good cause for not doing so, SSA will find that person not disabled. In contrast, applicants for VBA benefits are required to undergo functional assessment without their UEPs.

8-6. When determining whether an applicant meets or medically equals a listing related to hearing impairment, SSA considers only the individual's ability to hear without hearing aids. VBA adjudicators also test disability applicants without the use of hearing aids.

8-7. Consideration of hearing-related products and technologies in the private disability insurance sector focuses on the provision of these devices to facilitate return to work as a claimant's impairment will allow.

8-8. SSA evaluates applicants on their ability to produce speech by any means, including "mechanical or electronic devices that improve voice or articulation." VBA applicants using speech-related products or technologies are assessed based on the underlying conditions leading to their impairments. The VBA does not consider speech-generating devices or other speech-related technologies when impairments are assessed.

Conclusion

8-1. The mission of a disability benefits program affects the extent to which the program provides (or "helps beneficiaries to obtain") assistive products and technologies and related services designed to facilitate their ability to work.

REFERENCES

Flohr, B. 2016. *Veterans Benefits Administration impact of assistive devices on disability benefits*. Presentation to the Committee on the Use of Selected Assistive Devices in Eliminating or Reducing the Effects of Impairments, Washington, DC, September 27.

Government of Canada. 2015a. *Annual report of the Canada Pension Plan 2014-2015*. https://www.canada.ca/en/employment-social-development/programs/pensions/reports/annual-2015.html (accessed December 22, 2016).

Government of Canada. 2015b. *Canada Pension Plan adjudication framework*. https://www.canada.ca/en/employment-social-development/programs/disability/benefits/framework.html (accessed February 17, 2017).

Government of Canada. 2017a. *Canada pension plan disability benefit—how much could you receive*. https://www.canada.ca/en/services/benefits/publicpensions/cpp/cpp-disability-benefit/benefit-amount.html (accessed January 5, 2017).

Government of Canada. 2017b. *Canada Pension Plan disability benefit—what you need before you start*. http://www.esdc.gc.ca/en/cpp/disability/before_applying.page (accessed January 6, 2017).

Government of Canada. 2017c. *Canada Pension Plan disability benefits*. https://www.canada.ca/en/employment-social-development/programs/pensions/reports/disability-benefits.html (accessed January 5, 2017).

Government of Canada. 2017d. *Service Canada*. https://www.canada.ca/en/employment-social-development/corporate/portfolio/service-canada.html (accessed January 5, 2017).

IOM (Institute of Medicine). 2007. *A 21st century system for evaluating veterans for disability benefits*. Washington, DC: The National Academies Press.

IOM. 2015. *Psychological testing in the service of disability determination*. Washington, DC: The National Academies Press.

Jackson, M. C. 2016. *Unum utilization of assistive products and technology*. Presentation to the Committee on the Use of Selected Assistive Devices in Eliminating or Reducing the Effects of Impairments, Washington, DC, September 27.

Kidd, M. A. 2016. *Service Canada: Canada Pension Plan.* Presentation to the Committee on the Use of Selected Assistive Devices in Eliminating or Reducing the Effects of Impairments, Washington, DC, September 27.

Owen, III., J. E. 2009. *Disability determination services and their workload.* https://www.ssa.gov/oidap/Documents/Social%20Security%20Administration.%20Disability%20Determination%20Ser.pdf (accessed January 6, 2017).

Prudential Financial. 2015. *Disability program: Statutory agents and financial services associates.* http://hrre.prudential.com/media/managed/2015-Disability-Program-SPD-Statutory-Agents-FSAs.pdf (accessed April 5, 2017).

Prudential Financial. 2016. *Group disability insurance: Employee statement.* https://www.prudential.com/media/managed/100-ClaimPkg-A.pdf (accessed January 6, 2017).

Prudential Financial. 2017. *Prudential disability insurance and absence management: The numbers tell the story.* https://www.prudential.com/employers/group-insurance/products/disability-insurance (accessed February 13, 2017).

QTC (Quality Timeliness Customer Service). 2012. *Who we are.* http://www.qtcm.com/Pages/home.aspx (accessed December 22, 2016).

SSA (U.S. Social Security Administration). 2003. *DI 24535.015 Evaluation of speech impairments.* https://secure.ssa.gov/poms.nsf/lnx/0424535015 (accessed December 22, 2016).

SSA. 2012a. *DI 24505.001 Individual must have a medically determinable severe impairment.* https://secure.ssa.gov/apps10/poms.nsf/lnx/0424505001 (accessed December 22, 2016).

SSA. 2012b. *DI 25020.005 Physical limitations.* https://secure.ssa.gov/poms.nsf/lnx/0425020005 (accessed December 22, 2016).

SSA. 2015a. *Annual statistical supplement to the Social Security Bulletin, 2015.* https://www.ssa.gov/policy/docs/statcomps/supplement/index.html (accessed December 22, 2016).

SSA. 2015b. *DI 23022.000 Processing Quick Disability Determination (QDD) and Compassionate Allowance (CAL) in the Disability Determination Services (DDS).* https://secure.ssa.gov/apps10/poms.nsf/lnx/0423022000 (accessed December 22, 2016).

SSA. 2016a. *Agency financial report: Fiscal year 2016.* https://www.ssa.gov/finance/2016/Full%20FY%202016%20AFR.pdf (accessed January 25, 2017).

SSA. 2016b (unpublished). *Background for IOM on SSA policy and processes related to assistive devices and workplace accommodations.* Baltimore, MD: SSA.

SSA. 2016c. *DI 24501.001 The Disability Determination Services (DDS) Disability Examiner (DE), Medical Consultant (MC), and Psychological Consultant (PC) team, and the role of the Medical Advisor (MA).* https://secure.ssa.gov/poms.nsf/lnx/0424501001 (accessed December 22, 2016).

SSA. 2016d. *DI 24505.015 Finding disability based on the Listing of Impairments.* https://secure.ssa.gov/poms.nsf/lnx/0424505015 (accessed September 15, 2016).

SSA. 2016e. *Revisions to rules regarding the evaluation of medical evidence.* https://www.regulations.gov/document?D=SSA-2012-0035-0001 (accessed April 5, 2017).

SSA. 2017a. *Annual statistical supplement to the Social Security Bulletin, 2016.* https://www.ssa.gov/policy/docs/statcomps/supplement/2016 (accessed January 5, 2017).

SSA. 2017b. *Substantial gainful activity.* https://www.ssa.gov/oact/cola/sga.html (accessed January 5, 2017).

SSA. n.d.-a. *Disability evaluation under social security: 1.00 musculoskeletal system—adult.* https://www.ssa.gov/disability/professionals/bluebook/1.00-Musculoskeletal-Adult.htm (accessed December 22, 2016).

SSA. n.d.-b. *Disability evaluation under social security: 2.00 special senses and speech—Adult.* https://www.ssa.gov/disability/professionals/bluebook/2.00-SpecialSensesandSpeech-Adult.htm (accessed December 22, 2016).

SSA. n.d.-c. *Disability evaluation under social security: Part II—Evidentiary requirements.* https://www.ssa.gov/disability/professionals/bluebook/evidentiary.htm (accessed January 5, 2017).

SSA. n.d.-d. *Disability evaluation under social security: Part III—Listing of impairments.* https://www.ssa.gov/disability/professionals/bluebook/listing-impairments.htm (accessed February 16, 2017).

Tugman, K., and J. Kramschuster. 2016. *The use of assistive technology in return-to-work.* Presentation to the Committee on the Use of Selected Assistive Devices in Eliminating or Reducing the Effects of Impairments, Washington, DC, September 27.

Unum. 2016. *Long term disability claim form.* http://forms.unum.com/StreamPDF.aspx?strURL=/FMS_101699-10.pdf&strAudience=EMPLOYER (accessed January 6, 2017).

Unum. 2017a. *Unum difference.* http://www.unum.com/Employees/UnumDifference (accessed February 14, 2017).

Unum. 2017b. *Unum—Employees and families: FAQ Glossary.* http://www.unum.com/Employees/FAQs/FAQGlossary (accessed April 5, 2017).

VA (U.S. Department of Veterans Affairs). 2013. *Adjudication manual: M21-1, Part III, Subpart IV, Chapter 5—Evaluating evidence and making a decision.* http://www.knowva.ebenefits.va.gov/system/templates/selfservice/va_ss/#!portal/554400000001018/article/554400000014203/M21-1-Part-III-Subpart-iv-Chapter-5-Evaluating-Evidence-and-Making-a-Decision (accessed January 23, 2017).

VA. 2015. *Veterans Benefits Administration evidence requirements.* http://www.benefits.va.gov/compensation/evidence.asp (accessed December 22, 2016).

VA. 2016a. *FY 2015 Summary of Performance and Financial Information (SPFI).* https://www.va.gov/performance/docs/2015spfi.PDF (accessed December 22, 2016).

VA. 2016b. *Veterans Benefits Administration annual benefits report fiscal year 2015: Compensation.* http://www.benefits.va.gov/REPORTS/abr/ABR-Compensation-FY15-05092016.pdf. (accessed December 22, 2016).

VA. 2016c. *Veterans Benefits Administration, compensation, benefit description.* http://www.benefits.va.gov/compensation/ (accessed February 15, 2017).

VA. 2016d. *Veterans Benefits Administration, compensation, disability compensation.* http://www.benefits.va.gov/COMPENSATION/types-disability.asp (accessed February 15, 2017).

VA. 2017. *Veterans Benefits Administration.* http://www.benefits.va.gov/benefits (accessed January 6, 2017).

VBA (Veterans Benefits Administration). 2017. *Veterans Benefits Administration (VBA), U.S. Department of Veterans Affairs.* https://www.facebook.com/pg/VeteransBenefits/about/?ref=page_internal (accessed January 5, 2017).

VR&E (Vocational Rehabilitation and Employment Services). 2016. *What is the Vocational Rehabilitation and Employment Program?* Chapter 31 (fact sheet). http://www.benefits.va.gov/BENEFITS/factsheets/serviceconnected/Ch31FactSheet.pdf (accessed January 23, 2017).

Wixon, B., and A. Strand. 2013. *Identifying SSA's sequential disability determination steps using administrative data.* https://www.ssa.gov/policy/docs/rsnotes/rsn2013-01.html (accessed January 23, 2017).

CHAPTER 8 ANNEX TABLE BEGINS ON THE NEXT PAGE

ANNEX TABLE 8-1
Comparison of U.S. Social Security Administration and Similar Programs

	Social Security Administration	Veterans Benefits Administration
Size of Program	Fiscal year 2015: Social Security Disability Insurance (SSDI): 10,806,466 (including dependents); Supplemental Security Income (SSI): 8,309,564	Fiscal year 2015: 4,168,774 veterans
Disability focus (vocational versus personal)/mission	Vocational (inability to engage in any substantial gainful activity due to physical or mental impairment)	Personal (compensation for service-related disability)
Binary vs. graduated rating system	Binary	Graduated
Wheeled and Seated Mobility Devices		
Factor in consideration of severity	No	No
Factor in consideration of function/vocation	No	No
Upper-Extremity Prostheses		
Factor in consideration of severity	No	No
Factor in consideration of function/vocation	Yes (may be considered in residual functional capacity [RFC] assessment)	No
Hearing-Related Products/Technologies		
Factor in consideration of severity	No	No
Factor in consideration of function/vocation	Yes (considered in RFC assessment)	No
Speech-Related Products/Technologies		
Factor in consideration of severity	Yes (ability to produce speech by any means, which includes devices that improve voice/articulation)	No
Factor in consideration of function/vocation	Yes	No

	Service Canada	Private Insurance	
		Prudential	Unum
	Fiscal year 2014: 329,000 Canada Pension Plan (CPP) beneficiaries with disabilities (83,000 dependents)	5,600 employers (clients); 3.4 million participants	80,000 employers (clients); more than 17 million participants
	Vocational (inability regularly to pursue any substantially gainful occupation due to a medical condition)	Vocational/return to work (inability to perform the material and substantial duties of one's occupation because of sickness or injury)	Vocational/return to work (inability to perform the material and substantial duties of one's occupation because of sickness or injury)
	Binary	Policy dependent	Policy dependent
	No	No	No
	Not specifically (CPP considers impact of treatment)	Yes (may provide some types of wheeled and seated mobility devices [WSMDs] to facilitate return to work)	Yes (may provide some types of WSMDs to facilitate return to work)
	No	No	No
	Not specifically (CPP considers impact of treatment)	Unknown	Unknown
	No	No	No
	Not specifically (CPP considers impact of treatment)	Yes (may provide some types of hearing assistive technologies to facilitate return to work)	Yes (may provide some types of hearing assistive technologies to facilitate return to work)
	No	No	No
	Not specifically (CPP considers impact of treatment)	Unknown	Unknown

9

Overall Conclusions[1]

This chapter presents overall conclusions derived from the chapter-specific findings and conclusions detailed throughout the report.

OVERALL CONCLUSIONS

The committee's chapter-specific findings and conclusions (summarized in the next section) served as the basis for the following nine overall conclusions.

The Promise of Assistive Products and Technologies

The committee's review of the literature and the expert opinions of its members and others who provided input for this study made clear that appropriate-quality assistive products and technologies in all four categories examined may mitigate the impact of impairments sufficiently to allow people with disabilities to work. In some cases, however, environmental and personal factors create barriers to employment despite the impairment-mitigating effects of these products and technologies. For instance, work settings that are not accessible to wheeled and seated mobility devices (WSMDs) for entry and exit and maneuverability create barriers to employment. Likewise, the fit and function of a prosthesis and thus its impairment-mitigating effects may be impacted by such environmental factors

[1]This chapter does not include references. Citations to support the text and conclusions herein are provided in prior chapters of the report.

as exposure to moisture, heat, and dirt. And working in a noisy office with cubicles can create barriers to effective use of a hearing aid.

Maximal user performance requires that individuals receive the appropriate devices for their needs, proper fitting of and training in the use of the devices, and appropriate follow-up care. Even if these conditions are met, moreover, and even given relevant technological advances, assistive products and technologies may not fully mitigate the effects of impairments or associated activity limitations. The committee emphasizes that environmental, societal, and personal factors are as important in determining individuals' overall functioning with respect to employment. Even for people who are able to obtain upper-extremity prostheses (UEPs), for example, rejection rates are high, in part because of discomfort with wearing the devices, limited ability of the devices to meet individual needs, a lack of training in their use, and limited durability. For these reasons, the committee drew the following conclusions:

1. **Assistive products and technologies hold promise for partially or completely mitigating the impacts of impairments and enhancing work participation when appropriate products and technologies are available, when they are properly prescribed and fitted, when the user receives proper training in their use and appropriate follow-up, and when societal and environmental barriers are limited.**
2. **When matching individuals with appropriate assistive products and technologies, it is important to understand the complexity of factors that must be optimized to enhance function. Selecting, designing, or modifying the correct device for an individual and providing training in its use, as well as appropriate follow-up, are complex but necessary elements for maximizing function among users of assistive products and technologies.**

Access to and Coverage of Assistive Products and Technologies

Financial access to appropriate assistive products and technologies as well as qualified providers varies significantly across reimbursement and funding sources in the United States. Numerous pathways exist for accessing these assistive products and technologies and related services, but different coverage sources vary in their missions, their eligibility requirements, and the types of products and technologies and related services they cover. As discussed in Chapter 7, differences in funding policies among various programs affect access to these devices and services for some individuals. In addition, the provision of UEPs is contingent largely on reimbursement policy rather than patient need. The variation among reimbursement and funding sources in the United States also has a significant impact on the types of WSMDs individuals receive. Coverage of hearing aids varies by funding source as well; Medicare and some private health insurers, for example, do not cover hearing aids at all. In some cases, a mismatch exists between the products and technologies covered and those that would best meet the needs of users to enhance their participation in work and other life roles.

In some cases, there also exists a shortage or geographic imbalance of qualified providers and clinics with the knowledge, skill, and expertise to properly evaluate, fit, and train people in the use of assistive products and technologies. As discussed in Chapters 3 and 5, the distribution of providers and clinics with appropriate expertise to evaluate, prescribe, and train people in the use of WSMDs and hearing devices varies greatly throughout the United States. In addition, there is a need for more qualified providers (including physicians, prosthetists, and therapists) and clinics with expertise in the use of UEPs. Similarly, access to speech-language pathologists and other professional members of an augmentative and alternative communication (AAC) team with relevant knowledge, skills, and expertise is necessary and currently limited.

In addition, socioeconomic status and education levels may affect access to coverage for assistive products and technologies and related services. Health literacy is associated with a variety of factors, including educational level. Acquisition of assistive devices may be promoted by people's knowledge of their needs, device and coverage options, and means to pursue the device(s) they need. Moreover, loss of access and coverage among youth of transition age is a significant impediment to their independent living, transition to work, vocational readiness, or further education. The committee drew the following conclusions with respect to access and coverage:

3. **Access to appropriate assistive products and technologies and to qualified providers and teams with the knowledge, skill, and expertise necessary to properly evaluate, fit, train, and monitor people in the use of those products and technologies is frequently limited and varies considerably from case to case, state to state, district to district, urban to rural and frontier areas, and funding source to funding source.**
4. **The variability of coverage for assistive products, technologies, and related services is an important impediment to optimizing function and maintaining gainful employment among transitioning youth and adults with impairments.**

Information and Policy Concerning Assistive Products and Technologies

Individuals' knowledge about assistive product and technology options, their needs, their coverage options, and the means available to them to pursue the products and technologies they need will either promote or hinder their acquisition of the devices. The committee found, for example, that representation by an attorney or advocate who is experienced in health law could help individuals secure Medicaid or Medicare coverage and approval of various medical supplies, equipment, and assistive devices. However, the distribution of knowledge about available assistive products and technologies varies greatly. Socioeconomic status, education level, and a variety of personal factors—including ethnic, cultural, and language barriers—may affect access to assistive products and technologies and related services even when they are covered. The committee therefore drew the following conclusion:

5. **Education regarding the availability of assistive products and technologies and knowledge and training that empower users to self-advocate or have a significant other (e.g., family member, friend, or professional) advocate for them are important elements in achieving successful access to appropriate assistive products and technologies and related services.**

The provision of assistive products and technologies such as WSMDs, UEPs, and AAC devices is contingent largely on reimbursement policy rather than patient need. In some cases, the products and technologies that are covered by Medicare and other insurers as medically necessary are not those that would best meet the needs of users to enhance their participation in life roles. Medicare and other insurers may reject payment for devices and components that are new technologies or that they do not consider medically necessary even if prescribed by a trained professional. For example, Medicare's policy limiting coverage of WSMDs to those needed for home use is an impediment to achieving gainful employment. The variability in reimbursement for UEPs and related rehabilitation services also creates unequal access, particularly for new technologies. Similar limitations exist for users of hearing aids and communication devices. In addition, the relatively small numbers and/or variable distribution of providers and clinics qualified to provide relevant assistive technology services limit access to those services independently of funding or reimbursement considerations. Accordingly, the committee drew the following conclusion:

6. **Assistive products and technologies are advancing at a much faster rate relative to clinician education, regulations, and reimbursement systems, which may limit access to these devices and/or access to training in their use.**

The mission of funding sources and benefit programs affects the extent to which they provide, or help beneficiaries to obtain, appropriate assistive products and technologies and related services designed to facilitate their ability to work. Some private disability insurers provide certain assistive products and technologies in support of occupational functioning and return to work. Unum, for example, utilizes assistive products and technologies in support of occupational functioning in its private insurance disability determinations. Prudential Financial is another private disability insurer that supports assistive products and technologies used primarily for return-to-work purposes, most commonly musculoskeletal aids such as modified workstations, chairs, or mobility devices. State vocational rehabilitation agencies may provide or facilitate the acquisition of assistive products and technologies and related services to enable eligible individuals to prepare for, retain, or regain work based on their personal vocational goals. The Veterans Health Administration is an integrated health care system that provides high-quality, comprehensive, interdisciplinary care and assistive products and technologies to veterans. In addition, a few private health insurers provide integrated health care plans through which covered individuals receive clinical care, prescription drugs, and assistive products and technologies. Based on its review of selected monetary disability benefit programs and funding sources for assistive products and technologies, the committee drew the following conclusion:

7. **Some coverage and disability benefit models, such as those of the Veterans Health Administration, state vocational rehabilitation agencies, some private disability insurance carriers, and a few private health insurers, are more holistic than others, providing access to a greater range of assistive products and technologies and related services that can be appropriate to meeting individuals' needs and facilitating their ability to work.**

Evaluation of Ability to Work

The concept of disability has evolved to reflect a biopsychosocial model in which disability is perceived as the interaction between an individual's functional capacity and relevant social and physical environmental and personal factors. Although assistive products and technologies may mitigate the impacts of impairments sufficiently to allow a person to work, personal factors such as gender, race/ethnicity, age, socioeconomic status, insurance coverage, education, and previous work experience can influence how an individual experiences disability. In addition, the individual experience of disability is influenced by such environmental factors as the job market, workplace attitudes, geographic location, and the built environment. Although the committee found that a complete evaluation of a person's functioning would include the assistive products and technologies he or she normally uses, that finding needs to be tempered by the following conclusion:

8. **Professionals involved in disability determinations cannot assume that because an individual uses a particular assistive product or technology, this device is always effective for that person, that it mitigates the impact of the person's impairment, or that it enables the person to work. Environmental, societal, and personal factors also must be taken into account.**

Data on the Use and Effectiveness of Assistive Products and Technologies

The committee found that data on the prevalence of use of the assistive products and technologies discussed in this report and the extent to which they mitigate the impacts of impairments are fragmented and limited. At this time, it is difficult to quantify the impact of assistive products and technologies and related services on impairment mitigation and employability because of contextual/environmental, societal, and personal factors that affect device use and job function; the lack of data on occupational success; and unequal access to relevant products and technologies and training. The committee recognizes that limited or lack of evidence about the impact of assistive products and technologies and related rehabilitative services on activity and participation may affect decisions by funding sources about which devices and services to cover. Information from outcomes research could contribute to studies on the effectiveness or cost-effectiveness of various assistive products and technologies and thereby help to inform the development of rational resource utilization, including coverage decisions by insurers and other funding sources. Accordingly, the committee drew the following conclusion:

9. **Additional research is needed to understand how the specifications for and use of assistive technologies and products and related services impact inclusion in society and work participation for individuals with disabilities. Such research may not**

only enhance knowledge in these areas but also inform the development of rational resource utilization, including informing cost-benefit analyses and coverage for devices and related services.

SUPPORTING EVIDENCE FOR THE COMMITTEE'S OVERALL CONCLUSIONS

Box 9-1 shows the links between the overall conclusions presented above and the most relevant chapter-specific findings and conclusions that support them.[2]

[2]The committee's chapter-specific findings and conclusions are numbered according to the chapter in which they appear.

BOX 9-1
Overall Conclusions and Supporting Evidence

1. Assistive products and technologies hold promise for partially or completely mitigating the impacts of impairments and enhancing work participation when appropriate products and technologies are available, when they are properly prescribed and fitted, when the user receives proper training in their use and appropriate follow-up, and when societal and environmental barriers are limited.

Findings

3-8. Even though wheelchairs are ubiquitous, they do not replace all of the complex functions of the lower extremities; in addition, proper fitting and training are complex but necessary elements of maximizing users' performance, work potential, and health maintenance.

4-6. Currently available UEPs cannot replace the complex functions of the missing limb because of limitations inherent in their control and design, their lack of sensory feedback, and the methods required to suspend them onto the residual limb.

4-9. The fit and function of the prosthesis and thus its impairment-mitigating effects may be impacted by environmental factors that may change over time, such as exposure to moisture, heat, and dirt. The consistency of impairment mitigation also depends on the condition and volume of the residual limb, which impact socket fit and comfort.

5-7. Compared with the prevalence of hearing loss, the prevalence of hearing aid use is low in the United States.

Conclusions

3-5. A higher level of certification/training than the current assistive technology professional credential could improve the qualifications of providers in terms of the knowledge, skill, and expertise necessary to properly evaluate, prescribe, and train people in the use of WSMDs. The degree requirement from an accredited program and certification process for prosthetists and orthotists could serve as a good model for WSMD suppliers and technicians.

4-13. At this time, it is difficult to quantify fully the impact of UEPs on impairment mitigation and employability because of a lack of research on contextual/environmental factors that impact device use and job function and a lack of data on occupational success. Even as UEPs have the potential to improve functional capacity in work participation, their impact is limited by unequal access to the devices and training in their use.

5-3. Even with advances in technology, hearing aids and other hearing assistive devices may help but do not fully mitigate impairments or restrictions on participation caused by hearing loss. Environmental and personal factors are as important in determining the overall communicative functioning of individuals with hearing loss.

6-3. Although great progress has been achieved in AAC systems, use of an SGD [speech-generating device] does not fully mitigate the impact of a severe communication impairment. In addition, even when provided with optimal assessment, funding resources, AAC systems, interventions, and supports, individuals may not achieve their potential because of any number of environmental and personal factors that influence communication performance in employment contexts.

2. When matching individuals with appropriate assistive products and technologies, it is important to understand the complexity of factors that must be optimized to enhance function. Selecting, designing, or modifying the correct device for an individual and providing training in its use, as well as appropriate follow-up, are complex but necessary elements for maximizing function among users of assistive products and technologies.

Findings

3-14. There are limited data showing the relationship between individual users' medical conditions and health (e.g., comorbidities) and/or sociodemographic characteristics and the specific types of WSMDs they use.

4-2. Regardless of the type of prosthetic device used, a well-fitting and comfortable socket is essential to successful use of a prosthesis.

Conclusions

3-6. Information showing the relationship between individual users' medical conditions and health and/or sociodemographic characteristics and the specific types of WSMDs they use would be useful for payers, providers, and consumers to support future planning for treatment programs, the production of technologies, the training of providers, and the allocation of resources for these assistive devices.

4-5. Even for people who are able to obtain UEPs, rejection rates are high, in part because of discomfort with wearing the devices, limited ability of the devices to meet their needs, a lack of training in their use, and limited durability.

5-2. Proper fitting and training are complex but necessary elements of maximizing performance among users of hearing devices. Consumers who work with providers trained in the use of properly prescribed and fitted hearing devices can expect better results than those who use off-the-shelf products.

3. Access to appropriate assistive products and technologies and to qualified providers and teams with the knowledge, skill, and expertise necessary to properly evaluate, fit, train, and monitor people in the use of those products and technologies is frequently limited and varies considerably from case to case, state to state, district to district, urban to rural and frontier areas, and funding source to funding source.

continued

BOX 9-1 Continued

Findings

3-6. Access to WSMDs varies significantly across reimbursement and funding sources in the United States.

3-7. A mismatch exists between the types of WSMDs covered by Medicare and those required to maximize individuals' functioning based on their diagnosis and treatment.

3-10. The distribution of providers and clinics with the knowledge, skill, and expertise to properly evaluate, prescribe, and train people in the use of WSMDs varies greatly throughout the United States.

5-1. The distribution of providers and clinics with the knowledge, skill, and expertise to properly evaluate, prescribe, and train people in the use of hearing devices varies greatly throughout the United States.

5-10. The cost for hearing aids is usually covered under a bundled model that includes the costs of the devices and of the professional services required to fit them properly and follow up for rehabilitation.

6-19. School districts that have provided AAC systems for children often retain the devices; as a result, children transitioning from school into postsecondary/vocational settings must navigate the transition while completing the AAC assessment, funding, and new learning processes. Some children may even have to learn entirely new language representation, messaging, and access methods before they can engage in essential communication.

7-6. Individuals' acquisition of assistive devices may be promoted by their knowledge of their device options, their needs, their coverage options, and their means of pursuing the device(s) they need.

7-11. Health literacy, which may include knowledge about assistive products and technologies, varies greatly among adults in the United States, although individuals at lower socioeconomic levels generally demonstrate lower average health literacy.

Conclusions

3-1. The variation in reimbursement and funding sources and access to qualified professionals in the United States has a significant impact on the types of WSMDs individuals receive.

3-4. More qualified providers and clinics with the knowledge, skill, and expertise to properly evaluate, prescribe, and train people in the use of WSMDs are needed.

4-10. The provision of UEPs is contingent largely on reimbursement policy rather than patient need. In many cases, a mismatch exists between the UEPs covered by Medicare and other insurers as medically necessary and the products or technologies that would best meet the needs of users to enhance their participation in life roles.

4-11. There is a need for more qualified providers (including physicians, prosthetists, and therapists) and clinics with the knowledge, skill, and expertise to properly evaluate, prescribe, fit, and train people in the use of UEPs.

5-1. Qualified providers and clinics with the knowledge, skill, and expertise to properly evaluate, prescribe, and train people in the use of hearing devices are needed.
6-4. Access to SLPs [speech-language pathologists] and other professional members of an AAC team with relevant knowledge, skills, and expertise is necessary and currently limited.
6-6. Differences in funding policies among various programs significantly limit access to AAC technology and clinical services.

4. The variability of coverage for assistive products, technologies, and related services is an important impediment to optimizing function and maintaining gainful employment among transitioning youth and adults with impairments.

Findings

7-9. Loss of coverage of and access to assistive products and technologies and related services among youth of transition age is a significant impediment to their successful transition to work, vocational readiness, or further education.
3-5. The variable dependability and availability of WSMDs impact individuals' functioning and activity and their ability to be employed.
5-7. Compared with the prevalence of hearing loss, the prevalence of hearing aid use is low in the United States.

Conclusions

7-7. Ensuring continued access to appropriate assistive products and technologies and related services is vital to promoting a successful transition from high school to pathways to employment.
3-2. Medicare's policy limiting coverage of WSMDs to those needed for home use is an impediment to achieving gainful employment.
4-10. The provision of UEPs is contingent largely on reimbursement policy rather than patient need. In many cases, a mismatch exists between the UEPs covered by Medicare and other insurers as medically necessary and the products or technologies that would best meet the needs of users to enhance their participation in life roles.
5-5. The widespread lack of insurance coverage for hearing devices and related services is an impediment to optimizing communicative functioning and maintaining gainful employment among adults with hearing loss.
6-4. Access to SLPs and other professional members of an AAC team with relevant knowledge, skills, and expertise is necessary and currently limited.

5. Education regarding the availability of assistive products and technologies and knowledge and training that empower users to self-advocate or have a significant other (e.g., family member, friend, or professional) advocate for them are important elements in achieving successful ac-

continued

BOX 9-1 Continued

cess to appropriate assistive products and technologies and related services.

Findings

3-11. Providers of WSMDs vary in their level of knowledge, skills, and expertise.

6-20. Required education for preprofessional SLPs is limited, as a number of university programs still do not have a required AAC course.

7-6. Individuals' acquisition of assistive devices may be promoted by their knowledge of their device options, their needs, their coverage options, and their means of pursuing the device(s) they need.

7-7. Representation by an attorney or advocate who is experienced in health law could help individuals secure Medicaid or Medicare coverage and approval of various medical supplies, equipment, and assistive devices.

7-11. Health literacy, which may include knowledge about assistive products and technologies, varies greatly among adults in the United States, although individuals at lower socioeconomic levels generally demonstrate lower average health literacy.

Conclusions

3-4. More qualified providers and clinics with the knowledge, skill, and expertise to properly evaluate, prescribe, and train people in the use of WSMDs are needed.

4-11. There is a need for more qualified providers (including physicians, prosthetists, and therapists) and clinics with the knowledge, skill, and expertise to properly evaluate, prescribe, fit, and train people in the use of UEPs.

5-1. Qualified providers and clinics with the knowledge, skill, and expertise to properly evaluate, prescribe, and train people in the use of hearing devices are needed.

6-4. Access to SLPs and other professional members of an AAC team with relevant knowledge, skills, and expertise is necessary and currently limited.

7-3. Individuals of low socioeconomic status are limited in their access to coverage for assistive products and technologies and related services, as well as in their ability to obtain the devices and services when they are covered.

7-4. A variety of personal factors, including ethnic, cultural, and language barriers, may affect access to assistive products and technologies and related services when they are covered.

7-8. Knowledge and training that empower users to self-advocate or have a significant other (e.g., family member, friend, or professional) advocate for them can lead to successful access to appropriate assistive products and technologies and related services.

6. **Assistive products and technologies are advancing at a much faster rate relative to clinician education, regulations, and reimbursement systems, which may limit access to these devices and/or access to training in their use.**

Findings

3-10. The distribution of providers and clinics with the knowledge, skills, and expertise to properly evaluate, prescribe, and train people in the use of WSMDs varies greatly throughout the United States.

5-1. The distribution of providers and clinics with the knowledge, skill, and expertise to properly evaluate, prescribe, and train people in the use of hearing devices varies greatly throughout the United States.

6-22. High equipment costs and continual technology developments result in limited availability of AAC systems for use in the assessment, equipment trial, and intervention processes in clinical settings.

Conclusions

3-2. Medicare's policy limiting coverage of WSMDs to those needed for home use is an impediment to achieving gainful employment.

3-4. More qualified providers and clinics with the knowledge, skills, and expertise to properly evaluate, prescribe, and train people in the use of WSMDs are needed.

4-9. Reimbursement for UEPs and related rehabilitation services is highly variable, which creates unequal access, particularly for new technologies.

4-11. There is a need for more qualified providers (including physicians, prosthetists, and therapists) and clinics with the knowledge, skill, and expertise to properly evaluate, prescribe, fit, and train people in the use of UEPs.

5-1. Qualified providers and clinics with the knowledge, skill, and expertise to properly evaluate, prescribe, and train people in the use of hearing devices are needed.

6-4. Access to SLPs and other professional members of an AAC team with relevant knowledge, skills, and expertise is necessary and currently limited.

7. **Some coverage and disability benefit models, such as those of the Veterans Health Administration, state vocational rehabilitation agencies, some private disability insurance carriers, and a few private health insurers, are more holistic than others, providing access to a greater range of assistive products and technologies and related services that can be appropriate to meeting individuals' needs and facilitating their ability to work.**

Findings

8-1. Unum utilizes assistive products and technologies in support of occupational functioning in its private insurance disability determinations.

continued

BOX 9-1 Continued

8-2. Prudential specified that assistive products and technologies—most commonly musculoskeletal aids such as modified workstations, chairs, or mobility devices—were covered primarily for return-to-work purposes.

8-7. Consideration of hearing-related products and technologies in the private disability insurance sector focuses on the provision of these devices to facilitate return to work as a claimant's impairment will allow.

Conclusions

8-1. The mission of a disability benefits program affects the extent to which the program provides (or "helps beneficiaries to obtain") assistive products and technologies and related services designed to facilitate their ability to work.

8. Professionals involved in disability determinations cannot assume that because an individual uses a particular assistive product or technology, this device is always effective for that person, that it mitigates the impact of the person's impairment, or that it enables the person to work. Environmental, societal, and personal factors also must be taken into account.

Findings

2-3. Likewise, based on the *International Classification of Functioning, Disability and Health* model, understanding a person's ability to participate in work includes not only the person's functional capacity but also relevant environmental and personal factors.

Conclusions

2-1. Assistive products and technologies may mitigate the impact of an impairment sufficiently to allow a person to work. In some cases, however, environmental and personal factors create barriers to employment despite those impairment-mitigating effects.

9. Additional research is needed to understand how the specifications for and use of assistive technologies and products and related services impact inclusion in society and work participation for individuals with disabilities. Such research may not only enhance knowledge in these areas but also inform the development of rational resource utilization, including informing cost-benefit analyses and coverage for devices and related services.

Findings

3-14. There are limited data showing the relationship between individual users' medical conditions and health (e.g., comorbidities) and/or sociodemographic characteristics and the specific types of WSMDs they use.

4-15. The only U.S. data available on vocational reintegration following upper-extremity amputation come from the military health care system. The committee could find no other studies examining the impact of prosthetic devices and rehabilitation strategies on work participation in the United States.

5-4. Research investigating the impact of audiometric hearing function and/or hearing devices on real-world communicative functioning is extremely limited.

6-10. Established measures of real-world communicative functioning are sparse, and research investigating the impact of AAC products and technologies on real-world communicative functioning is extremely limited.

Conclusions

3-6. Information showing the relationship between individual users' medical conditions and health and/or sociodemographic characteristics and the specific types of WSMDs they use would be useful for payers, providers, and consumers to support future planning for treatment programs, the production of technologies, the training of providers, and the allocation of resources for these assistive devices.

4-7. Comprehensive efforts to study the impact of upper-limb loss, prosthesis use, and amputation rehabilitation on activity and participation, including work participation, are needed. Such research may not only enhance knowledge in these areas but also inform the development of rational resource utilization, including informing cost–benefit analyses and coverage for devices and related services.

4-13. At this time, it is difficult to quantify fully the impact of UEPs on impairment mitigation and employability because of a lack of research on contextual/environmental factors that impact device use and job function and a lack of data on occupational success. Even as UEPs have the potential to improve functional capacity in work participation, their impact is limited by unequal access to the devices and training in their use.

5-4. The establishment of objective measures of real-world communicative functioning is vital to promoting a better understanding of the effects on this functioning of audiometric hearing function and hearing devices.

6-1. Data on the prevalence and use of AAC systems by adults are fragmented and limited, resulting in incomplete knowledge of employability, vocational effectiveness, and overall employment outcomes.

Appendix A

Public Session Agendas

MEETING 1: PUBLIC SESSION

Hosted by the Committee on the Use of Selected Assistive Products and Technologies in Eliminating or Reducing the Effects of Impairments

March 31, 2016

Keck Center of the National Academies
Room 101
500 Fifth Street, NW
Washington, DC 20001

Agenda

10:00 a.m. **Welcome and Introductions**
Alan Jette, Committee Chair

10:10 a.m. **U.S. Social Security Administration (SSA) Presentations Relevant to the Committee's Task**

10:30 a.m. **Discussion of Statement of Task**
Committee Members and SSA Staff

11:30 a.m. **Close Morning Session**
Alan Jette, Committee Chair

1:00 p.m. **Presentations and Discussion with Committee**

- **SSA policy on assistive devices and GAO reports**
  Patricia M. Owens, M.P.A., Consultant on Health and Disability Policy and Programs
- **Assistive devices pertaining to hearing**
  Ryan McCreery, Ph.D., Director of the Center for Audiology, Boys Town National Research Hospital
- **Assistive devices pertaining to communication and speech recognition**
  Laura J. Ball, Ph.D., Director of Research, Hearing and Speech Center, Children's National Medical Center

3:35 p.m. **Summary and Closing Remarks**
Alan Jette, Committee Chair

3:30 p.m. **Adjourn**

MEETING 2: PUBLIC SESSION

Hosted by the Committee on the Use of Selected Assistive Products and Technologies in Eliminating or Reducing the Effects of Impairments

May 16, 2016

Keck Center of the National Academies
Room 101
500 Fifth Street, NW
Washington, DC 20001

Agenda

9:00 a.m. **Welcome and Introductions**
Alan Jette, Committee Chair

9:10 a.m. **Wheeled and seated mobility devices—presentation and discussion**
Mark Schmeler, Assistant Professor, University of Pittsburgh School of Health and Rehabilitation Sciences

10:00 a.m. **Upper-extremity prostheses—presentation and discussion**
Gerald Stark, Senior Upper Limb Clinical Specialist, Ottobock

10:50 a.m.	**Workplace accommodations—presentation and discussion** *Susanne M. Bruyère, Director, K. Lisa Yang and Hock E. Tan Institute on Employment and Disability, Cornell University*
11:55 a.m.	**Close Morning Session** *Alan Jette, Committee Chair*
1:00 p.m.	**Disability statistics—presentation and discussion** *William A. Erickson, Research Specialist, K. Lisa Yang and Hock E. Tan Institute on Employment and Disability, Cornell University*
1:50 p.m.	**Veterans Affairs—presentation and discussion** *Penny Nechanicky, National Director, Prosthetic and Sensory Aids Service, U.S. Department of Veterans Affairs*
2:40 p.m.	**Private disability—presentation and discussion** *Michelle C. Jackson, Assistant Vice President, Workforce Solutions Group, Unum*
3:25 p.m.	**Summary and Closing Remarks** *Alan Jette, Committee Chair*
3:30 p.m.	**Adjourn**

MEETING 3: PUBLIC SESSION

Hosted by the Committee on the Use of Selected Assistive Products and Technologies in Eliminating or Reducing the Effects of Impairments

July 18, 2016

National Academy of Sciences Building
Members' Room
2101 Constitution Avenue, NW
Washington, DC 20418

Agenda

9:00 a.m.	**Welcome and Introductions** *Alan Jette, Committee Chair*

9:10 a.m.	**Veterans Benefits Administration—presentation and discussion** *Brad Flohr, Compensation Service, U.S. Department of Veterans Affairs*
10:00 a.m.	**Vocational Rehabilitation Services—presentation and discussion** *Jo Anne Materkowski, Office of Field Services, Maryland Division of Rehabilitation Services* *Melissa Day, Workforce and Technology Center, Maryland Division of Rehabilitation Services* *Justin Creamer, Workforce and Technology Center, Maryland Division of Rehabilitation Services*
10:55 a.m.	**Break**
11:05 a.m.	**Medicare coverage for selected assistive products and technologies—presentation and discussion** *Susan M. Miller, M.D., Coverage and Analysis Group, Centers for Medicare & Medicaid Services*
12:00 p.m.	**Close Morning Session** *Alan Jette, Committee Chair*
1:00 p.m.	**Private health insurance industry—presentation and discussion** *Daniel E. Kubrin, M.S.H.A., M.B.A., PMP, Benefits Policy, Design and Implementation, Kaiser Permanente*
2:00 p.m.	**Transition from high school—presentations and panel discussion** *Colleen Thoma, Ph.D., Counseling and Special Education, Virginia Commonwealth University School of Education* *Amy S. Goldman, M.S., Institute on Disabilities, Temple University* *Megan Conway, Ph.D., Center on Disability Studies, University of Hawai'i at Mánoa*
2:50 p.m.	**Break**
3:00 p.m.	**Transition from high school—panel discussion (continued)**

3:50 p.m. **Summary and Closing Remarks**
Alan Jette, Committee Chair

4:00 p.m. **Adjourn**

TELECONFERENCE WITH REPRESENTATIVES OF SERVICE CANADA AND PRUDENTIAL

Hosted by the Committee on the Use of Selected Assistive Products and Technologies in Eliminating or Reducing the Effects of Impairments

September 27, 2016

J. Erik Jonsson Conference Center, Carriage House
314 Quissett Avenue
Woods Hole, MA 02543

Agenda

9:00 a.m. **Welcome and Introductions**
Alan Jette, Committee Chair

9:05 a.m. **Service Canada, Canada Pension Plan—presentation and discussion**
Michael Kidd, Service Canada, Canada Pension Plan

9:35 a.m. **Private disability insurance—presentation and discussion**
John Kramschuster, M.S., CRC, Vocational Services, Prudential
Kristin Tugman, Ph.D., CRC, LPC, Health and Productivity Analytics and Consulting Practice, Prudential

12:00 p.m. **Adjourn**
Alan Jette, Committee Chair

Appendix B

Glossary

Accessible design:
(1) Specialized design based on accepted dimensional requirements that is added to or used in lieu of typical everyday products, spaces, and technologies to remove barriers to people with specific types of disabilities (Sanford, 2012).
(2) "A design process in which the needs of people with disabilities are specifically considered. *Accessibility* sometimes refers to the characteristic that products, services, and facilities can be independently used by people with a variety of disabilities" (DO-IT, 2015).

Activity: "The execution of a task or action by an individual. It represents the individual perspective of functioning" (WHO, 2001, p. 213).

Adaptive devices: "Any structure, design, instrument, contrivance, or equipment that enables a person with a disability" to improve function (Mosby, 2009). "Adaptive device" is synonymous with "personal assistive device," "assistive technology," and "assistive technology device."

Assistive technology: "[T]echnology designed to be utilized in an assistive technology device or assistive technology service."[1]

Assistive technology device: "[A]ny item, piece of equipment, or product system, whether acquired commercially, modified, or customized, that is

[1]Assistive Technology Act of 2004, Public Law 108-364, § 3(3), 118 Stat. 1710 (2004).

used to increase, maintain, or improve functional capabilities of individuals with disabilities."[2]

Assistive technology service: "The term 'assistive technology service' means any service that directly assists an individual with a disability in the selection, acquisition, or use of an assistive technology device."[3]

Augmentative and alternative communication devices: Computer- and non-computer-based electronic or nonelectronic technologies "that provide individuals whose natural speech is not functional with a means of communication" (AAC Institute, 2015).

Body functions: "The physiological functions of body systems, including psychological functions. 'Body' refers to the human organism as a whole, and thus includes the brain. Hence, mental (or psychological) functions are subsumed under body functions. The standard for these functions is considered to be the statistical norm for humans" (WHO, 2001, p. 213).

Body structures: "The structural or anatomical parts of the body such as organs, limbs and their components classified according to body systems. The standard for these structures is considered to be the statistical norm for humans" (WHO, 2001, p. 213).

Cognitive assistive technologies: A subclass of assistive technology "that is designed to 'increase, maintain, or improve functional capabilities' for individuals whose cognitive [abilities] limit their effective participation in daily activities" (adapted from Scherer et al., 2005, p. 197).

Disability:
(1) *International Classification of Functioning, Disability and Health* definition: "An umbrella term for impairments, activity limitations and participation restrictions. It denotes the negative aspects of the interaction between an individual (with a health condition) and that individual's contextual factors (environmental and personal factors)" (WHO, 2001, p. 213).
(2) U.S. Social Security Administration (SSA) definition: In adults, "the inability to engage in any substantial gainful activity . . . by reason of any medically determinable physical or mental impairment(s) which can be expected to result in death or which has lasted or can be expected to last for a continuous period of not less than 12 months" (SSA, n.d., see also SSA, 2012).

[2]Assistive Technology Act of 2004, Public Law 108-364, § 3(4), 118 Stat. 1710 (2004).
[3]Assistive Technology Act of 2004, Public Law 108-364, § 3(5), 118 Stat. 1710 (2004).

(3) Americans with Disabilities Act (ADA) definition: "The ADA defines a person with a disability as a person who has a physical or mental impairment that substantially limits one or more major life activity. This includes people who have a record of such an impairment, even if they do not currently have a disability. It also includes individuals who do not have a disability but are regarded as having a disability. The ADA also makes it unlawful to discriminate against a person based on that person's association with a person with a disability" (ADA National Network, 2017).
(4) U.S. Centers for Disease Control and Prevention definition: "Any condition of the body or mind (impairment) that makes it more difficult for the person with the condition to do certain activities (activity limitation) and interact with the world around them (participation restrictions)" (CDC, 2016).
(5) State vocational rehabilitation definition: "State vocational rehabilitation (VR) offices define a person with a disability to be eligible for VR services if he or she has a physical or mental impairment that constitutes or results in a 'substantial impediment' to employment for the applicant" (DOL, 2017).

Durable medical equipment:
(1) Medicare definition: "[Durable medical equipment] meets these criteria: durable (can withstand repeated use), used for a medical reason, not usually useful to someone who isn't sick or injured, used in your home, [and] has an expected lifetime of at least 3 years" (CMS, 2017).
(2) SSA Program Operations Manual System definition: "Durable medical equipment is equipment which can withstand repeated use, . . . *and* is primarily and customarily used to serve a medical purpose, . . . *and* generally is not useful to a person in the absence of an illness or injury, . . . *and* is appropriate for use in the home" (SSA, 2014).

Environmental modifications: Any "alterations, adjustments, or additions to the . . . environment through the use of specialized, customized, off-the-shelf, or universally designed technologies; low- or high-tech equipment, products, hardware controls and cues, finishes, and furnishings; and other features that affect the layout and structure" of the built environment (adapted from AOTA, 2016).[4]

Health care disparities: Differences in access to or availability of facilities and services.

---

[4]Adapted from the American Occupational Therapy Association definition of "home" modifications (i.e., "environment" replaced the word "home"), which was proposed by Fagan and Sanford (2004).

Health inequalities: Differences in health status or in the distribution of health determinants among different population groups.

Health status disparities: Variation in rates of disease occurrence and disabilities among socioeconomic and/or geographically defined population groups.

Hearing assistive technologies: "Encompasses a wide range of products—from traditional hearing aids regulated as medical devices to consumer-technology products and hearing assistive technologies—with the overall goal of enabling the user to hear and communicate better in their homes (e.g., television), in public spaces (e.g., movies and lectures), and through phones or other communications products and systems" (NASEM, 2016, p. 149).

Impairment: "A loss or abnormality in body structure or physiological function (including mental functions). Abnormality here is used strictly to refer to a significant variation from established statistical norms (i.e., as a deviation from a population mean within measured standard norms) and should be used only in this sense" (WHO, 2001, p. 213).

Orthoses: Externally applied devices "used to stabilize or unload joints, normalize motion and stresses on tissue, substitute for muscle weakness or paralysis, and assist in normal growth, development and function. Orthoses can be applied to the head, neck, trunk, or limbs" (adapted from University of Pittsburgh, 2017).

Participation: "A person's involvement in a life situation. It represents the societal perspective of functioning" (WHO, 2001, p. 213).

Personal assistive device: Any device that improves or compensates for loss of body function to improve the capacity of persons with disabilities. "Any device designed or adapted to help people with physical or emotional disorders perform actions, tasks, and activities" (*Assistive device*, n.d.).

Prostheses: Artificial limbs "used to replace missing limbs or portions of limbs, and to restore more normal function of the upper or lower extremities" (University of Pittsburgh, 2017).

Surgically implanted devices: "Medical implants are devices or tissues that are placed inside or on the surface of the body. Many implants are prosthetics, intended to replace missing body parts. Other implants deliver medication, monitor body functions, or provide support to organs and tissues. Some implants are made from skin, bone or other body tissues. Others are made from metal, plastic, ceramic or other materials. Implants can be placed permanently or they can be removed once they are no longer needed" (FDA, 2015). Cochlear implants are an example of a surgically implanted device.

Transition: A coordinated set of activities for a child with a disability that (1) is designed to be within a results-oriented process and is focused on improving the academic and functional achievement of the child to facilitate movement from school to postschool activities, including postsecondary education, vocational education, integrated employment (including supported employment), continuing and adult education, adult services, independent living, or community participation; (2) is based on the individual child's needs, taking into account his or her strengths, preferences, and interests; and (3) includes instruction, related services, community experiences, the development of employment and other postschool adult living objectives, and if appropriate, acquisition of daily living skills and functional vocational evaluation.

Universal design: The design of all products and environments "to be usable by all people to the greatest extent possible" without the need for adaptation or specialized design (adapted from Mace et al., 1991, p. 156).

Wheelchair: A "wheeled mobility device with a seating support system for a person with impaired mobility, intended to provide mobility in a seated position as its primary function. Includes manual and power wheelchairs. Excludes: Devices such as prone mobility carts that provide mobility in a non-seated position" (Waugh, 2013, p. 20).

Wheeled mobility devices: Medical devices with wheels that are intended to provide mobility and function to persons with restricted or no ability to ambulate without assistance from technology.

Workplace reasonable accommodations: "The term *reasonable accommodation* means: (i) modifications or adjustments to a job application process that enable a qualified applicant with a disability to be considered for the position such qualified applicant desires; or (ii) modifications or adjustments to the work environment, or to the manner or circumstances under which the position held or desired is customarily performed, that enable an individual with a disability who is qualified to perform the essential functions of that position; or (iii) modifications or adjustments that enable a covered entity's employee with a disability to enjoy equal benefits and privileges of employment as are enjoyed by its other similarly situated employees without disabilities."[5]

REFERENCES

AAC Institute. 2015. *What is AAC?* http://aacinstitute.org/what-is-aac (accessed January 26, 2017).

ADA National Network. 2017. *What is the definition of disability under the ADA?* https://adata.org/faq/what-definition-disability-under-ada (accessed January 27, 2017).

AOTA (American Occupational Therapy Association). 2016. *Home modifications and occupational therapy.* http://www.aota.org/about-occupational-therapy/professionals/rdp/homemods.aspx (accessed January 27, 2017).

Assistive device. n.d. *McGraw-Hill Concise Dictionary of Modern Medicine*, 2002. http://medical-dictionary.thefreedictionary.com/assistive+device (accessed January 30, 2017).

CDC (U.S. Centers for Disease Control and Prevention). 2016. *Disability overview.* https://www.cdc.gov/ncbddd/disabilityandhealth/disability.html (accessed March 21, 2017).

CMS (Centers for Medicare & Medicaid Services). 2017. *Medicare.gov: Durable medical equipment (DME) coverage.* https://www.medicare.gov/coverage/durable-medical-equipment-coverage.html (accessed January 27, 2017).

DO-IT (Disabilities, Opportunities, Internetworking, and Technology). 2015. *What is the difference between accessible, usable, and universal design?* http://www.washington.edu/doit/what-difference-between-accessible-usable-and-universal-design (accessed January 26, 2017).

DOL (U.S. Department of Labor). 2017. *Frequently asked questions.* https://www.dol.gov/odep/faqs/general.htm (accessed February 13, 2017).

Fagan, L. A., and J. A. Sanford. 2004. *Home modifications: Assessment, implementation, and innovation.* Presented at the 84th Annual Conference & Expo of the American Occupational Therapy Association, Minneapolis, MN, May.

FDA (U.S. Food and Drug Administration). 2015. *Implants and prosthetics.* http://www.fda.gov/MedicalDevices/ProductsandMedicalProcedures/ImplantsandProsthetics (accessed January 27, 2017).

Mace, R., G. Hardie, and J. Place. 1991. Accessible environments: Toward universal design. In *Design intervention: Toward a more humane architecture*, edited by W. E. Preiser, J. C. Vischer, and E. T. White. New York: Van Nostrand Reinhold Publishers. Pp. 155-175.

Mosby. 2009. *Mosby's Medical Dictionary*, 9th ed. St Louis, MO: Elsevier.

NASEM (National Academies of Sciences, Engineering, and Medicine). 2016. *Hearing health care for adults: Priorities for improving access and affordability.* Washington, DC: The National Academies Press.

Sanford, J. A. 2012. *Design for the ages: Universal design as a rehabilitation strategy.* New York: Springer.

Scherer, M. J., T. Hart, N. Kirsch, and M. Schulthesis. 2005. Assistive technologies for cognitive disabilities. *Critical Reviews in Physical and Rehabilitation Medicine* 17(3):195-215.

SSA (U.S. Social Security Administration). 2012. *DI 00115.015 Definitions of disability.* https://secure.ssa.gov/poms.nsf/lnx/0400115015 (accessed January 26, 2017).

SSA. 2014. *HI 00610.200 Definition of durable medical equipment.* https://secure.ssa.gov/apps10/poms.nsf/lnx/0600610200 (accessed January 27, 2017).

SSA. n.d. *Disability evaluation under social security; Part I—General information.* http://www.ssa.gov/disability/professionals/bluebook/general-info.htm (accessed January 26, 2017).

[5]29 CFR § 1630.2.

University of Pittsburgh. 2017. *Prosthetics & orthotics: About.* https://www.shrs.pitt.edu/po/about (accessed January 27, 2017).

Waugh, K. 2013. *Glossary of wheelchair terms and definitions, Version 1.0.* https://www.ncart.us/uploads/userfiles/files/glossary-of-wheelchair-terms.pdf (accessed January 27, 2017).

WHO (World Health Organization). 2001. *International Classification of Functioning, Disability and Health (ICF).* Geneva, Switzerland: WHO.

Appendix C

Medicare Data

METHODS

This study was a secondary analysis of Medicare claims data for the calendar years 2013-2014. We used a 5 percent random sample of Medicare beneficiaries' claims data that is available at the University of Texas Medical Branch, in the Research Identifiable Format, for those years.

Study Sample Population

The study sample population comprised all Medicare beneficiaries, irrespective of the type of plan (e.g., traditional fee-for-service or Medicare Advantage) in which they were enrolled during the study period. However, we selected only those beneficiaries aged 20 to 67 years so the sample would be representative of the beneficiaries of the U.S. Social Security Administration. No other inclusion/exclusion criterion were used for deriving the study sample cohort.

Data Sources and Characteristics

For this study, we used data from two data files that are part of the Medicare claims data resources. Detailed descriptions of these data files are provided in Table C-1.

TABLE C-1
Description of Data Files

Data File	Years	Description
Durable Medical Equipment (DME)	2013–2014	Two DME data files were used: the DME claim line file and the DME claims file. (For additional information related to these files, see ResDAC, n.d.-b.) • The DME claim line file comprised Berenson-Eggers type of service (BETOS) codes and Health Care Common Procedure Coding System (HCPCS) codes and all information related to processing the claims. • The DME claims file comprised individual-level information such as sociodemographic characteristics and diagnosis codes.
Master Beneficiary Summary File (MBSF)	2013–2014	The MBSF comprised individual-level characteristics such as age, gender, race/ethnicity, disability status, Medicare/Medicaid dual eligibility status, and Medicare Advantage participation. (For additional information related to these files, see ResDAC, n.d.-d.)

Data Extraction and Management Process

The primary criterion for selection of cases for this study was type of durable medical equipment (DME). We targeted three broad categories of DME: wheeled and seated mobility devices (WSMDs), speech-generating devices (SGDs), and upper-extremity prostheses (UEPs). We constructed three separate datasets comprising these DME categories. The data extraction for each type of DME was based on a combination of the Berenson-Eggers type of service (BETOS) codes and the Health Care Common Procedure Coding System (HCPCS) level II alphanumeric codes:

- BETOS codes were developed as a way to categorize the types of services provided to Medicare beneficiaries. There are seven categories for these codes: evaluation and management, procedures, imaging, tests, DME, other, and exception/unclassified. For example, BETOS codes for WSMDs are in the DME category. Table C-2 provides a detailed list of the BETOS codes (CMS, n.d.).
- The HCPCS is a combination of codes that indicate services, procedures, or products (e.g., DME) provided to Medicare beneficiaries or to individuals under other health plans (including private insurance). There are three levels of HCPCS codes. For this study, we utilized HCPCS level II alphanumeric codes to identify and define the types of DME that were provided. Tables C-3, C-4, and C-5,

respectively, list HCPCS level II alphanumeric codes associated with the WSMD, UEP, and SGD groups (ResDAC, n.d.-c).

After constructing the product database, we linked it with the Master Beneficiary Summary File (MBSF) to obtain sociodemographic and clinical characteristics (including diagnosis codes) and state of residence for individuals in these three categories who received DME. All the individual-level sociodemographic characteristics were extracted from the MBSF:

- For age we used four categories: 20-45, 46-55, 56-64, and 65-67.
- Gender was classified as male or female.
- Race/ethnicity was divided into white, black, Hispanic, and other.
- For Medicare Advantage enrollment, we determined the number of months a person was covered under Medicare health maintenance organization (HMO) plans, and those with "no" Medicare HMO enrollment for that year were classified as Medicare fee-for-service.

For classification of *International Classification of Diseases,* Ninth Revision (ICD-9) codes into diagnostic categories, we used a method suggested by the Centers for Medicare & Medicaid Services (CMS) as part of its release of public-use files for DME. Using that method, we could classify ICD-9 codes associated with provision of WSMDs, SGDs, and UEPs into such categories as diseases of the nervous system, diseases of the circulatory system, and diseases of the musculoskeletal system and connective tissue, among others. Table C-6 provides a full list of the ICD-9 codes and their

TABLE C-2
Berenson-Eggers Type of Service Codes: Durable Medical Equipment

Code	Service
D1A	Medical/surgical supplies
D1B	Hospital beds
D1C	Oxygen and supplies
D1D	Wheelchairs
D1E	Other Durable Medical Equipment
D1F	Prosthetic/orthotic devices
D1G	Drugs administered through Durable Medical Equipment

SOURCE: ResDAC, n.d.-a.

TABLE C-3
List of Healthcare Common Procedure Coding System (HCPCS) Codes for Wheeled and Seated Mobility Devices

HCPCS Code	Description
E0983	Manual wheelchair accessory, power add-on to convert manual wheelchair to motorized wheelchair, joystick control
E0986	Manual wheelchair accessory, push-rim activated power assist system
E1038	Transport chair, adult size, patient weight capacity up to and including 300 pounds
E1039	Transport chair, adult size, heavy-duty, patient weight capacity greater than 300 pounds
E1088	High-strength, lightweight wheelchair, detachable arms desk or full length, swing-away detachable elevating leg rests
E1130	Standard wheelchair, fixed full-length arms, fixed or swing-away detachable footrests
E1140	Wheelchair, detachable arms, desk or full length, swing-away detachable footrests
E1161	Manual adult-size wheelchair, includes tilt in space
K0001	Standard wheelchair
K0002	Standard hemi (low-seat) wheelchair
K0003	Lightweight wheelchair
K0004	High-strength, lightweight wheelchair
K0005	Ultralightweight wheelchair
K0006	Heavy-duty wheelchair
K0007	Extra-heavy-duty wheelchair
K0009	Other manual wheelchair/base
K0011	Standard—weight frame motorized/power wheelchair with programmable control parameters for speed adjustment, tremor dampening, acceleration control, and braking
K0014	Other motorized/power wheelchair base
K0800	Power-operated vehicle, group 1 standard, patient weight capacity up to and including 300 pounds
K0801	Power-operated vehicle, group 1 heavy-duty, patient weight capacity 301 to 450 pounds
K0802	Power-operated vehicle, group 1 very-heavy-duty, patient weight capacity 451 to 600 pounds
K0806	Power-operated vehicle, group 2 standard, patient weight capacity up to and including 300 pounds
K0807	Power-operated vehicle, group 2 heavy-duty, patient weight capacity 301 to 450 pounds

continued

TABLE C-3
Continued

HCPCS Code	Description
K0808	Power-operated vehicle, group 2 very-heavy-duty, patient weight capacity 451 to 600 pounds
K0814	Power wheelchair, group 1 standard, portable, captains chair, patient weight capacity up to and including 300 pounds
K0815	Power wheelchair, group 1 standard, sling/solid seat and back, patient weight capacity up to and including 300 pounds
K0816	Power wheelchair, group 1 standard, captains chair, patient weight capacity up to and including 300 pounds
K0820	Power wheelchair, group 2 standard, portable, sling/solid seat/back, patient weight capacity up to and including 300 pounds
K0821	Power wheelchair, group 2 standard, portable, captains chair, patient weight capacity up to and including 300 pounds
K0822	Power wheelchair, group 2 standard, sling/solid seat/back, patient weight capacity up to and including 300 pounds
K0823	Power wheelchair, group 2 standard, captains chair, patient weight capacity up to and including 300 pounds
K0824	Power wheelchair, group 2 heavy-duty, sling/solid seat/back, patient weight capacity 301 to 450 pounds
K0825	Power wheelchair, group 2 heavy-duty, captains chair, patient weight capacity 301 to 450 pounds
K0826	Power wheelchair, group 2 very-heavy-duty, sling/solid seat/back, patient weight capacity 451 to 600 pounds
K0827	Power wheelchair, group 2 very-heavy-duty, captains chair, patient weight capacity 451 to 600 pounds
K0829	Power wheelchair, group 2 extra-heavy-duty, captains chair, patient weight 601 pounds or more
K0835	Power wheelchair, group 2 standard, single power option, sling/solid seat/back, patient weight capacity up to and including 300 pounds
K0837	Power wheelchair, group 2 heavy-duty, single power option, sling/solid seat/back, patient weight capacity 301 to 450 pounds
K0838	Power wheelchair, group 2 very-heavy-duty, single power option sling/solid seat/back, patient weight capacity 451 to 600 pounds
K0839	Power wheelchair, group 2 very-heavy-duty, single power option sling/solid seat/back, patient weight capacity 451 to 600 pounds
K0840	Power wheelchair, group 2 extra-heavy-duty, single power option, sling/solid seat/back, patient weight capacity 601 pounds or more
K0841	Power wheelchair, group 2 standard, multiple power option, sling/solid seat/back, patient weight capacity up to and including 300 pounds
K0843	Power wheelchair, group 2 heavy-duty, multiple power option, sling/solid seat/back, patient weight capacity 301 to 450 pounds

continued

TABLE C-3
Continued

HCPCS Code	Description
K0848	Power wheelchair, group 3 standard, sling/solid seat/back, patient weight capacity up to and including 300 pounds
K0849	Power wheelchair, group 3 standard, captains chair, patient weight capacity up to and including 300 pounds
K0850	Power wheelchair, group 3 heavy-duty, sling/solid seat/back, patient weight capacity 301 to 450 pounds
K0851	Power wheelchair, group 3 heavy-duty, captains chair, patient weight capacity 301 to 450 pounds
K0853	Power wheelchair, group 3 very-heavy-duty, captains chair, patient weight capacity 451 to 600 pounds
K0854	Power wheelchair, group 3 extra-heavy-duty, sling/solid seat/back, patient weight capacity 601 pounds or more
K0855	Power wheelchair, group 3 extra-heavy-duty, captains chair, patient weight capacity 601 pounds or more
K0856	Power wheelchair, group 3 standard, single power option, sling/solid seat/back, patient weight capacity up to and including 300 pounds
K0857	Power wheelchair, group 3 standard, single power option, captains chair, patient weight capacity up to and including 300 pounds
K0858	Power wheelchair, group 3 heavy-duty, single power option, sling/solid seat/back, patient weight 301 to 450 pounds
K0860	Power wheelchair, group 3 very-heavy-duty, single power option, sling/solid seat/back, patient weight capacity 451 to 600 pounds
K0861	Power wheelchair, group 3 standard, multiple power option, sling/solid seat/back, patient weight capacity up to and including 300 pounds
K0862	Power wheelchair, group 3 heavy-duty, multiple power option, sling/solid seat/back, patient weight capacity 301 to 450 pounds
K0870	Power wheelchair, group 4 heavy-duty, sling/solid seat/back, patient weight capacity 301 to 450 pounds
K0877	Power wheelchair, group 4 standard, single power option, sling/solid seat/back, patient weight capacity up to and including 300 pounds
K0880	Power wheelchair, group 4 very-heavy-duty, single power option, sling/solid seat/back, patient weight 451 to 600 pounds
K0884	Power wheelchair, group 4 standard, multiple power option, sling/solid seat/back, patient weight capacity up to and including 300 pounds
K0886	Power wheelchair, group 4 heavy-duty, multiple power option, sling/solid seat/back, patient weight capacity 301 to 450 pounds

SOURCE: CMS, 2016.

TABLE C-4
Healthcare Common Procedure Coding System (HCPCS) Codes for Upper-Extremity Prostheses

Prosthetic Devices	HCPCS Codes
Body-Powered Devices	'L6620' 'L6621' 'L6623' 'L6624' 'L6625' 'L6637' 'L6640' 'L6641' 'L6642' 'L6645' 'L6646' 'L6647' 'L6799' 'L6700' 'L6704' 'L6705' 'L6706' 'L6707' 'L6708' 'L6709' 'L6710' 'L6711' 'L6712' 'L6713' 'L6714' 'L6720' 'L6721' 'L6722' 'L6723' 'L6725' 'L6730' 'L6804' 'L6845' 'L6850' 'L6855' 'L6860' 'L6865' 'L6867' 'L6868' 'L6870' 'L6872' 'L6873' 'L6875' 'L7610' 'L7611' 'L7612' 'L7613' 'L7614' 'L7621' 'L7622'
Myoelectric Devices	'L6611' 'L6621' 'L6628' 'L6629' 'L6638' 'L6648' 'L6681' 'L6682' 'L6881' 'L6882' 'L6920' 'L6925' 'L6930' 'L6935' 'L6940' 'L6945' 'L6950' 'L6955' 'L6960' 'L6965' 'L6970' 'L6975' 'L7007' 'L7008' 'L7009' 'L7040' 'L7045' 'L7170' 'L7180' 'L7181' 'L7185' 'L7186' 'L7190' 'L7191' 'L7260' 'L7261' 'L7360' 'L7362' 'L7364' 'L7366' 'L7367' 'L7368'
Other	NA

NOTE: NA = not applicable.

SOURCE: Etter et al., 2015.

TABLE C-5
Healthcare Common Procedure Coding System (HCPCS) Codes for Speech-Generating Devices

Speech-Generating Device	HCPCS Code
Speech-generating device, digitized speech, using prerecorded messages, greater than 8 minutes but less than or equal to 20 minutes recording time	E2502
Speech-generating device, synthesized speech, permitting multiple methods of message formulation and device access	E2510

SOURCE: ASHA, n.d.

classification in these diagnosis categories, while Table C-7 lists the ICD-9 codes associated with the distribution of diagnosis categories for upper-extremity amputation.

DATA LIMITATIONS

The data used for this study were Medicare claims for the years 2013-2014. These data are "claims processing" data and not typically intended

TABLE C-6
International Classification of Diseases, Ninth Revision (ICD-9) Codes and Diagnostic Categories

Diagnostic Category	ICD-9 Codes
Infectious and parasitic diseases	001-139
Neoplasms	140-239
Endocrine, nutritional, and metabolic diseases and immunity disorders	240-279
Diseases of the blood and blood-forming organs	280-289
Mental disorders	290-319
Diseases of the nervous system	320-359
Diseases of the sense organs	360-389
Diseases of the circulatory system	390-459
Diseases of the respiratory system	460-519
Diseases of the digestive system	520-579
Diseases of the genitourinary system	580-629
Complications of pregnancy, childbirth, and the puerperium	630-679
Diseases of the skin and subcutaneous tissue	680-709
Diseases of the musculoskeletal system and connective tissue	710-739
Congenital anomalies	740-759
Certain conditions originating in the perinatal period	760-779
Symptoms, signs, and ill-defined conditions	780-799
Injury and poisoning	800-999
External causes of injury and supplemental classification	E and V codes
Mental disorders	290-319

SOURCE: CMS, 2010.

for use in research studies. They lack the information necessary for creating a health/disability profile of patients to match with the types of DME that were prescribed. Thus, the information presented in this report cannot be used to determine the appropriateness of the provision of DME. In addition, the data are based on a random 5 percent sample of Medicare beneficiaries. That sample yielded a small study sample for the SGD and UEP groups, which limited the presentation of granular information based on individual-level characteristics. In future analyses, use of a 20 percent random sample and/or more years of data is needed. The age criterion used for selection of the study cohort (ages 20-67 years) also is underrepresented in Medicare claims data. This is another reason for the small study sample

TABLE C-7
Distribution of Diagnosis Categories for Upper-Extremity Amputation Using *International Classification of Diseases,* Ninth Revision (ICD-9) Codes

Amputation Category	ICD-9 Codes
Below Elbow	'8870' '8871' 'V4965' '24930' '25900' '25905' '25907' '25909' '25915' '8405' 'V4963' '25927' '25931' '8403' 'V4964' '25920' '25924' '8404'
Above Elbow	'8872' '8873' '8406' 'V4966' '24900' '24920' '24925' '24931' '24935' '24940' '8407'
Level/Side Unspecified	'8874' '8875' '8876' '8877' 'V4960' 'V520' 'V528'
Thumb/Finger	'885' '8850' '8851' '886' '8860' '8861' 'V4961' 'V4962'

SOURCE: Etter et al., 2015.

for the SGD and UEP groups. It is important as well to acknowledge the coding errors that occurred in the course of the claims processing and are part of these data and could not be detected or eliminated in the data extraction process.

Despite these limitations, however, the Medicare DME files are a valuable resource in the absence of universal data developed specifically to study the prescription and utilization of assistive devices. These data represent a good resource for determining the use of these devices among older adults and individuals with disabilities.

REFERENCES

ASHA (American Speech-Language-Hearing Association). n.d. *Medicare coverage policy on speech-generating devices.* http://www.asha.org/practice/reimbursement/medicare/sgd_policy (accessed March 3, 2017).

CMS (Centers for Medicare & Medicaid Services). 2010. *CMS 2010 basic stand alone (BSA) DME line items public use file (PUF) data dictionary and codebook.* https://www.cms.gov/Research-Statistics-Data-and-Systems/Statistics-Trends-and-Reports/BSAPUFS/Downloads/2010_DME_DataDictionary.pdf (accessed January 24, 2017).

CMS. 2016. *Medicare referring provider DMEPOS data CY2014.* https://www.cms.gov/Research-Statistics-Data-and-Systems/Statistics-Trends-and-Reports/Medicare-Provider-Charge-Data/DME2014.html (accessed March 6, 2017).

CMS. n.d. *Berenson-Eggers type of service (BETOS) codes.* https://www.cms.gov/Research-Statistics-Data-and-Systems/Statistics-Trends-and-Reports/MedicareFeeforSvcPartsAB/downloads/betosdesccodes.pdf (accessed January 23, 2017).

Etter, K., M. Borgia, and L. Resnik. 2015. Prescription and repair rates of prosthetic limbs in the VA healthcare system: Implications for national prosthetic parity. *Disability and Rehabilitation: Assistive Technology* 10(6):493-500.

ResDAC (Research Data Assistance Center). n.d.-a. *BETOS table*. https://www.resdac.org/sites/resdac.umn.edu/files/BETOS%20Table.txt (accessed March 6, 2017).

ResDAC. n.d.-b. *Durable medical equipment RIF*. https://www.resdac.org/cms-data/files/dme-rif/data-documentation (accessed January 23, 2017).

ResDAC. n.d.-c. *Health care common procedure coding system*. https://www.resdac.org/cms-data/variables/Line-HCFA-Common-Procedure-Coding-System (accessed January 23, 2017).

ResDAC. n.d.-d. *Master beneficiary summary file*. https://www.resdac.org/cms-data/files/mbsf/data-documentation (accessed January 23, 2017).

Appendix D

Biographical Sketches of Committee Members

Alan M. Jette, P.T., Ph.D., M.P.H. (*Chair*), is professor of health law, policy, and management at Boston University School of Public Health. His research interests include late-life exercise; evaluation of rehabilitation treatment outcomes; and the measurement, epidemiology, and prevention of disability. Dr. Jette is an international expert in the development and dissemination of contemporary outcome measurement instruments for evaluation of health care quality and outcomes and has published more than 200 peer-reviewed articles on these topics. He currently directs a project entitled "Use of Computer Adaptive Testing to Assist with the Social Security Work Disability Determination Process." Dr. Jette also directs the Boston Rehabilitation Outcome Measurement Center, serves on the Executive Committee of the Boston Roybal Center for Active Lifestyle Interventions, and is project director of the New England Regional Spinal Cord Injury Center. He also is editor in chief of the journal *Physical Therapy*. For the past 15 years he has directed the Boston University Postdoctoral Fellowship Program in Outcomes Research, and from 1996 to 2004 he served as dean of Boston University's Sargent College of Health & Rehabilitation Sciences. Dr. Jette has served on multiple study committees for the former Institute of Medicine (now the National Academies of Sciences, Engineering, and Medicine's Health and Medicine Division), to which he was elected a member in 2013. He received a B.S. in physical therapy from the State University of New York at Buffalo in 1973 and an M.P.H. (1975) and a Ph.D. (1979) in public health from the University of Michigan.

Fabricio E. Balcazar, Ph.D., is a professor in the Department of Disability and Human Development at the University of Illinois at Chicago. His primary research interest is developing effective strategies for enhancing consumer empowerment and personal effectiveness among individuals with disabilities. Dr. Balcazar has conducted research over the past 25 years in several disability-related areas, such as the development of systematic approaches for the effective involvement of people with disabilities in consumer advocacy organizations; the development and evaluation of a model service-delivery approach to increase consumers' empowerment in the vocational rehabilitation service-delivery system; the development of interventions for helping Latino youth with disabilities who have dropped out of high school return to education and/or find jobs they can keep; the development of interventions to help minority students with disabilities transition into employment (including the development of entrepreneurial skills and start-ups for small businesses) and career development; and the promotion of cultural competence in rehabilitation services. He has published more than 70 peer-reviewed journal articles and recently co-edited a book entitled *Race, Culture and Disability: Issues in Rehabilitation Research and Practice*. Dr. Balcazar is a fellow of the American Psychological Association.

Laura J. Ball, Ph.D., is director of hearing and speech research at Children's National Health System in Washington, DC, and a professor in the Department of Pediatrics at the School of Medicine and Health Sciences, The George Washington University. She completed her Ph.D. at the University of Nebraska–Lincoln with a specialization in augmentative and alternative communication (AAC) and complex communication disorders and has more than 35 years of experience as a clinical speech-language pathologist. Her research focus is on individuals with complex neuromotor speech disorders across the life span, with particular interest in examining functional communication and participation; AAC assessment and implementation; and neurological speech-language and swallowing impairments resulting from neuromuscular, neurogenetic, and white matter disease. Her current research is examining advanced neural decoders for communication interfaces (i.e., brain–computer interface), functional communication for adolescents with Fragile X transitioning from school to vocational environments, and improving patient–provider communication for individuals from minority populations with severe communication impairments. Dr. Ball served on the Massachusetts General Hospital Committee for Assistive Communication and Technology and is currently active in the Global Leukodystrophy Initiative Standardization of Care Task Force. She has been a member of the Medicare Implementation Team, an Ad Hoc Committee for AAC Funding Advocacy, since 1999.

Rory A. Cooper, Ph.D., earned B.S. and M.Eng. degrees in electrical engineering from California Polytechnic State University and a Ph.D. in electrical and computer engineering with a concentration in bioengineering from the University of California, Santa Barbara. He is FISA Foundation and Paralyzed Veterans of America chair and distinguished professor in the Department of Rehabilitation Science and Technology and professor of bioengineering, physical medicine and rehabilitation, and orthopedic surgery at the University of Pittsburgh. Dr. Cooper is founding director and the U.S. Department of Veterans Affairs (VA) senior research career scientist at the Human Engineering Research Laboratories, a VA Rehabilitation R&D Center of Excellence. He has authored or co-authored more than 300 peer-reviewed journal publications and two books, and he has 20 patents awarded or pending. He is an elected fellow of the National Academy of Inventors as well as several other professional societies. He has been a distinguished speaker for several organizations and an honorary professor at Hong Kong Polytechnic University and Xi'an Jiatong University. Dr. Cooper has been involved with Paralympics for a number of years and served with numerous governmental and nongovernmental organizations focused on disability and rehabilitation. He also has actively collaborated with the Indian Spinal Injuries Centre on increasing access to quality services and devices for people with disabilities in India and throughout developing countries. Dr. Cooper is a U.S. Army veteran with a spinal cord injury and a director of the Paralyzed Veterans of America Research Foundation as well as a civilian aide to the secretary of the Army. He currently serves as a member of the Honorary Board of Advisors for Student Veterans of America; the National Science Foundation Advisory Committee for Education and Human Resources; the Command Council, Staff Sergeant Donnie D. Dixon Center for Military and Veterans Community Services; and the World Health Organization Global Cooperation on Assistive Technology (GATE) Committee.

Janna L. Friedly, M.D., is a board-certified physiatrist and associate professor in the Department of Rehabilitation Medicine at the University of Washington, Seattle. She is also the medical director for the Limb Preservation and Amputation Rehabilitation Services and the outpatient Rehabilitation Medicine clinics at Harborview Medical Center. Dr. Friedly conducts outcomes research related to back pain treatments in the Comparative Effectiveness, Cost and Outcomes Research Center at the University of Washington. She has received numerous awards and grants for her research related to back pain. She received her undergraduate degree from Stanford University and her medical degree from Oregon Health Sciences University. She completed her residency training in physical medicine and rehabilitation at the University of Washington and a Rehabilitation

Medicine Scientist Training Program K12 fellowship in 2008. She has been a clinician scientist with the University of Washington since 2008. Dr. Friedly is actively involved in administration at the University of Washington. She has served as rehabilitation medicine representative on the Medical Quality Improvement Committee at Harborview Medical Center for the past 8 years and as a member at large of the center's Medical Executive Committee and a past medical staff president. She is currently serving as an at-large member and on the Executive Committee of the University of Washington Physicians Board of Trustees. She is listed among "The Best Doctors in America," and received the Top Doctors Award from *Seattle Metropolitan Magazine* in 2014, 2015, and 2016.

Walter R. Frontera, M.D., Ph.D., is a professor in the Department of Physical Medicine, Rehabilitation, and Sports Medicine and the Department of Physiology at the University of Puerto Rico School of Medicine. He is former inaugural chair and professor of physical medicine and rehabilitation at Vanderbilt University School of Medicine, where he served as medical director of rehabilitation services. He is a former dean of the Medical School at the University of Puerto Rico. In 1996, he was recruited to Harvard Medical School to establish the Department of Physical Medicine and Rehabilitation (PM&R), and he was appointed Earle P. and Ida S. Charlton professor and chairman of the Department of PM&R at Harvard Medical School and Spaulding Rehabilitation Hospital. He was also chief of service at the Massachusetts General Hospital and the Brigham and Women's Hospital. Dr. Frontera's main research interest is the mechanisms underlying muscle atrophy and weakness in the elderly and the development of rehabilitative interventions for sarcopenia. He has authored more than 220 scientific publications, including more than 95 peer-reviewed articles and 16 edited books. Currently, he serves as editor in chief of the *American Journal of PM&R* and is president elect of the International Society of PM&R. He has received several awards for his contributions to the field of PM&R. In 2008, he was elected a member of the National Academy of Medicine. Dr. Frontera completed his M.D. and residency in PM&R at the University of Puerto Rico and his Ph.D. in applied anatomy and physiology at Boston University.

Katya Hill, Ph.D., CCC-SLP, is an internationally recognized speaker and advocate in the field of AAC and assistive technology (AT), evidence-based practice, and performance measurement. She obtained her Ph.D. in the School of Health and Rehabilitation Sciences at the University of Pittsburgh, where she is currently an associate professor in the Department of Communication Science and Disorders, with a secondary appointment in the Department of Rehabilitation Sciences and Technology. As a speech-language pathologist, she has more than 30 years of AAC and AT clinical experience. Her clinical experiences led to a keen desire to conduct research to develop methods for measuring AAC performance and outcomes. Dr. Hill's research has been in the area of AAC language activity monitoring, AAC language transcription and analysis, performance measurement, and brain–computer interfaces. Her research has led to the development of AAC software analysis tools, standards for definitions for measuring AAC communication performance, systematic approaches to evaluating AAC technologies, and several patents. Her career reflects her mission of improving the quality of life for individuals who rely on AAC by advocating for the most effective communication possible. Dr. Hill is also co-founder of the AAC Institute and ICAN Talk Clinic, nonprofit charitable organizations dedicated to advancing professional practices in AAC/AT and the life experience of people who use AAC/AT and their families.

Barbara L. Kornblau, J.D., OTR/L, is executive director of the Coalition for Disability Health Equity and serves on the faculty in the Division of Occupational Therapy, School of Allied Health, Florida A&M University. She also serves as a consultant to the United Spinal Association's Pathways to Employment Program. Ms. Kornblau is past president of the American Occupational Therapy Association, a former Robert Wood Johnson Foundation health policy fellow in the Offices of Senators Harkin and Rockefeller, an attorney, a certified disability management specialist, a certified pain educator, and a person with a disability. She is recognized as an expert in disability policy, return-to-work issues, assistive technology, and reasonable accommodations under the Americans with Disabilities Act and the Rehabilitation Act.

Frank R. Lin, M.D., Ph.D., is an associate professor of otolaryngology-head and neck surgery, geriatric medicine, mental health, and epidemiology at Johns Hopkins University. He completed his medical education, residency in otolaryngology, and Ph.D. in clinical investigation at Johns Hopkins, and further otologic fellowship training in Lucerne, Switzerland. Dr. Lin's clinical practice is dedicated to otology and the medical and surgical management of hearing loss. His epidemiologic research focuses on how hearing loss impacts the health and functioning of older adults and the role of hearing rehabilitative strategies in potentially mitigating these effects. In particular, his research group has demonstrated that hearing loss in older adults is strongly and independently associated with the risk of cognitive decline, incident dementia, impairments in physical functioning and mobility, and greater health care resource utilization in multiple epidemiologic studies. He collaborates extensively with researchers across multiple fields including gerontology, cognitive neuroscience, audiology, and epidemiology, and has collaborative working relationships with individuals in industry, government, and nonprofit advocacy organizations.

Laura A. Miller, Ph.D., CP, is a research scientist/prosthetist for the Center for Bionic Medicine at the Shirley Ryan AbilityLab (previously known as the Rehabilitation Institute of Chicago). She is a board-certified and Illinois-licensed prosthetist. Her clinical interests include high-level upper-limb prosthetic fittings. Dr. Miller is also an associate professor in physical medicine and rehabilitation at Northwestern University and works as a research prosthetist with the AbilityLab's Center for Bionic Medicine. She is particularly interested in the application of pattern recognition as a method for controlling upper-extremity powered prostheses. She received her B.S. summa cum laude from Tulane University and an M.S. and a Ph.D. in biomedical engineering from Northwestern University, where she also completed a certificate program in prosthetics. She completed her prosthetics residency at the Rehabilitation Institute of Chicago. Dr. Miller has multiple publications in the areas of normal gait and lower-limb prosthetics as well as high-level upper-limb prosthetic fittings. She serves as a member of the board and treasurer of the U.S. Chapter of the International Society for Prosthetics and Orthotics.

Kenneth J. Ottenbacher, Ph.D., OTR, holds the Russell Shearn Moody Distinguished Chair in Neurological Rehabilitation at the University of Texas Medical Branch at Galveston. He serves as director of the Division of Rehabilitation Sciences in the School of Health Professions as well as associate director for the Sealy Center on Aging. Dr. Ottenbacher received his Ph.D. from the University of Missouri-Columbia and is a licensed occupational therapist. His research interests include rehabilitation outcomes, with a focus on functional assessment, disability, and frailty in older adults. He has published more than 320 scientific/technical articles in refereed journals and is the author, co-author, or editor of four textbooks. Dr. Ottenbacher's research has been supported by continuous federal funding since 1984. His current research is examining hospital readmission and quality-of-care indicators across post-acute care settings.

Linda J. Resnik, P.T., Ph.D., is a research career scientist at the Providence VA Medical Center and a professor in the Department of Health Services, Policy, and Practice at Brown University. As a member of the Executive Committee of the Providence VA Medical Center's Rehabilitation Research-funded Center of Excellence on Neurorestoration and Neurotechnology, she leads a focus area on Restoring Limb Function. She is also the principal investigator of the Center on Health Services Training and Research, a multi-institutional research and training center funded by the Foundation for Physical Therapy. Dr. Resnik is currently the principal investigator of a U.S. Department of Defense–funded national study of veterans and service members with upper-limb amputation. She has also led the VA's studies to optimize the DEKA arm and is currently the principal investigator of a VA-funded home study of this device. Dr. Resnik is an active collaborator on several other research studies evaluating the usability and outcomes of new prosthetic controls and technologies. She served as an editorial board member for the journal *Physical Therapy* for more than a decade and is the author of more than 75 peer-reviewed manuscripts, more than one-third of which pertain to persons with upper-limb amputation. She completed her postdoctoral training in health services research at Brown University and received her Ph.D. in physical therapy from Nova Southeastern University; her M.S. in physical therapy from Sargent College, Boston University; and her B.S. from Hampshire College.

Jon A. Sanford, M.Arch., is director of the Center for Assistive Technology and Environmental Access and professor of industrial design at Georgia Institute of Technology. He was a research architect at the Rehabilitation R&D Center at the Atlanta VA Medical Center for 28 years. Mr. Sanford is one of the few architecturally trained researchers engaged in the design and usability of products, technologies, and environments for older adults and people with disabilities. He is internationally recognized for his expertise in universal design, workplace accommodations, and home modifications and is principal investigator for the Rehabilitation Engineering Research Center on Technologies for Successful Aging with Disability (RERC TechSAge), a 5-year grant from the Department of Health and Human Services' Administration for Community Living. He also served as co-principal investigator for the RERC on workplace accommodations from 2003 to 2013. His current work focuses on promoting universal design through the integration of digital technologies into physical products. He has more than 300 presentations and publications and recently authored the book *Design for the Ages: Universal Design as a Rehabilitation Strategy.*

Stephanie Sjoblad, Au.D., is a professor at the University of North Carolina (UNC) at Chapel Hill Division of Speech and Hearing Sciences. She has served as clinical coordinator since 2001 and is clinic director for the UNC Hearing and Communication Center. Dr. Sjoblad also teaches graduate courses and supervises students in the clinic. A consumer of hearing instrument technology from childhood, she offers a unique perspective to patients and students alike. She has served on the board for the American Academy of Audiology-North Carolina, most recently as past president; for a division of the North Carolina Speech and Hearing Association; and on the Coding and Reimbursement Committee for the American Academy of Audiology.

She served for 8 years as president of the board of directors of Beginnings for Parents of Children who are Deaf or Hard of Hearing, Inc. Dr. Sjoblad and the team at the UNC Hearing and Communication Center are leading the way in national efforts to make hearing care more accessible through unbundled and itemized fee structures while utilizing best practices as outlined by the American Academy of Audiology.

Lawrence C. Vogel, M.D., has been chief of pediatrics at the Chicago Shriners Hospitals for Children since 1981 and medical director of the Spinal Cord Injury program since its inception in 1983. He received his B.A. with distinction from Northwestern University and his medical degree from the University of Illinois. He served as a pediatric resident at Yale-New Haven Hospital and subsequently completed a fellowship in pediatric infectious diseases at Michael Reese Hospital and the University of Chicago. Dr. Vogel is a diplomate of the American Board of Pediatrics and is certified in the subspecialty of spinal cord injury medicine. He is a professor of pediatrics at Rush Medical College and an adjunct professor of biomedical engineering at Marquette University, and he is a member of several professional societies focused on spinal cord injury. Dr. Vogel is past president of the Chicago Pediatric Society, the board of directors of the American Paraplegia Society, and the American Spinal Injury Association. Over the past three decades, he has dedicated his time to the care of children and adolescents with spinal cord injuries. A major interest is in long-term follow-up of children and adolescents with spinal cord injuries. He has authored more than 150 articles in peer-reviewed journals, 24 book chapters, more than 350 presentations or posters, and 20 instructional courses at national and international medical meetings and co-edited one book.